T0180700

Pediatric Dialysis Case Studies

Bradley A. Warady • Franz Schaefer
Steven R. Alexander
Editors

Pediatric Dialysis Case Studies

A Practical Guide to Patient Care

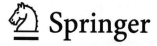 Springer

Editors
Bradley A. Warady
Division of Pediatric Nephrology
University of Missouri
Kansas City School of Medicine
Children's Mercy Hospital
Kansas City, MO, USA

Franz Schaefer
Division of Pediatric Nephrology
Center for Pediatrics and Adolescent
  Medicine
University of Heidelberg
Heidelberg, Germany

Steven R. Alexander
Division of Pediatric Nephrology
Department of Pediatrics
Stanford University School of Medicine
Lucile Packard Children's Hospital Stanford
Stanford, CA, USA

ISBN 978-3-319-85579-0   ISBN 978-3-319-55147-0   (eBook)
DOI 10.1007/978-3-319-55147-0

Printed on acid-free paper

This Springer imprint is published by Springer Nature
The registered company is Springer International Publishing AG
The registered company address is: Gewerbestrasse 11, 6330 Cham, Switzerland

Preface

The management of chronic dialysis therapy in children is a complex, all-consuming, and ultimately rewarding discipline. As members of a small, yet international subspecialty, pediatric dialysis practitioners have learned to turn to one another for clinical advice when faced with difficult clinical problems. It is, in fact, the clinical experience of our colleagues that continues to be a truly invaluable resource. Whereas bedside rounds remain the "gold standard" of clinically based instruction, writing about clinical situations using real-life cases employs the same teaching technique by directly applying clinical management principles at the patient level.

The worldwide success of *Pediatric Dialysis* and its second edition, which remain the only textbooks available that are entirely devoted to dialysis in children, led us to consider a companion text in which cases would be used to reinforce the material contained in those publications. To that end, we have had the great pleasure of working with a team of international experts in pediatric dialysis care to develop the book *Pediatric Dialysis Case Studies*. In this unique text, each chapter is introduced by a case presentation that serves as the basis for key learning points that are clinically applicable and presented in a succinct manner by authors who have a wealth of knowledge and clinical expertise. Whereas some chapters address frequently noted complications with evidence-based recommendations for prevention and treatment, other chapters highlight less common events and provide unique perspectives on disease management. The topics that we have included in *Pediatric Dialysis Case Studies* cover virtually all aspects of pediatric dialysis care and, in turn, represent the efforts of individuals with firsthand clinical expertise in virtually every discipline that is represented in the pediatric dialysis team.

As was the case in the development of the first and second editions of *Pediatric Dialysis*, the goal of this book is to create a resource that is worthy of a place on the bookshelves of all busy dialysis clinicians and would be frequently consulted for some "bedside" expertise. In *Pediatric Dialysis Case Studies*, we believe that we have achieved that goal.

We conclude by sincerely thanking our co-authors, all of whom are experts in their own right, and all of our patients and their families who are our best teachers. We also want to thank Springer developmental editor Michael Wilt for his patient guidance and unfailing support. Together, we have created what we believe is a special textbook about clinical challenges associated with pediatric dialysis that we all have encountered or will likely encounter in the future. Most importantly, we hope that this textbook becomes a resource that will lead to improved outcomes for the sometimes complex, but always special, patients we care for.

Kansas City, MO, USA   Bradley A. Warady
Heidelberg, Germany   Franz Schaefer
Stanford, CA, USA   Steven R. Alexander

Contents

Contributors

Steven R. Alexander, MD Division of Pediatric Nephrology, Department of Pediatrics, Stanford University School of Medicine, Lucile Packard Children's Hospital Stanford, Stanford, CA, USA

Talal Alfaadhel, MD Division of Nephrology, Sunnybrook Health Sciences Centre, University of Toronto, Toronto, ON, Canada

Walter S. Andrews, MD, FACS, FAAP Department of Pediatric Surgery, Children's Mercy Hospital, Kansas City, MO, USA

Klaus Arbeiter Department of Pediatrics and Adolescent Medicine, Medical University of Vienna, Vienna, Austria

David J. Askenazi, MD Department of Pediatrics, University of Alabama at Birmingham, Children's Hospital of Alabama, Birmingham, AL, USA

Christoph Aufricht, MD Department of Pediatrics and Adolescent Medicine, Medical University of Vienna, Vienna, Austria

Rose M. Ayoob, MD Nationwide Children's Hospital, Division of Nephrology, The Ohio State University, Columbus, OH, USA

Sevcan A. Bakkaloglu, MD Division of Pediatric Nephrology, Gazi University School of Medicine, Ankara, Turkey

Nathan T. Beins, MD Division of Pediatric Nephrology, University of Missouri, Kansas City School of Medicine, Children's Mercy Hospital, Kansas City, MO, USA

Lorraine E. Bell, MDCM, FRCPC Division of Nephrology, Department of Pediatrics, McGill University Health Centre, Montreal Children's Hospital, Montreal, QC, Canada

Dagmara Borzych-Duzalka, MD, PhD Department of Pediatrics, Nephrology and Hypertension, Medical University of Gdansk, Gdansk, Poland

Mary L. Brandt, MD Division of Pediatric Surgery, Michael E. DeBakey Department of Surgery, Baylor College of Medicine, Houston, TX, USA

Patrick D. Brophy, MD Stead Family Department of Pediatrics and Division of Pediatric Nephrology, University of Iowa Stead Family Children's Hospital, Iowa City, IA, USA

Timothy E. Bunchman, MD Department of Pediatric Nephrology, Virginia Commonwealth University, Richmond, Virginia, USA

Rainer Büscher, MD, MME Department of Pediatric Nephrology, University Children's Hospital, Essen, Germany

Francisco J. Cano Faculty of Medicine, University of Chile, Santiago, Chile

Luis Calvo Mackenna Children's Hospital, Santiago, Chile

Vimal Chadha, MD Division of Pediatric Nephrology, University of Missouri, Kansas City School of Medicine, Children's Mercy Hospital, Kansas City, MO, USA

Eugene Y.H. Chan, MRCPCH, FHKAM(Paed) Princess Margaret Hospital, Hong Kong, China

Annabelle N. Chua, MD Duke University, Department of Pediatrics/Division of Pediatric Nephrology, Durham, NC, USA

Pierre Cochat, MD Reference Center for Rare Renal Diseases Nephrogones, Hospices Civils de Lyon & Université Claude-Bernard Lyon 1, Lyon, France

Elisa Colombini, MD Dialysis Unit, Department of Pediatrics, "Bambino Gesù" Children's Research Hospital, Rome, Italy

Dagmar Csaicsich Department of Pediatrics and Adolescent Medicine, Medical University of Vienna, Vienna, Austria

Meredith Cushing, MS, MSHSE Division of Nephrology, British Columbia Children's Hospital, Vancouver, BC, Canada

Joseph T. Flynn, MD, MS University of Washington School of Medicine, Division of Nephrology, Seattle Children's Hospital, Seattle, WA, USA

Aviva M. Goldberg, MD, MA, FRCPC Section of Nephrology, Departments of Pediatric and Child Health, Max Rady College of Medicine, Winnipeg, Manitoba, Canada

Stuart L. Goldstein, MD Center for Acute Care Nephrology, Pheresis Service, Cincinnati Children's Hospital Medical Center, Cincinnati, OH, USA

University of Cincinnati College of Medicine, Cincinnati, OH, USA

Paul C. Grimm, MD Division of Pediatric Nephrology, Department of Pediatrics, Stanford University School of Medicine, Lucile Packard Childrens Hospital Stanford, Stanford, CA, USA

Lyndsay A. Harshman, MD Stead Family Department of Pediatrics and Division of Pediatric Nephrology, University of Iowa Stead Family Children's Hospital, Iowa City, IA, USA

Elizabeth Harvey, MD, FRCPC Department of Pediatrics, Division of Nephrology, Hospital for Sick Children, University of Toronto, Toronto, ON, Canada

Hiroshi Hataya, MD Department of Nephrology, Tokyo Metropolitan Children's Medical Center, Tokyo, Japan

Richard J. Hendrickson, MD, FACS, FAAP Department of Pediatric Surgery, Children's Mercy Hospital, Kansas City, MO, USA

Michelle A. Hladunewich, MD, MSc, FRCP Divisions of Nephrology and Obstetric Medicine, Department of Medicine, Sunnybrook Health Sciences Centre, University of Toronto, Toronto, ON, Canada

Masataka Honda, MD, PhD Department of Nephrology, Tokyo Metropolitan Children's Medical Center, Tokyo, Japan

Daljit K. Hothi, MBBS, MRCPCH, MD Department of Pediatric Nephrology, Great Ormond Street Hospital for Children Foundation Trust, London, UK

Rebecca J. Johnson, PhD, ABPP Division of Developmental and Behavioral Sciences, Children's Mercy Hospital, Kansas City, MO, USA

John D. Mahan, MD Nationwide Children's Hospital, Division of Nephrology, The Ohio State University, Columbus, OH, USA

Mignon I. McCulloch, MBBCh, FRCPCH, FCP Red Cross Children's Hospital, Department of Paediatric Nephrology and Paediatric ICU, Cape Town, South Africa

Joseph L. Mills, MD Division of Vascular Surgery, Michael E. DeBakey Department of Surgery, Baylor College of Medicine, Houston, TX, USA

Mark M. Mitsnefes, MD, MS Cincinnati Children's Hospital Medical Center, Division of Nephrology and Hypertension, Cincinnati, OH, USA

Alicia M. Neu, MD Department of Pediatrics, The Johns Hopkins University School of Medicine, Baltimore, MD, USA

Shari K. Neul, PhD Department of Neurosciences, University of California San Diego, La Jolla, CA, USA

Stefano Picca, MD Dialysis Unit, Department of Pediatrics, "Bambino Gesù" Children's Research Hospital, Rome, Italy

Nonnie Polderman, BSc Division of Nephrology, British Columbia Children's Hospital, Vancouver, BC, Canada

Lesley Rees, MD, FRCPCH Great Ormond Street Hospital for Children NHS Foundation Trust, London, UK

Rebecca L. Ruebner, MD, MSCE Department of Pediatrics, The Johns Hopkins University School of Medicine, Baltimore, MD, USA

Thomas Sacherer-Mueller Department of Pediatrics and Adolescent Medicine, Medical University of Vienna, Vienna, Austria

Betti Schaefer, MD Division of Pediatric Nephrology, Center for Pediatrics and Adolescent Medicine, University of Heidelberg, Heidelberg, Germany

Franz Schaefer, MD Division of Pediatric Nephrology, Center for Pediatrics and Adolescent Medicine, University of Heidelberg, Heidelberg, Germany

Claus Peter Schmitt Division of Pediatric Nephrology, Center for Pediatrics and Adolescent Medicine, University of Heidelberg, Heidelberg, Germany

Christine B. Sethna, MD, EdM Division of Pediatric Nephrology, Cohen Children's Medical Center of New York, Queens, NY, USA

Department of Pediatrics, Hofstra Northwell School of Medicine, Hempstead, NY, USA

Vanessa Shaw, MA, FBDA Great Ormond Street Hospital for Children NHS Foundation Trust, London, UK

Rukshana Shroff, MD, PhD Great Ormond Street Hospital for Children, Nephrology Unit, London, UK

Kate Sinnott, BSc (Hons) Department of Pediatric Nephrology, Great Ormond Street Hospital for Children Foundation Trust, London, UK

Sarah J. Swartz, MD Department of Pediatrics, Baylor College of Medicine, Houston, TX, USA

Jordan M. Symons, MD Department of Pediatrics, University of Washington School of Medicine, Seattle, WA, USA

Division of Nephrology, Seattle Children's Hospital, Seattle, WA, USA

Enrico Eugenio Verrina, MD Giannina Gaslini Children's Hospital, Dialysis Unit, Genoa, Italy

Enrico Vidal, MD, PhD Nephrology, Dialysis and Transplant Unit, Department of Women's and Children's Health, University-Hospital of Padova, Padova, Italy

Bradley A. Warady, MD Division of Pediatric Nephrology, University of Missouri, Kansas City School of Medicine, Children's Mercy Hospital, Kansas City, MO, USA

Aaron Wightman, MD, MA University of Washington School of Medicine, Seattle, WA, USA

Hui-Kim Yap, MBBS, MMed, FRCPCH Department of Pediatrics, Yong Loo Lin School of Medicine, National University of Singapore, Singapore, Singapore

Joshua J. Zaritsky, MD, PhD Nemours/A.I. duPont Hospital for Children, Wilmington, DE, USA

Chapter 1
Peritoneal Access

Richard J. Hendrickson and Walter S. Andrews

Case Presentation

A previously healthy one-year-old male presented to the emergency room with a several day history of decreased oral intake, cough, and decreased urine output. His past medical history was significant for poor oral intake with failure to thrive being evaluated for surgical gastrostomy placement. He had no past surgical history. After a comprehensive evaluation and initial fluid resuscitation in the emergency room, he was admitted to the pediatric intensive care unit with dehydration and septic shock. He was intubated for respiratory insufficiency and diagnosed with rhino/enterovirus infection. He remained hemodynamically stable after initial fluid resuscitation. His initial laboratory values demonstrated an elevated creatinine of 8.0 mg/dL. His electrolytes were maintained within normal ranges with medical therapy.

Despite aggressive fluid resuscitation, he remained anuric, consistent with acute kidney injury (AKI). Due to persistent anuria and worsening anasarca over the next 24 h, nephrology was consulted for further management. Despite continued maximal medical therapy, his renal function did not improve, and a surgical consult was obtained for dialysis access. At our center, we prefer peritoneal dialysis (PD) as the initial mode for both acute and chronic dialysis. If urgent dialysis is needed, hemodialysis may be instituted temporarily and possibly continuous renal replacement therapy (CRRT) if the patient cannot tolerate hemodialysis. Once stabilized, we convert to PD if possible.

R.J. Hendrickson, MD, FACS, FAAP (✉) • W.S. Andrews, MD, FACS, FAAP
Department of Pediatric Surgery, Children's Mercy Hospital, Kansas City, MO, USA
e-mail: rjhendrickson@cmh.edu

© Springer International Publishing AG 2017
B.A. Warady et al. (eds.), *Pediatric Dialysis Case Studies*,
DOI 10.1007/978-3-319-55147-0_1

Once this patient was stable, he was taken to the operating room for PD catheter placement. In addition, as he had been scheduled to have a gastrostomy tube inserted in the near future, this procedure was added to PD catheter placement. In the OR, cefazolin and fluconazole were given within 60 min before incision, and the patient's abdomen was prepped. The PD catheter that was selected was a double-cuffed, curled, swan neck catheter (Argyle™, Peritoneal Dialysis Catheters, Covidien, Mansfield, MA). The catheter was sized by measuring the distance between the umbilicus and the symphysis pubis. The location of the exit site of the catheter was marked on the patient's right side, halfway between the midclavicular and anterior axillary lines and lateral and inferior to the initial incision located just lateral to the umbilicus.

The catheter was inserted laparoscopically with the curled portion positioned deep in the pelvis. No skin exit site sutures were used. A MIC-KEY (Ballard Medical Products, Draper, UT) gastrostomy tube was then inserted laparoscopically utilizing the LEFT upper quadrant access port incision, and the stomach wall was secured to the anterior abdominal wall with internal retention absorbable sutures. Catheter function and the absence of leaks were confirmed intraoperatively by using two passes of 10 cc/kg of dialysate. Low-volume dialysis was initiated postoperatively and over the next several days was increased to full volume without incident.

One month later, his renal function returned and his PD treatment was held. During this time off PD, his PD catheter was routinely inspected with regular dressing changes and flushing of the catheter.

Two months later his renal function deteriorated and he required PD treatment again. Unfortunately, the PD catheter would not flush easily and did not drain. An abdominal radiograph demonstrated the PD catheter to be in the pelvis. Therefore, a surgical consult was obtained and the patient was taken to the operating room for laparoscopic evaluation where intraluminal fibrin plugs were identified and removed. His PD catheter continues to function well, and the patient is undergoing evaluation for kidney transplantation.

Clinical Questions

1. What are the available modalities for pediatric dialysis?
2. When PD is the preferred method, what PD catheters are available for pediatric patients?
3. What antibiotics are routinely used for PD catheter insertion or revision?
4. How are the PD catheters surgically inserted?
5. What are the options if a PD catheter does not drain satisfactorily?

Diagnostic Discussion

1. In acute situations, hemodialysis or PD may be used to help stabilize the patient who requires fluid and toxin removal. If it is apparent that the patient will require chronic treatment, PD is the preferred modality in our center.
2. There are various types of pediatric PD catheters available (Tenckhoff single and dual cuff, Tenckhoff curl catheter, Tenckhoff Swan Neck, Tenckhoff Swan Neck curl catheter) which come in various lengths. We currently prefer Argyle catheters (Argyle™, Peritoneal Dialysis Catheters. Covidien. Mansfield, MA) (Fig. 1.1). We routinely use the dual cuff Swan Neck curl catheter for both acute (e.g. patients who have Hemolytic Uremic Syndrome) and chronic dialysis situations.

Pediatric Swan Neck Curl Cath Catheters

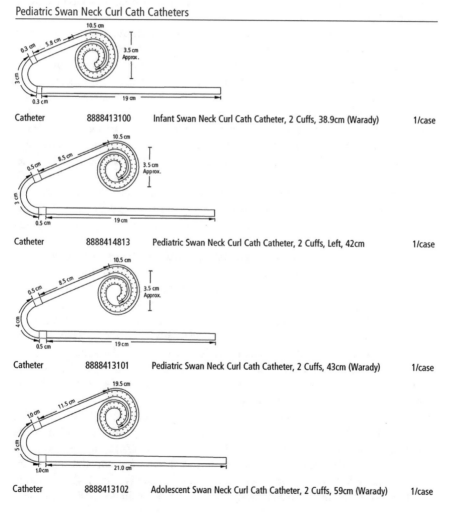

Catheter	8888413100	Infant Swan Neck Curl Cath Catheter, 2 Cuffs, 38.9cm (Warady)	1/case
Catheter	8888414813	Pediatric Swan Neck Curl Cath Catheter, 2 Cuffs, Left, 42cm	1/case
Catheter	8888413101	Pediatric Swan Neck Curl Cath Catheter, 2 Cuffs, 43cm (Warady)	1/case
Catheter	8888413102	Adolescent Swan Neck Curl Cath Catheter, 2 Cuffs, 59cm (Warady)	1/case

Fig. 1.1 Various types of PD catheters available for pediatric patients (Image copyright © 2016 Medtronic. All rights reserved. Used with the permission of Medtronic)

3. When a PD catheter is inserted or revised, we routinely use perioperative administration of a first-generation cephalosporin such as cefazolin, per ISPD guideline 2.2 [1]. Vancomycin is an alternative in patients hypersensitive to
   cephalosporins. Of note, if a gastrostomy tube will be placed simultaneously, an
   antifungal agent such as fluconazole is administered perioperatively as well, per
   ISPD guideline 7.4 [1].
4. We routinely gain access to the peritoneum via the umbilicus with a 5 mm STEP
   (STEP™ Instruments, Medtronic, Covidien. Mansfield, MA) port and establish
   a pneumoperitoneum of 12–15 mm Hg with carbon dioxide. Laparoscopy allows
   for a complete inspection of the peritoneal cavity for any pathology and to also
   identify patent internal inguinal rings that should be repaired prior to initiation of
   PD treatment to avoid development of inguinal hernias. Preexisting inguinal hernias can be repaired at this point via an open or laparoscopic technique at the
   discretion of the surgeon.

   An additional 5 mm port is placed in the LEFT upper quadrant to help facilitate visualization, as the camera can be switched between these two ports.
   Additionally, a 5 mm instrument can be utilized with the additional port.

   Next, we perform an omentectomy in an attempt to prevent the omentum from
   clogging the side holes of the PD catheter. The available omentum is retrieved
   via the umbilicus and sequentially ligated with Vicryl ties and electrocautery
   (Fig. 1.2). We are reluctant to perform an omentopexy (i.e., fixation of the omentum to the anterior abdominal wall) for fear of a potential midgut volvulus [2].

   Next, we select the appropriate length dual cuff swan neck curl catheter based
   upon the patient's size. The ideal catheter length should be approximated by
   placing the internal cuff lateral and 1 cm above the umbilicus and then measuring
   to the level of the symphysis pubis. We usually place the exit site on the RIGHT
   side of the abdomen, since some of these patients may need a gastrostomy tube
   in the LEFT upper quadrant.

   After marking out the anticipated catheter track on the skin of the abdomen,
   an incision is made in the skin to the RIGHT of midline, and the dissection is
   carried down to the anterior fascia of the rectus muscle where a transverse incision is made. A purse-string monofilament suture is placed in the anterior fascia.
   Next, a STEP access needle and sheath are inserted through this opening and
   carefully advanced to the preperitoneal space with laparoscopic guidance. The
   sheath is tilted and carefully advanced in the preperitoneal space downward
   toward the pelvis where it is allowed to enter the peritoneum just above the dome
   of the bladder (Fig. 1.3). Once fully deployed within the peritoneal cavity, the
   needle is removed and the sheath left in place.

   Ultimately, a peel-away introducer sheath set (Peel Away® Intoducer Set.
   Cook Medical; Bloomington, IN) is inserted, starting with placment of the
   included guidewire through the STEP sheath and advancing it into the pelvis
   under direct visualization. The STEP sheath is removed and the dilator and
   sheath advanced over the guidewire down into the pelvis (Fig. 1.4). The guidewire and dilator are removed leaving the 20 French sheath down in the pelvis.

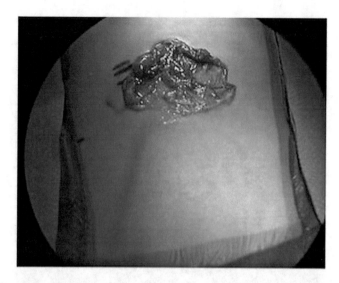

Fig. 1.2 Omentum retrieved via the umbilicus. Pen markings show anticipated medial incision to the RIGHT of the umbilicus and the more LATERAL and DOWNWARD incision for the EXIT site

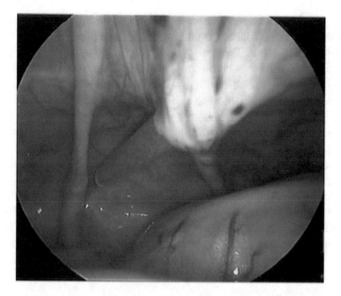

Fig. 1.3 STEP needle and sheath in a preperitoneal tunnel entering the deep pelvis above the dome of the bladder

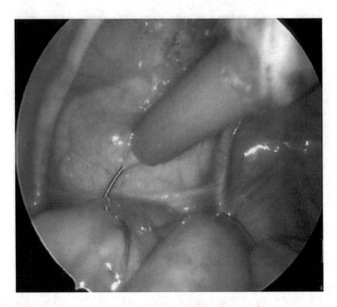

Fig. 1.4 Peel-away sheath with dilator and guide wire down deep in the pelvis

Next, the PD catheter is inserted and advanced through the peel-away sheath. When the first cuff is under the anterior fascia level, the PD catheter is usually curled within the pelvis. The peel-away sheath is then removed while holding the cuff with a pair of forceps below the level of the anterior rectus sheath. Once the sheath is removed, the cuff will remain below the rectus muscle. If needed, a 5 mm instrument can be used to steer the curl end of the PD catheter into an optimal position (Fig. 1.5). Laparoscopy is used to confirm that the radiopaque stripe is not twisted and that the inner cuff has not migrated into the peritoneum.

Next, a second incision is made out LATERAL and INFERIOR to the initial incision so that the second cuff will be positioned within the tunnel about 2 cm from the exit site, and the catheter is facing in a DOWNARD position. The catheter is then tunneled from the first or medial incision, out toward the DOWNWARD and LATERAL incision, ensuring the radiopaque strip is not twisted (Fig. 1.6).

We routinely have a dialysis nurse in the operating room to flush our newly placed PD catheter. We watch the peritoneum fill and then drain under direct laparoscopic visualization. A dwell and drain are also performed without insufflation to ensure proper function.

Once good flow is documented, the anterior fascia purse string suture is tied around the catheter to help anchor the cuff under the anterior rectus sheath to prevent leakage. The subcutaneous tissue is closed in layers followed by skin closure. The LEFT upper quadrant 5 mm incision is closed as well to ensure no leakage. Of note, this incision can be used for a gastrostomy tube placement if needed, as described in this case. The umbilical port is removed last, and the

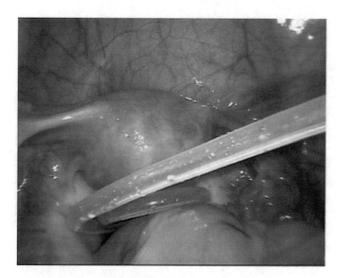

Fig. 1.5 PD catheter curl in satisfactory position deep in the pelvis

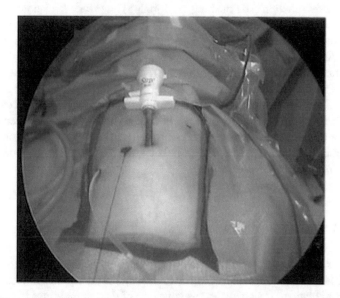

Fig. 1.6 PD catheter EXIT site is LATERAL and DOWNWARD facing. The RIGHT medial incision has the anterior fascia purse string and a 5 mm STEP port within the umbilicus. Also note the 5 mm incision in the LEFT upper quadrant where a 5 mm STEP port was utilized

fascia and skin closed in layers. NO sutures are placed at the PD catheter exit site.

Once the sterile drapes are removed, the PD catheter exit site is dressed by the dialysis nurse.

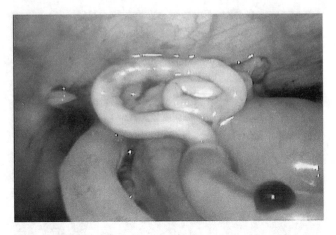

Fig. 1.7 Intraluminal fibrin plug occluding the PD catheter

5. If a peritoneal catheter is not functioning after all medical attempts to reestablish PD catheter function (i.e., flushing, positioning) have failed, a laparoscopic revision is warranted. Entrance is gained via the umbilicus, and an additional 5 mm port can be placed in the LEFT upper quadrant to help facilitate the operation. If the catheter has "flipped" out of the pelvis, it can be repositioned and tested for function. If the catheter has been encased in a fibrous peel, it can be dissected free, repositioned, and tested. If the internal lumen of the catheter is clogged (Fig. 1.7), it can be grasped via the umbilical incision and externalized to help remove the debris; note the camera will need to be in the LEFT upper quadrant port for this maneuver. If none of these maneuvers help restore function, or if the patient has outgrown the initial PD catheter, then removal and replacement can be performed as described above.

Clinical Pearls

1. Laparoscopy via the umbilicus allows for excellent peritoneal visualization for PD catheter insertion, avoiding injury to surrounding structures such as the intestines and bladder. It also allows visualization of the internal rings to ensure they are closed. If the internal rings are patent, they can be repaired with either an open or laparoscopic approach.
2. Omentectomy is routinely performed to help prevent clogging of the side holes within the catheter. Omentopexy, which is described in adults, is not our common practice for fear of a midgut volvulus.
3. STEP needle and sheath tunneling along the posterior sheath allows for deeper placement of the guide wire and sheath for the PD catheter.

4. Creation of a preperitoneal tunnel from the anterior fascia incision to the midline cephalad to the bladder helps prevent catheter dislodgement.
5. Utilization of an additional 5 mm port in the left upper quadrant helps facilitate proper catheter placement into the pelvis and omental removal. This incision can also be used for laparoscopic placement of a gastrostomy tube if needed.
6. Intraoperative testing of the peritoneal dialysis catheter with the dialysis nursing staff is very beneficial to ensure satisfactory dwell and drainage prior to leaving the operating room.
7. If PD catheters are not used for treatment, weekly inspection, and regular dressing changes and catheter flushing will help ensure continued catheter patency.

References

1. Warady BA, Bakkaloglu S, Newland J, et al. Consensus guidelines for the prevention and treatment of catheter-related infections and peritonitis in pediatric patients receiving peritoneal dialysis: 2012 update. Perit Dial Int. 2012;32(Suppl 2):S32–86.
2. Crabtree JH, Fishman A. Selective performance of prophylactic omentopexy during laparoscopic implantation of peritoneal dialysis catheters. Surg Laparosc Endosc Percutan Tech. 2003;13(3):180–4.

Chapter 2
Peritoneal Equilibration Testing and Application

Francisco J. Cano

Case Presentation

FW, a recently diagnosed patient with CKD Stage 5, is a 6-year-old boy who has been recommended to initiate chronic dialysis. His primary renal disorder is renal dysplasia. His nutritional evaluation reveals a weight of 18.1 kg (SDS −1.08), height 102 cm (SDS −2.64), and BSA 0.8 m^2. His residual renal Kt/V is 0.3. A pre-dialysis biochemical evaluation showed BUN 70 mg/dl, creatinine 6.5 mg/dl, hemoglobin 9.4 g/dl, serum calcium 9.2 mg/dl, phosphorus 7.7 mg/dl, PTH 580 pg/ml, 25(OH)D_3 14.5 ng/ml, and serum albumin 3.8 g/L; electrolytes were Na 138 meq/L, K 5.4 meq/L, Cl 101 meq/L, and serum CO_2 19.2 meq/L. Echocardiography showed a left ventricular mass index (LVMI) value of 45 $g/m^{2.7}$.

Peritoneal dialysis (PD) was initiated several weeks after PD catheter placement, with the fill volume reaching 700 ml/exchange (900 ml/m^2) 3 weeks after dialysis initiation. The PD modality used was continuous ambulatory peritoneal dialysis (CAPD), and FW's initial dialysis prescription consisted of Dianeal® 1.5%, four exchanges per day, with each exchange lasting 6 h. During the second month of PD, a 4-h peritoneal equilibration test (PET) was performed.

During the night prior to the test, an 800 ml (1,100 ml/m^2) exchange of 2.5% dextrose dialysis solution was instilled for 8 h. On the day of the test, the overnight exchange was drained, and another exchange with Dianeal 2.5% was infused. Dialysate samples for creatinine and glucose were obtained at 0, 2, and 4 h of dwell time, and a blood sample for creatinine was obtained at 2 h. The 4-h results were as follows:

F.J. Cano (✉)
Faculty of Medicine, University of Chile, Santiago, Chile

Luis Calvo Mackenna Children's Hospital, Santiago, Chile
e-mail: fcanosch@gmail.com

© Springer International Publishing AG 2017
B.A. Warady et al. (eds.), *Pediatric Dialysis Case Studies*,
DOI 10.1007/978-3-319-55147-0_2

11

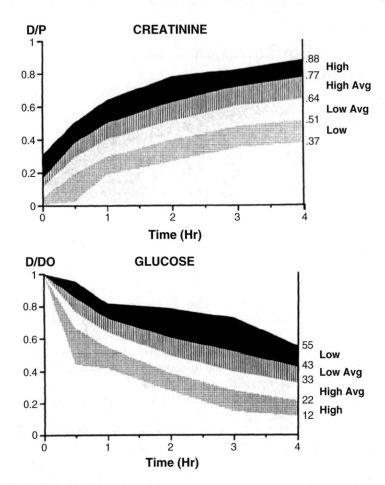

Fig. 2.1 Peritoneal equilibration test categories

D/P creatinine, 0.64, and D/D_0 glucose, 0.38. These results were compatible with a high-average transporter status (Fig. 2.1).

In view of these PET results, the PD modality was changed to nocturnal intermittent PD (NIPD). The prescription consisted of seven, 1-h exchanges nightly, with an 800 ml fill volume using Dianeal 1.5% peritoneal dialysis solution. Over the initial 18 months of PD, the patient experienced a single episode of peritonitis with a good response to antibiotic treatment. The PET was not repeated after this peritonitis episode.

After 2 years of PD, the patient's blood pressure was 110/76 mmHg (95th percentile), and the residual renal Kt/V decreased to a value of 0.2. Echocardiography demonstrated an increased LVMI with a value of 54 $g/m^{2.7}$. As a result of the clinical evidence of hypervolemia and the desire to provide the best PD prescription for both solute and fluid management, a repeat PET was performed. The treating physician chose not to conduct a short PET. Results showed a 4-h D/P creatinine of 0.45 and a 4-h D/Do glucose of 0.58, findings now compatible with a low transporter status. Based on this result, FW had his PD prescription changed to a long dwell PD schedule, specifically the use of CAPD with a 1,000-ml fill volume and four, 6-h exchanges daily.

Clinical Questions

1. Is the PET a useful tool in pediatric peritoneal dialysis?
2. What is the importance of the duration of the exchange preceding the PET?
3. What is the importance of the fill volume in the PET?
4. How should the results of the PET be used to help select the PD modality and prescription?
5. Are both the Short PET and the Classical PET appropriate for use in children?
6. When should the PET be repeated?

Diagnostic Discussion

1. The success of peritoneal dialysis therapy is based on the ability of the peritoneal membrane to serve as a semipermeable membrane for solute transport and ultrafiltration. The properties of this membrane are also key determinants of the patient's outcome [1–4].

   The peritoneal equilibration test (PET) represents a semiquantitative means to assess the peritoneal membrane permeability in dialyzed patients, and the resultant data aids in the individualized prescription of peritoneal dialysis therapy. In pediatrics, a considerable experience with the PET has been accumulated during the past 20 years [4, 5]. The PET helps tailor the PD prescription to meet the specific needs of the patient in terms of

   (a) Fill volume
   (b) Length of each exchange
   (c) Number of daily cycles
   (d) Dextrose concentration of peritoneal dialysis solution

   - *The PET is performed in children in the following manner:*

     1. An overnight 3–8h exchange is performed.
     2. The overnight exchange is drained upon arrival to the PD unit the following morning.
     3. A transfer Y-type set is installed.
     4. A 1,100-ml/m$_2$ fill volume, 2.5% glucose peritoneal dialysis solution is infused, and patient is rolled from side to side during the infusion.

5. After concluding the infusion, dialysis solution is maintained in the peritoneal cavity for a 2- (short PET) or 4-h (classical PET) dwell time.
6. Dialysate samples are taken at 0, 2, and 4 h for the classical PET. A 10-ml volume is sent for glucose and creatinine measurement.
7. A serum sample is obtained at the midpoint of the PET (at 1 or 2 h, dependent on length of PET).
8. The dialysate to plasma (D/P) hour 2 if short PET, hour 4 if classical PET for creatinine, and dialysate hour 2 (if short PET) or hour 4 (if classical PET) to dialysate hour 0 (D2-4/D0) glucose ratios are calculated.

- *Interpretation of the PET*

Patients are categorized as low, low-average, high-average, or high transporters according to the PET results [6].

A low transport state is diagnosed when the D/P creatinine ratio is below −1 standard deviation (SD), and the glucose D/D_0 ratio is above +1 SD of the mean normative value; a low-average transport capacity corresponds to a D/P creatinine ratio between the mean and −1 SD and a D/D_0 glucose ratio between the mean and +1 SD; a high-average transport capacity is diagnosed when the D/P creatinine ratio is between the mean and +1 SD and the D/D_0 glucose is between the mean and −1 SD; and a high transport capacity corresponds to a D/P creatinine ratio more than +1 SD and a D/D_0 glucose ratio less than −1 SD of the mean value. Pediatric reference PET data have been published [7].

2. The importance of the long-dwell exchange prior to the PET relates to the desire to obtain plasma-peritoneal solute equilibrium. In the original description of the PET, the dwell time of the preceding exchange was approximately 8 h [6]. Whereas this long-dwell exchange is easily performed in CAPD patients, pediatric patients are often prescribed automated peritoneal dialysis (APD); therefore, a nocturnal long-dwell exchange represents an important change in their dialysis regimen. In turn, Lilaj et al. [8] subsequently showed that the absence of a prior long exchange had a significant influence on the D/P ratios of small solutes, urea, creatinine, and proteins. Twardowski et al. [9] confirmed that a prior exchange with a dwell time between 3 and 8 h results in only a small and nonsignificant influence on the D/P ratios of creatinine and urea, as well as on the D/Do glucose. Therefore, each center should define a standard preceding exchange duration prior to the PET test and implement it uniformly in order to be able to draw conclusions and compare results [10].

3. The peritoneal membrane surface area in children has been determined to be twice as large as the surface area in adults when expressed per kg body weight. In contrast, the peritoneal membrane surface areas of children and adults are more comparable when the scaling factor is body surface area (BSA). In turn, when weight is used to calculate fill volume, infants and children with low body weight will receive less dialysate in proportion to their peritoneal surface area, and the PET results will give the artifactual impression of a high peritoneal membrane transport capacity because of rapid equilibration of solutes between plasma and dialysate in the setting of a small fill volume. As shown by Warady et al. [11], this phenomenon is explained by the concept of "geometry of diffusion." Therefore,

the PET fill volume in children should be prescribed in terms of BSA to avoid a diagnosis of functional hyperpermeability and to provide the most accurate information upon which to base the dialysis prescription [12].

4. The optimal dialysis prescription in terms of solute and fluid removal will differ according to the peritoneal transporter type. In the case of fast transporters, short-dwell time exchanges should be prescribed to obtain adequate ultrafiltration and urea purification.

   Clinically, a patient with a high peritoneal membrane transport capacity using long-duration dwell times will limit ultrafiltration and will show signs of volume overload, such as edema, hypertension, and cardiovascular deterioration.

   Conversely, in slow transporters, long-dwell exchanges and large fill volumes are required to optimize solute clearance. At the same time, the slow transport results in maintenance of the glucose gradient and the achievement of adequate ultrafiltration.

   Therefore, APD regimens are indicated for fast transporters, and CAPD is often the best PD modality choice for patients with low peritoneal membrane transport capacity [13–15].

   High-average and low-average transporters will benefit from the use of a mixed dialysis regimen, such as with the use of CCPD, using short-time dwells during the night and keeping 1 or 2 long-dwell exchanges during the day.

5. Twardowski et al. [9, 16] previously measured D/P creatinine and D/D_0 glucose during a 2-h (short) and a 4-h (classical) PET. Those authors found that for both solutes, equilibration curves were almost identical irrespective of test duration. Thus, the short PET was considered a valid study to classify membrane characteristics as established in the original PET study.

   In pediatrics, Warady et al. [17] characterized peritoneal membrane transport capacity comparing a 2- vs 4-h D/P creatinine and 2- vs 4-h D/D_0 glucose values in a retrospective experience in 20 children on PD. Results were consistent with the previous adult findings indicating that the short and classical PET provide equal characterizations of peritoneal membrane transport capacity. These conclusions were supported in a prospective multicenter pediatric study of 84 PET studies in 74 PD patients [18].

   Together, these data suggest that, like in adult patients, a short version of the PET can be applied to the pediatric population.

6. The K-DOQI Guidelines on peritoneal dialysis adequacy [14] are one of the most comprehensive set of recommendations published to date on the care of patients receiving peritoneal dialysis. For adults patients, the recommendations suggest that total urea Kt/V (dialysis Kt/V + residual renal Kt/V) and peritoneal transport characteristics should be measured 1 month after starting PD. Whereas there is no need to routinely repeat the PET since peritoneal transport is stable over time in most patients, the PET should be repeated when one of the following situations arises:

   - Unexplained volume overload
   - Edema, hypertension, or increased LVMI
   - Unexplained decreasing drain volume
   - Unexplained worsening of uremia symptoms

- Changes in Kt/V
- Increasing needs for hypertonic dialysis solution to maintain ultrafiltration

The findings generated by the PET in these settings will assist the care provider in appropriately modifying the patient's dialysis prescription in terms of fill volume, exchange duration, and dextrose concentration of the dialysis solution [1, 2, 4, 15, 19].

Clinical Pearls

1. The peritoneal equilibration test (PET) has been validated to be the best method to evaluate peritoneal membrane transport capacity in children and adults.
2. The PET permits patients to be categorized as low, low-average, high-average, or high transporters which, in turn, helps determine the best PD prescription characteristics in terms of fill volume, length of each exchange, and dextrose concentration of the dialysis solution.
3. Changes in peritoneal transport should be evaluated with a repeat PET when there is clinical evidence of changes in dialysis efficiency, especially when the changes have the potential of influencing cardiovascular morbidity and mortality in uremic children.

References

1. Schaefer F, Warady B. Peritoneal dialysis in children with end-stage renal disease. Nat Rev Nephrol. 2011;7:659–68.
2. Fischbach M, Stefanidis CJ, Watson AR. Guidelines by an ad hoc European committee on adequacy of the pediatric peritoneal dialysis prescription. Nephrol Dial Transplant. 2002;17:380–2.
3. Fischbach M, Warady B. Peritoneal dialysis prescription in children: bedside principles for optimal practice. Pediatr Nephrol. 2009;24:1633–42.
4. Schmitt CP, et al. Peritoneal dialysis tailored to pediatric needs. Int J Nephrol. 2011;2011:1–9.
5. Verrina E, et al. Selection of modalities, prescription, and technical issues in children on peritoneal dialysis. Pediatr Nephrol. 2009;24:1453–64.
6. Twardowski ZJ, Nolph KD, Khanna R, Prowant BF, Ryan LP, Moore HL. Peritoneal equilibration test. Perit Dial Bull. 1987;7:138–47.
7. Warady BA, Alexander SR, Hossli S, Vonesh E, Geary D, Watkins S, Salusky IB, Kohaut EC. Peritoneal membrane transport function in children receiving long-term dialysis. J Am Soc Nephrol. 1996;7:2385–91.
8. Lilaj T, Vychytil A, Schneider B, Hörl WH, Haag-Weber M. Influence of the preceding exchange on peritoneal equilibration test results: a prospective study. Am J Kidney Dis. 1999;34:247–53.
9. Twardowski Z, Prowant F, Moore H, Lou C, White E, Farris K. Short peritoneal equilibration test: impact of preceding dwell time. Adv Perit Dial. 2003;19:53–8.
10. Figueiredo AE, Conti A, de Figueiredo CE. Influence of the preceding exchange on peritoneal equilibration test results. Adv Perit Dial. 2002;18:75–7.

11. Warady BA, Alexander SR, Hossli S, Vonesh E, Geary D, Kohaut EC. The relationship between intraperitoneal volume and solute transport in pediatric patients. J Am Soc Nephrol. 1995;5:1935–9.
12. Kohaut EC, Waldo FB, Benfield MR. The effect of changes in dialysate volume on glucose and urea equilibration. Perit Dial Int. 1994;14:236–9.
13. Fischbach M, Dheu C, Seuge-Dargnies L, Delobbe JF. Adequacy of peritoneal dialysis in children: consider the membrane for optimal prescription. Perit Dial Int. 2002;27(Suppl 2):S167–70.
14. KDOQI clinical practice guidelines and clinical practice recommendations for 2006 updates: hemodialysis adequacy, peritoneal dialysis adequacy and vascular access. Am J Kidney Dis. 2006;48(Suppl 1):S1–S322.
15. Brimble K, et al. Meta-analysis: peritoneal membrane transport, mortality, and technique failure in peritoneal dialysis. J Am Soc Nephrol. 2006;17:2591–8.
16. Twardowski ZJ, Nolph KD, Khanna R, et al. Peritoneal equilibration test. Perit Dial Bull. 1987; Short peritoneal equilibration test 58 7:138–147.
17. Warady B, et al. The short PET in pediatrics. Perit Dial Int. 2007;27:441–5.
18. Cano F, et al. The short peritoneal equilibration test in pediatric peritoneal dialysis. Pediatr Nephrol. 2010;25:2159–4.
19. Schaefer F, Klaus G, Mehls O. Mid-European Pediatric Peritoneal Dialysis Study Group. Peritoneal transport properties and dialysis dose affect growth and nutritional status in children on chronic peritoneal dialysis. J Am Soc Nephrol. 1999;10:1786–92.

Chapter 3
Peritoneal Dialysis Prescription

Nathan T. Beins and Bradley A. Warady

Case Presentation

A 3-year-old patient was diagnosed at birth with posterior urethral valves and associated chronic kidney disease (CKD) and subsequently developed end-stage renal disease at 13 months of age. He was started on peritoneal dialysis (PD) and was gradually advanced to his current automated PD prescription consisting of a fill volume of 900 mL/m^2, dwell time of 50 min, and 10 cycles occurring overnight with a daytime fill volume of 400 mL/m^2. A peritoneal equilibration test (PET) conducted 5 weeks following PD initiation revealed the patient to be a high-average transporter. His weekly total Kt/V_{urea} was 2.7 approximately 6 months ago. His initial prescription included the use of 1.5% dextrose peritoneal dialysis solution, as he did not require substantial ultrafiltration because of the presence of residual kidney function. Recently, however, he has been experiencing a gradual reduction in his residual kidney function, and a repeat assessment of clearance revealed a total weekly Kt/V_{urea} measurement of only 1.6 with a 24-h urine collection demonstrating less than 100 mL of urine output. Over the past several months, he has also developed increasing evidence of "underdialysis" as reflected by rising blood urea nitrogen (BUN) and serum creatinine levels, moderate secondary hyperparathyroidism, and a decreased appetite. His anemia has remained well managed. Noteworthy is the fact that he has only had a single episode of peritonitis.

N.T. Beins (✉) • B.A. Warady
Division of Pediatric Nephrology, University of Missouri, Kansas City School of Medicine, Children's Mercy Hospital, Kansas City, MO, USA
e-mail: ntbeins@cmh.edu

© Springer International Publishing AG 2017
B.A. Warady et al. (eds.), *Pediatric Dialysis Case Studies*,
DOI 10.1007/978-3-319-55147-0_3

As a result of the finding of a Kt/V_{urea} below the KDOQI target and the associated clinical/laboratory evidence of decreased solute removal, the patient underwent a repeat PET which demonstrated low-average transporter status with a dialysis to plasma creatinine ratio of 0.56 at 2 h. Based upon these results and the use of the PD Adequest modeling program, his dialysis prescription was adjusted to 1.5% dextrose, 90-min dwell time, and eight cycles nightly. His fill volume was increased to 1,100 mL/m^2 with good tolerance. Despite a reduction in cycle number and a lower urine output, UF on the new prescription was sufficient to maintain a stable fluid balance with 1.5% dextrose. Repeat weekly Kt/V_{urea} testing a few weeks following these adjustments was 2.2, with an improved appetite and decreased BUN and serum creatinine values. He remained active on the deceased donor transplant waiting list.

Clinical Questions

1. What is peritoneal dialysis "adequacy" in children?
2. What are the components of the peritoneal dialysis prescription?
3. What options are available for peritoneal dialysis solutions?
4. What are the peritoneal dialysis modality options?
5. What tools are available to assist with individualizing the PD prescription?

Diagnostic Discussion

1. Guidelines for the determination of peritoneal dialysis adequacy predominantly focus on small solute clearance in the form of Kt/V_{urea}. While small solute clearance provides a useful target for standardized guidelines, the determination of dialysis adequacy involves many other facets of clinical care. The adequacy of a patient's dialysis care must also incorporate consideration of fluid status, nutrition and growth, anemia, control of calcium-phosphate balance, and preservation of residual renal function. However, solute clearance can serve as a useful calculated indicator regarding the sufficiency of the dialysis prescription. Current national pediatric guidelines recommend ensuring a weekly urea clearance divided by the volume of distribution (Kt/V_{urea}) of 1.8 or more, including both dialysis and renal clearance [1–3]. These guidelines and the associated evidence are based predominantly upon adult studies, and most experts recommend that the small solute clearance in children should meet or exceed the adult standards [1–5]. Most guidelines recommend assessment of dialysis adequacy within 1 month of dialysis initiation and at least every 6 months thereafter.

   Calculation of the weekly Kt/V_{urea} involves the collection of a 24-h timed collection of dialysate and any residual urine output for calculation of urea clearance. The Kt/V_{urea} for dialysis is the dialysate/plasma urea concentration ratio divided by the volume of distribution of urea, which is assumed to be equal to total body water. For patients with residual renal output, the dialysis associated Kt/V_{urea} should be considered in addition to the renal urea clearance as demonstrated by the formula below:

$$\frac{\left(\text{Dialysate urea concentration} / \text{plasma urea concentration} \times \text{daily dialysate volume} \times 7\right)}{\text{Total body water}}$$
$$+ \frac{\text{Renal urea clearance in } mL / \min \times 1,440 \min/ day \times 7}{1,000 mL \times V} = \text{Weekly} Kt / V_{urea}$$

2. The overarching goal of peritoneal dialysis is to achieve adequate ultrafiltration and solute clearance. To achieve that goal, the peritoneal dialysis prescription should be individualized with reference to the peritoneal fill volume, dwell time, total session duration, and dialysate composition. Most dialysate composition is determined by preformed manufacturer solutions (see Table 3.1). The vast majority of patients on peritoneal dialysis utilize an automated cycling machine with nocturnal cycles with or without a prolonged daytime dwell [6].

   The peritoneal fill volume is typically 1,000–1,200 mL/m² in children [5]. Body surface area (BSA) is used as the scaling factor because of the direct relationship between peritoneal surface area and BSA. Younger children (less than 2 years) will often not tolerate a high intraperitoneal volume (due to discomfort, increased risk of hernia formation, and leakage), and thus their prescription is based more upon patient tolerance than an ideal clearance-based approach. Most young children will tolerate an intraperitoneal volume between 600 and 800 mL/m². The target intraperitoneal volumes for children have been developed based upon the proposed volume necessary to fully recruit the peritoneal membrane and to avoid excessive intraperitoneal pressure which may result in patient discomfort [7]. Daytime exchanges, when prescribed, usually consist of a lower fill volume (approximately 50% of the nocturnal fill volume), while the nocturnal volumes used can be larger due to the lower intraperitoneal pressure associated with a supine position.

   The prescribed peritoneal dwell time is strongly influenced by the peritoneal membrane solute transport characteristics and ultrafiltration capacity. Patients with a high membrane transport capacity per the PET evaluation (see below) will characteristically be prescribed a relatively short dwell time to achieve adequate ultrafiltration due to the rapid loss of the osmotic gradient between dialysate and the patient. In contrast, those patients with a low membrane solute transport capacity will require fewer cycles per session to achieve adequate ultrafiltration because of their maintenance of the osmotic gradient. However, they may require an increased fill volume to achieve the desired solute removal.

3. Most patients receiving chronic peritoneal dialysis receive standard commercially available peritoneal dialysis solutions. Regardless of the commercial

Table 3.1 Composition of commercially available peritoneal dialysis solutions

	Balance	Gambrosol 10/40	Dianeal	Physioneal	BicaVera	Extraneal (icodextrin)
Sodium (mmol/L)	134	132	132	132	132	132
Chloride (mmol/L)	100.5	95/96	96	95	104.5	96
Calcium (mmol/L)	1.25/1.75	1.35/1.75	2.5/3.5	1.25	1.75	1.75
Magnesium (mmol/L)	0.5	0.25	0.5	0.25	0.5	0.25
Glucose (%)	1.5/2.3/4.25	1.5/2.5/4.0	1.5/2.5/4.25	1.36/2.27/3.86	1.5/2.3/4.25	7.5% icodextrin
Osmolarity (mOsm/L)	356–509	353–492	346–485	344–484	358–511	284
pH	7.0	5.5	5.5	7.4	7.4	5.5
Lactate (mmol/L)	35	40	40	15	0	40
Bicarbonate	0	0	0	25	34	0

Adapted from Ref. [8]

solution selected, the majority of solutions consist of a mildly hyponatremic, hyperosmolar solution utilizing dextrose as the primary active osmolar agent. Much of the decision regarding the selection of a peritoneal dialysis solution focuses on the glucose/dextrose concentration and the calcium content. Commercially available solutions usually provide dextrose concentrations of 1.5%, 2.5%, and 4.25%. Whereas higher concentrations of dextrose enhance ultrafiltration by increasing the osmotic gradient between the patient and the dialysis solution, a strategy that has been used in "high transporters," the hypertonic solutions increase exposure to glucose degradation products (GDPs) and the risk of subsequent impaired function of the peritoneal membrane. Icodextrin is a glucose polymer that exerts a colloidal osmotic effect that can serve as an effective and likely safer alternative to hypertonic solutions in many patients. Commercially available solutions also provide high and low calcium content options, allowing for higher calcium administration to infants and young children with higher needs to maintain linear growth. Newer biocompatible dialysis solutions have been developed that incorporate more neutral pH, bicarbonate buffering, and decreased production of GDPs and are available in many countries, but not in the US. Table 3.1 summarizes the composition of several commercially available solutions (traditional and biocompatible) including the available dextrose and calcium options.

4. Peritoneal dialysis can be performed with an automated cycler (automated peritoneal dialysis, APD) or with manual exchanges (continuous ambulatory peritoneal dialysis, CAPD). The vast majority of children on peritoneal dialysis are now treated with APD, especially in areas where it is not limited by cost constraints [6]. CAPD is performed via multiple daytime manual exchanges (usually 3–5 exchanges) and a prolonged nocturnal dwell. Due to the ambulatory nature of CAPD, it necessitates the utilization of smaller intraperitoneal fill volumes due to patient tolerance [8]. While patients can achieve adequate clearance on CAPD, especially those with residual renal function, it is often overly burdensome for children because of the need for daytime exchanges.

APD offers numerous benefits to children on peritoneal dialysis, including flexibility with lifestyle choices and the ability to attend school without the need for daytime exchanges. Nightly intermittent peritoneal dialysis (NIPD) is characterized by several short nocturnal dwells with a dry peritoneum during the day. NIPD is often the first regimen adopted due to its ease of implementation, especially in those patients with residual renal function. However, due to the short nocturnal dwells there is often limited solute clearance (primarily middle-sized molecules) and patients with low or low-average peritoneal transport capacity will often have inadequate clearance on an NIPD schedule. Continuous cycling peritoneal dialysis (CCPD) slightly modifies the NIPD schedule with the addition of a prolonged daytime exchange. This daytime dwell volume allows for further middle-sized molecule clearance and allows for further flexibility regarding fluid status and ultrafiltration.

Tidal PD is another modification of an APD regimen that maintains a residual volume of dialysate within the peritoneum during drainage cycles. The maintenance

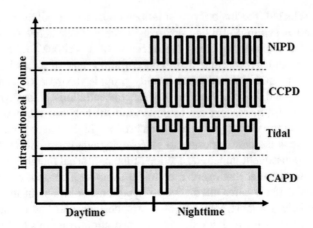

Fig. 3.1 Peritoneal dialysis regimens

of a "reserve" volume of dialysate within the peritoneum ensures continued contact with the peritoneal membrane, allowing for improved solute removal. Tidal PD also can be beneficial in patients who suffer from discomfort/pain with drain cycles or those patients who have frequent cycler alarms. The volumes required in Tidal PD must be individualized in each patient to identify the "breakpoint," or the time at which the catheter drainage flow rate decreases, as that point can serve to indicate the necessary remaining intraperitoneal volume to ensure adequate solute transport (Fig. 3.1).

5. Unlike hemodialysis, where the semipermeable membrane is standardized, children utilizing the peritoneal membrane for dialysis can have wide variations in the characteristics and function of their peritoneal membrane. In turn, formal testing of the peritoneal membrane transport characteristics with the peritoneal equilibration test (PET) can facilitate individualization of the dialysis prescription to optimize therapy. Current expert recommendations call for the assessment of peritoneal membrane transport characteristics at the initiation of peritoneal dialysis and anytime there is evidence of decreased ultrafiltration capacity or decreased solute clearance, both of which can occur after repeated episodes of peritonitis [3, 9].

The standard PET is performed with a standardized procedure including the use of 2.5% dextrose dialysis solution and a fill volume of 1,100 mL/m^2 body surface area. Dialysate and plasma concentrations of solutes and glucose are measured at initiation, 2 h, and 4 h. Dialysate to plasma (D/P) ratio of solutes and glucose should be calculated at each time interval, and the resulting curve is compared to the standardized reference data (Fig. 3.2) to determine the transport characteristics of the peritoneal membrane [10]. A shorter 2-h PET is also validated for use in children with similar results [11]. Patients with high transporter status will often experience limited ultrafiltration (due to rapid glucose absorption) whereas those with low transporter status will typically have successful

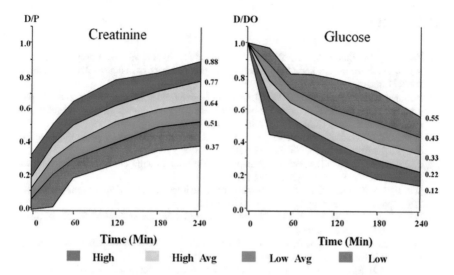

Fig. 3.2 Peritoneal transport characteristics according to the standardized peritoneal equilibration test (Republished with permission of Warady et al. [10]. Permission conveyed through Copyright Clearance Center, Inc.)

ultrafiltration because of maintenance of the osmotic gradient between dialysate and plasma, but may have considerable difficulty achieving adequate solute clearance targets.

Clinical Pearls

1. Dialysis adequacy is a complex determination involving solute clearance (measured with weekly Kt/V_{urea}), fluid status, nutrition/growth, and residual renal function. Weekly Kt/V_{urea} should be >1.8 and measured at least every 6 months, more frequently if there is a progressive loss of residual renal function.
2. The components of the peritoneal dialysis prescription include the intraperitoneal fill volume, the dwell time, and the composition of the peritoneal dialysate, with particular reference to the dextrose concentration.
3. Standard commercial, lactate-buffered peritoneal dialysate solutions are commonly used, but result in increased glucose degradation products and an increased risk of direct peritoneal membrane toxicity. Newer, biocompatible solutions with bicarbonate buffering are available in certain locales, but are associated with increased expense.
4. Most children on peritoneal dialysis will utilize an automated peritoneal dialysis regimen utilizing a cycler with a nocturnal, intermittent or continuous cycling regimen.
5. The peritoneal equilibration test is the most common test used to evaluate peritoneal membrane function and can provide valuable information for individualizing a dialysis prescription.

References

1. Fischbach M, Stefanidis CJ, Watson AR. Guidelines by an ad hoc European committee on adequacy of the pediatric peritoneal dialysis prescription. Nephrol Dial Transplant. 2002;17:380–5.
2. National Kidney Foundation. KDOQI clinical practice guidelines and clinical practice recommendations for 2006 updates. Hemodialysis adequacy, peritoneal dialysis adequacy and vascular access. Am J Kidney Dis. 2006;28(Suppl 1):S1.
3. White CT, Gowrishanker M, Feber J, et al. Clinical practice guidelines for pediatric peritoneal dialysis. Pediatr Nephrol. 2006;21:1059–66.
4. Fischbach M, Warady BA. Peritoneal dialysis prescription in children: bedside principles for optimal practice. Pediatr Nephrol. 2009;24:1633–42.
5. Warady BA, Neu AM, Schaefer F. Optimal care of the infant, child, and adolescent on dialysis: 2014 update. Am J Kidney Dis. 2014;64(1):128–42.
6. North American Pediatric Renal Trials and Collaborative Studies (NAPRTCS). Annual dialysis report. Rockville: Emmes Corp.; 2011.
7. Fischbach M, Haraldsson B. Dynamic changes of total pore area available for peritoneal exchange in children. J Am Soc Nephrol. 2001;12:1524–9.
8. Schmitt CP, Bakkaloglu SA, Klaus G, et al. Solutions for peritoneal dialysis in children: recommendations by the European Pediatric Dialysis Working Group. Pediatr Nephrol. 2011;26(7):1137–47.
9. Morgenstern B. Peritoneal dialysis and prescription monitoring. In: Warady BA, Schaefer FS, Fine RN, Alexander SR, editors. Pediatric dialysis. Dordrecht: Kluwer Academic; 2004. p. 147–61.
10. Warady BA, Alexander SR, Hossli S, et al. Peritoneal membrane transport function in children receiving long-term dialysis. J Am Soc Nephrol. 1996;7:2385–91.
11. Warady BA, Jennings J. The short PET in pediatrics. Perit Dial Int. 2007;27:441–5.

Additional Resources

Cho Y, Johnson DW, Craig JC, et al. Biocompatible dialysis fluids for peritoneal dialysis. Cochrane Database Syst Rev. 2014;3:Art. No.: CD007554
Fischbach M, Zaloszyc A, Schaefer B, et al. Optimizing peritoneal dialysis prescription for volume control: the importance of varying dwell time and dwell volume. Pediatr Nephrol. 2014;29:1321–7.
Honda M. Peritoneal dialysis prescription suitable for children with anuria. Perit Dial Int. 2008;28(suppl 3):S153–8.
Johnson DW, Brown FG, Clarke M, et al. Effects of biocompatible versus standard fluid on peritoneal dialysis outcomes. J Am Soc Nephrol. 2012;23:1097–107.
McIntyre CW. Update on peritoneal dialysis solutions. Kidney Int. 2007;71:486–90.
Schaefer F, Langebeck D, Heckert KH, et al. Evaluation of peritoneal solute transfer by the peritoneal equilibration test in children. Adv Perit Dial. 1992;8:410–5.
Schaefer F, Haraldsson B, Haas S, et al. Estimation of peritoneal mass transport by three-pore model in children. Kidney Int. 1998;54:1372–9.
Tam P, Sheldrake P, Ng A, et al. Peritoneal equilibration testing: correcting the correction factor. Perit Dial Int. 2009;29:352–5.
Verrina E, Cappelli V, Perfumo F. Selection of modalities, prescription, and technical issues in children on peritoneal dialysis. Pediatr Nephrol. 2009;24:1453–64.

Chapter 4
Dialysis During Infancy

Joshua J. Zaritsky and Bradley A. Warady

Case Presentation

A 38-week gestation male infant was born and quickly intubated due to the presence of severe respiratory distress. The prenatal history was notable for oligohydramnios. Prenatal ultrasound conducted at 30 weeks revealed bilateral hydronephrosis with echogenic renal parenchyma. On initial postnatal exam, the baby was noted to have a distended abdomen with absent abdominal musculature and undescended testes. An abdominal ultrasound revealed dysplastic kidneys with grossly dilated ureters and a dilated bladder with a thickened wall.

Over the next 7 days the respiratory status improved, but the infant developed progressive fluid overload despite the repeated use of diuretics. Although nutrition had been limited as a result of prescribed fluid restriction because of the presence of oliguria, the infant was relatively hyperkalemia (K=6.5 mmol/L) with an elevated BUN (85 mg/dL). The serum creatinine also steadily increased over the first week of life to 4.2 mg/dL. Discussions occurred daily involving the family, attending neonatologist and nephrologist, during which time information was provided about the child's overall status and ultimately about the dialysis process, its risks potential complications and likely long-term outcome. Subsequent to meeting with multiple additional members of the neonatal multidisciplinary team, the dialysis social worker and nurse, and extended family members, the child's parents agreed with the plan for placement of a peritoneal dialysis catheter along with a gastrostomy tube in preparation for the initiation of chronic dialysis.

J.J. Zaritsky, MD, PhD (✉)
Nemours/A.I. duPont Hospital for Children, Wilmington, DE, USA
e-mail: Joshua.zaritsky@nemours.org

B.A. Warady, MD
Division of Pediatric Nephrology, University of Missouri, Kansas City School of Medicine, Children's Mercy Hospital, Kansas City, MO, USA

© Springer International Publishing AG 2017
B.A. Warady et al. (eds.), *Pediatric Dialysis Case Studies*,
DOI 10.1007/978-3-319-55147-0_4

Clinical Questions

1. What is known about the incidence, prevalence, and etiology of end-stage renal disease (ESRD) during infancy?
2. What are some of the ethical issues that come into play when making a decision regarding the initiation of chronic dialysis during infancy?
3. What is the preferred chronic dialysis modality in the infant age group?
4. What are some of the nutritional considerations for an infant on dialysis?
5. What are the long-term outcome data for infants who receive chronic dialysis?

Diagnostic Discussion

1. Despite an increased awareness of the capacity to care for infants with end-stage renal disease (ESRD), the need for long-term renal replacement therapy (RRT) in this age group remains rare. Much of the published data examining the management of ESRD patients uses a rather broad age range of birth to 24 months. Carey et al. [1] using data from the dialysis registry of the NAPRTCS reported an incidence of 0.32 ESRD cases per 10,000 live births during the first 2 years of life. The United States Renal Data System (USRDS) reported an ESRD incidence of approximately ten cases per million population in the 0–4-year age group over the last decade and a point prevalence (dialysis and transplant) of 600 cases [2]. The incidence of ESRD resulting in chronic dialysis in infants also appears to vary regionally with a recent report of the International Pediatric Peritoneal Dialysis Network (IPPN) suggesting that centers in low-income countries (gross national income <$12,000) rarely offer PD to young patients, with only 8% of their dialysis patients being <3 years old [3].

Table 4.1 Primary renal disorders in infants with ESRD

Diagnosis	Age ≤ 1 month n (%)	Age > 1–24 months n (%)
Renal dysplasia	72 (37.3)	129 (25.5)
Obstructive uropathy	39 (20.2)	89 (15.8)
Autosomal recessive polycystic kidney disease	23 (11.9)	40 (7.9)
Congenital nephrotic syndrome	3 (1.5)	54 (10.7)
Other	56 (29)	202 (40.0)

Table adapted from Carey et al. [1]

The list of disorders that result in kidney disease requiring chronic dialysis in the infant is relatively short. Carey et al. [1] reported the most frequent disorders to be renal dysplasia and obstructive uropathy (Table 4.1). Prune-belly syndrome, diagnosed in the case above, is included in the obstructive uropathy category and is characterized by the clinical triad of (1) absent or deficient abdominal musculature, (2) severe urinary tract abnormalities, and (3) bilateral cryptorchidism in males.

2. Clearly, one of the most difficult issues that families and pediatric nephrology teams are confronted with is the decision regarding when and if chronic dialysis therapy should be initiated for the infant with ESRD (see also Chap. 6). Despite advances in dialysis technology and clinical expertise that now makes it possible to provide dialysis to this patient population safely and effectively, the concept of proceeding with a lifetime of ESRD care is unavoidably complex. Comorbidities such as neurocognitive delay, growth delay, the prospect of multiple hospitalizations, and the almost universal need for supplemental tube feeding contribute to the ethical dilemma experienced by many families and healthcare providers. Often complicating the situation is the presence of significant non-renal comorbidities, such as neurological abnormalities and/or pulmonary hypoplasia, which are present in up to one third of infants with ESRD and which are associated with an increased risk for mortality [4, 5]. In fact, the mortality rate of the youngest infants (0–2 years) who have received chronic dialysis has historically been quite poor, with 2-year mortality rates as high as 30%; however, more recent data has revealed significantly better outcomes (see below) [1, 6].

In adult patients, the four principles of medical ethics, autonomy, beneficence, non-maleficence, and justice are characteristically applied to decisions on whether to withhold or withdraw dialysis [7]. However, in the case of infants, the wishes of the parents, who are usually entitled to make decisions regarding the medical care their children receive, must also be taken into consideration. This ethical dilemma is not all that uncommon in the neonatal intensive care unit and occurs in other situations, such as in the case of the infant with hypoplastic left heart syndrome [8, 9]. Ideally, the decision of whether to provide or withhold dialysis represents a consensus opinion of the parents, nephrologist, neonatalogist, and other members of a multidisciplinary team. That decision should be determined only after a thorough review of the patient's clinical status, the family's dynamics, and a review of the limited data that exists within the medical literature on the outcome of young infants with ESRD. Despite the best efforts to this end, there remains substantial potential for disagreement regarding the best course of action to take because of the multiple patient and social factors that often exist, along with the different prior experiences of healthcare team members with similar patient scenarios. Whereas the nephrology team and family members most often come to a conclusion that is agreeable to all, on occasion, a hospital ethics committee may be consulted for their opinion.

More than a decade ago, Geary and colleagues surveyed the opinions of pediatric caregivers from around the globe regarding the decision process surrounding the initiation of chronic dialysis in infants <1 year of age [10]. In that survey, a substantial percentage (50%) of physicians responded that it was usually acceptable for parents to refuse dialysis for children less than 1 month of age, in contrast to the situation when children were 1–12 months of age at presentation, at which time dialysis refusal was deemed less acceptable. Factors felt to be most influential by the physicians with respect to their opinions regarding withholding dialysis were the presence of "coexistent serious medical abnormalities" and the "anticipated morbidity for the child." As a follow-up to that survey, Teh et al. reported on the results of a similar multination survey of both nephrologists and nephrology nurses on this topic to determine if the perspectives of healthcare providers had changed over the subsequent decade in association with the advances in care that had taken place [11]. Only 30% of the 270 nephrologists indicated that they offer chronic dialysis therapy to all children less than 1 month of age, and 50% reported that they do so to all children with ESRD aged 1–12 months. The figure of 30% was decreased from the figure of 41% reported in the prior survey. In the more recent assessment, a minority of physicians (27%) believed that the parents should not be given the option to refuse dialysis for infants less than 1 month of age, a figure which increased to 50% for children aged 1–12 months. Noteworthy was the finding that nurses were more likely than physicians to consider the presence of oliguria or anuria as a contraindication to initiating dialysis, and they placed more emphasis on the parent's right to decide.

3. Chronic PD is particularly advantageous compared to HD for the infant patient for a variety of reasons. Most importantly, long-term HD access in a neonate or infant consists of a central venous catheter, a practice that is accompanied by a high risk of infection. In addition, use of a HD catheter is associated with a significant potential for central venous stenosis and the resultant inability to create an arteriovenous fistula in the future for patients who face a lifetime of ESRD care [12, 13]. In contrast, a chronic PD catheter can be inserted in infants as young as newborns with few long-term complications of the procedure itself. The advantages of PD over HD in this population are reflected in the overwhelmingly preferred use of PD, with Carey et al. reporting PD to be the initial modality prescribed to greater than 91% of infants initiating chronic dialysis therapy [1].

Surgical expertise and antibiotic prophylaxis are keys to minimizing the risks associated with PD catheter insertion. When supplemental tube feeding is considered likely, the prior or concurrent placement of a gastrostomy tube/button at the time of PD catheter placement, with appropriate antibiotic and antifungal prophylaxis decreases the risk of bacterial or fungal infections that can occur soon after PD catheter placement [14].

Typically, initial dialysis fill volumes should be 10–20 mL/kg body weight (300–600 mL/m²) and are increased as clinically warranted and tolerated.

Accordingly, the recommended maintenance exchange fill volume for patients below age 2 years is limited by patient tolerance and is generally 600–800 ml/m² [15]. This is in contrast to a volume of approximately 1,200 ml/m² that is recommended for older children and adolescents [15]. The lower dialysate fill volume that is employed in the neonate generally necessitates the use of manual exchanges early in the course of PD, in contrast to an automated cycling device. Because these low volumes result in a rapidly diminished osmotic gradient and resultant limited ultrafiltration, dwell times of 1 h or less are frequently utilized. Dwell times as short as 20 min have been used in neonates when rapid removal of small solutes is desired, with recognition of the associated risk of hypernatremia as a result of sodium seiving [16]. In the chronic setting, an initial empiric dwell time of 1 h is often used in infants, although consideration has to be made for clearance of larger molecules (e.g., phosphorus) which would be favored by longer dwell times.

Meeting the nutritional needs of infants can be challenging (see below), especially for the severely oliguric/anuric patient who must receive formula volumes as high as 150 mL/kg of body weight per day. The relative ease with which the fluid status can be managed with PD on a daily basis precludes wide fluctuations of body fluid volume and blood pressure. Finally, PD promotes gradual expansion of the abdominal cavity in preparation for successful renal transplantation. This takes on added importance when one considers that parents of these young children often serve as living donors, a process that mandates insertion of an adult-sized kidney into a recipient who may have a body weight of only 10 kg. The lack of abdominal musculature in patients with prune belly syndrome, as was seen in our patient, is not associated with a higher rate of PD related complications [17].

4. In the setting of ESRD during infancy, the provision of adequate nutrition takes on particular importance because the neonatal/infant period is typically characterized by accelerated brain growth and a linear growth rate of nearly 25 cm/year. Remarkably, ½ of postnatal brain growth takes place in the first year of life, and 1/3 of the normal final adult height is achieved during the initial 2 years of life [18, 19]. Most noteworthy is the fact that this early period of growth is primarily dependent upon the provision of optimal nutrition, with the growth hormone/insulin-like growth factor (IGF) axis having less importance when compared to later in life.

There are several nutritional considerations that need to be addressed when PD is conducted. Specifically, neonates and infants can experience excessive losses of protein via PD with studies demonstrating average daily losses of 250 mg of protein per kg of body weight or almost twice the peritoneal protein losses seen in older children [20]. In order to avoid the negative consequences of protein depletion, current guidelines recommend an allowance for dietary protein of at least 1.8 g/kg/day for the first 6 months of life, taking into account the dietary reference intakes (DRI) and peritoneal losses [21].

Infants receiving PD also experience excessive sodium losses across the peritoneal membrane due to the need for high ultrafiltration rates in relation to body weight. Without adequate sodium supplementation (~3–5 mEq/kg/day), the consequences of the resultant hyponatremia and low intravascular volume can be catastrophic and include both blindness due to anterior ischemic optic neuropathy and cerebral edema (see also Chap. 5) [22, 23].

In most cases, the nutritional targets defined by the guidelines for neonates on PD (see also Chap. 21) are not achievable without the implementation of either nasogastric (NG) or gastrostomy tube feeding. Whereas historically NG tubes were preferentially used because of the simplicity of placement (although not necessarily considered "simple" from the perspective of the parent and patient), frequently associated complications of this approach to therapy, in addition to the unsightly appearance, include recurrent emesis, nasal trauma associated with tube replacement, and inhibition of the normal development of oral motor skills [24–26]. On the other hand, gastrostomy tubes/buttons are not as frequently associated with the development of altered oral motor skills, are not regularly associated with emesis, and are not visible. They also offer the advantage of being available for prolonged use into the post-renal transplant period where they can be essential to ensure proper hydration and enhance medication administration in the young infant [27].

As mentioned above, a gastrostomy tube/button should ideally be placed prior to or simultaneously with placement of the PD catheter. Ideally, percutaneous placement while on PD should not be performed due to the high risk of infection and mechanical failure [28]. Placement via an open Stamm gastrostomy procedure in the patient already on PD is, however, possible if sufficient precautions are taken, specifically the use of prophylactic antibiotic and antifungal therapy. Conversely, PD catheter placement is possible in the setting of a well-established gastrostomy tube/button with no increased risk of bacterial or fungal peritonitis [29–31].

5. Whereas mortality data have improved in children on dialysis over the past few decades, the highest mortality rates are seen in those patients who receive dialysis during the first year of life [32, 33]. The most recent NAPRTCS results, based on data collected from 2000–2012, show a 3-year patient survival of 78.6% and 84.6% for patients who initiate dialysis during the first month and first year of life, respectively [34]. Combined data from four other registries shows a slightly lower survival rate for those patients who initiated chronic dialysis within the first month of life with 2- and 5-year survival rates of 81% and 76%, respectively [5]. What persists, however, is the finding that the most important predictor of mortality in this PD patient age group remains the presence of non-renal disease [33, 35–37]. Wood et al., and later Van Stralen et al., clearly showed that comorbidities such as anuria, neurological complications, and pulmonary hypoplasia were associated with the greatest risk of mortality in infants undergoing dialysis [5, 35]. A recent publication of the IPPN exam-

ining 1,830 patients aged 0–19 years found that the presence of at least one comorbidity was associated with a 4-year survival of 73% versus 90% survival in those without a comorbidity ($p < 0.001$) [4]. Data on the influence of comorbidities on survival is likely impacted by regional differences, as countries with a lower gross national income appear to be more restrictive in terms of making PD available to very young patients and those with significant extra-renal complications [3].

Clinical Pearls

1. Peritoneal dialysis (PD) has long been considered the modality of choice when treating neonates and infants with end-stage renal disease (ESRD) needing chronic renal replacement therapy. Its popularity and success largely derive from its simplicity and effectiveness in even the smallest patients.
2. PD during infancy helps meet the nutritional demands of patients through the effective removal of solute and fluid. The substantial nutritional needs of this patient population are intended to address the marked increases in height, weight and brain development that the young infant should be experiencing.
3. Over the last decade, there has been steady improvement in survival rates with recent studies showing excellent survival 1 year after therapy initiation, even in patients who first receive dialysis when they are less than 1 month of age. Nevertheless, ethical issues/concerns pertaining to the provision of dialysis remain present, especially when extrarenal comorbidities exist.

References

1. Carey WA, et al. Outcomes of dialysis initiated during the neonatal period for treatment of end-stage renal disease: a North American Pediatric Renal Trials and Collaborative Studies special analysis. Pediatrics. 2007;119(2):e468–73.
2. Atlas of ESRD: United States Renal Data System (USRDS) [cited 7/8/2010]. Available from: http://www.usrds.org/2010/pdf/v2_08.pdf. 2010.
3. Schaefer F, et al. Impact of global economic disparities on practices and outcomes of chronic PD in children: insights from the International Pediatric Peritoneal Dialysis Network (IPPN) Registry. Perit Dial Int. 2012;32(4):399–409.
4. Neu AM, et al. Co-morbidities in chronic pediatric peritoneal dialysis patients: a report of the International Pediatric Peritoneal Dialysis Network (IPPN). Perit Dial Int. 2012;32(4):410–8.
5. van Stralen KJ, et al. Survival and clinical outcomes of children starting renal replacement therapy in the neonatal period. Kidney Int. 2014;86(1):168–74.
6. Brunner FP, et al. Survival on renal replacement therapy: data from the EDTA registry. Nephrol Dial Transplant. 1988;3(2):109–22.

7. Beauchamp TL, Childress JF. Principles of biomedical ethics. 5th ed. Oxford; New York: Oxford University Press; 2001. p. 454.

8. Mavroudis C, et al. Informed consent, bioethical equipoise, and hypoplastic left heart syndrome. Cardiol Young. 2011;21(Suppl 2):133–40.

9. Zeigler VL. Ethical principles and parental choice: treatment options for neonates with hypoplastic left heart syndrome. Pediatr Nurs. 2003;29(1):65–9.

10. Geary DF. Attitudes of pediatric nephrologists to management of end-stage renal disease in infants. J Pediatr. 1998;133(1):154–6.

11. Jun Chuan Teh MLF, Sienna JL, Denis F. Geary, caregivers' attitude to management of end-stage renal disease in infants. Perit Dial Int. 2011;31(4):459–65.

12. Verrina E, et al. A multicenter experience on patient and technique survival in children on chronic dialysis. Pediatr Nephrol. 2004;19(1):82–90.

13. Rees L. Long-term peritoneal dialysis in infants. Perit Dial Int. 2007;27(Suppl 2):S180–4.

14. Warady BA, et al. Consensus guidelines for the prevention and treatment of catheter-related infections and peritonitis in pediatric patients receiving peritoneal dialysis: 2012 update. Perit Dial Int. 2012;32(Suppl 2):S32–86.

15. Clinical practice recommendations for peritoneal dialysis adequacy. Am J Kidney Dis. 2006;48(Suppl 1): S130–58.

16. Alarabi AA, et al. Continuous peritoneal dialysis in children with acute renal failure. Adv Perit Dial. 1994;10:289–93.

17. Wisanuyotin S, et al. Complications of peritoneal dialysis in children with Eagle-Barrett syndrome. Pediatr Nephrol. 2003;18(2):159–63.

18. Reed RB, Stuart HC. Patterns of growth in height and weight from birth to eighteen years of age. Pediatrics. 1959;24:904–21.

19. Lowrey G. Growth and development of children. 7th ed. Chicago: Year Book Medical Publishers; 1978.

20. Quan A, Baum M. Protein losses in children on continuous cycler peritoneal dialysis. Pediatr Nephrol. 1996;10(6):728–31.

21. KDOQI. Clinical Practice Guideline for Nutrition in Children with CKD: 2008 update. Executive summary. Am J Kidney Dis. 2009;53(3 Suppl 2):S11–104.

22. Lapeyraque AL, et al. Sudden blindness caused by anterior ischemic optic neuropathy in 5 children on continuous peritoneal dialysis. Am J Kidney Dis. 2003;42(5):E3–9.

23. Bunchman TE. Chronic dialysis in the infant less than 1 year of age. Pediatr Nephrol. 1995;9(Suppl):S18–22.

24. Dello Strologo L, et al. Feeding dysfunction in infants with severe chronic renal failure after long-term nasogastric tube feeding. Pediatr Nephrol. 1997;11(1):84–6.

25. Warady BA, et al. Nutritional and behavioural aspects of nasogastric tube feeding in infants receiving chronic peritoneal dialysis. Adv Perit Dial. 1990;6:265–8.

26. Warady BA, Weis L, Johnson L. Nasogastric tube feeding in infants on peritoneal dialysis. Perit Dial Int. 1996;16(Suppl 1):S521–5.

27. Wong H, et al. Caregiver attitudes towards gastrostomy removal after renal transplantation. Pediatr Transplant. 2005;9(5):574–8.

28. von Schnakenburg C, et al. Percutaneous endoscopic gastrostomy in children on peritoneal dialysis. Perit Dial Int. 2006;26(1):69–77.

29. Ledermann SE, et al. Gastrostomy feeding in infants and children on peritoneal dialysis. Pediatr Nephrol. 2002;17(4):246–50.

30. Ramage IJ, et al. Complications of gastrostomy feeding in children receiving peritoneal dialysis. Pediatr Nephrol. 1999;13(3):249–52.

31. Warady BA, Bashir M, Donaldson LA. Fungal peritonitis in children receiving peritoneal dialysis: a report of the NAPRTCS. Kidney Int. 2000;58(1):384–9.

32. Coulthard MG, Crosier J. Outcome of reaching end stage renal failure in children under 2 years of age. Arch Dis Child. 2002;87(6):511–7.

33. Shroff R, et al. Long-term outcome of chronic dialysis in children. Pediatr Nephrol. 2006;21(2):257–64.
34. Carey WA, Martz KL, Warady BA. Outcome of patients initiating chronic peritoneal dialysis during the first year of life. Pediatrics. 2015;136(3):e615–22.
35. Wood EG, et al. Risk factors for mortality in infants and young children on dialysis. Am J Kidney Dis. 2001;37(3):573–9.
36. Kari JA, et al. Outcome and growth of infants with severe chronic renal failure. Kidney Int. 2000;57(4):1681–7.
37. Ledermann SE, et al. Long-term outcome of peritoneal dialysis in infants. J Pediatr. 2000;136(1):24–9.

Chapter 5
Hypotension in Infants on Peritoneal Dialysis

Enrico Vidal

Case Presentation

A 10-month-old male with bilateral renal dysplasia and on peritoneal dialysis (PD) presented to a local emergency room in the late morning because of acute blindness.

He had been started on PD within the first month of life, and his automated PD dialysis regimen was based on an 11-h nocturnal intermittent schedule (NIPD). Diuresis was well preserved and he was treated with a fill volume of 700 ml/m², an exchange time of 30 min, using a 1.36% glucose solution. Enteral feeding with adequate amounts of fortified milk was administered via nasogastric tube. He was receiving low doses of potassium-chelating resins and calcium carbonate. His development was normal, without extrarenal comorbidities.

In the 24 h prior to admission, the boy had a sudden onset of gastroenteritis, with diarrhea and two episodes of vomiting. In the morning, after detachment from the PD cycler, the mother noticed that the child was unable to follow her gaze, and he began to move his eyes randomly. Moreover, he was pale, confused, and hyporesponsive. Admission followed 4 h after the first symptoms were noticed. The child presented with bilateral afferent pupillary defect and did not respond to visual threat. Upon admission, his blood pressure (BP) was 60/40 mmHg, with a pulse rate of 160 bpm. The patient showed signs of moderate dehydration, with a body weight of 0.7 kg (−8%) less than his normal body weight (8,000 g). Laboratory exams showed hemoglobin 13 g/dl, hematocrit 40%, and hyponatremia (122 mmol/L).

Immediately after admission, he received two consecutive boluses of 160 ml of normal saline, resulting in normalization of BP, followed by 600 ml normal saline for 12 h. Peritoneal dialysis was suspended for 24 h. Ophthalmological examination

E. Vidal (✉)
Nephrology, Dialysis and Transplant Unit, Department of Women's and Children's Health, University-Hospital of Padova, Via Giustiniani, 3, 35128 Padova, Italy
e-mail: enrico.vidal@inwind.it

© Springer International Publishing AG 2017
B.A. Warady et al. (eds.), *Pediatric Dialysis Case Studies*,
DOI 10.1007/978-3-319-55147-0_5

Table 5.1 Definition of hypotension according to Pediatric Advanced Life Support guidelines [3]

Age group	Systolic BP threshold
0 day–1 week	<60
1 week–1 month	<60
1 month–1 year	<70
1 year	72
2 years	74
3 years	76
4 years	78
5 years	80
6 years	82
7 years	84
8 years	86
9 years	88
≥10 years	90

revealed swollen and pale optic discs with blurred disc margins consistent with acute ischemic optic neuropathy (AION). Computed tomography and MRI scans of the brain were normal. The patient's vision improved within 24 h after admission, but on last examination, 1 year after the episode, recovery was found to be only partial with bilateral mild atrophy of the optic nerve and, using lenses, a Snellen visual acuity of 20/70 on the right eye and 20/100 on the left eye.

Clinical Questions

1. How is arterial hypotension defined in infants?
2. Why are infants on PD at risk of arterial hypotension?
3. What are the hypotension-related complications in infants on PD?
4. What are the treatment options during an acute hypotensive episode?
5. How can hypotension be prevented in infants on PD?

Diagnostic Discussion

1. Blood pressure physiologically increases by more than 30 mmHg from neonatal to adolescent age [1]. Pediatric nephrologists are usually well aware of this age dependence and use age-, gender-, and height-specific percentiles to diagnose hypertension in dialyzed children [2]. Much less attention tends to be paid to the lower end of the BP range, which is equally age dependent (Table 5.1). According to the American Heart Association's Pediatric Advanced Life Support guidelines, arterial hypotension is defined as a systolic BP lower than 60 mmHg in term

newborns (0–28 days), lower than 70 mmHg in infants (1–12 months), lower than 70 + (2 × the child's age in years) mmHg in children 1–10 years, and lower than 90 mmHg in children more than 10 years of age [3]. These thresholds are set just above the 5th percentile of systolic BP for age, sex, and height, which corresponds to a Z-score of −1.64.

2. Infants on PD are particularly prone to become salt depleted [4]. The subsequent decline in extracellular osmolality and loss of osmotic fluid into cells in turn lead to hyponatremic hypovolemia and chronic hypotension. The tendency toward sodium (Na) depletion in children on PD is multifactorial and depends mainly on the specific primary cause of end-stage renal disease (ESRD) and on the perito-neal membrane characteristics.

   Malformations of the kidneys and urinary tract are the most common cause of chronic renal failure in infants [5]. These disorders are characterized by impaired tubular function as a consequence of renal dysplasia, causing polyuria and sodium depletion even in ESRD. Urine output in affected children is typically 2–3 times normal, resulting in significant losses of free water and sodium. Hyponatremia may occur also in infants with oligo/anuric renal failure receiving PD, due to the substantial sodium losses related to the ultrafiltration necessary to maintain fluid balance while the patient is ingesting standard infant formula.

   Measurements of the mass transfer area coefficient have suggested that, as a consequence of both higher peritoneal permeability and a larger effective surface area of peritoneal membrane, solute transport capacity is relatively greater in infants than in older children and adults [6]. In infants, sodium removal from plasma is, in addition to diffusion, mainly a consequence of ultrafiltration-related convective transport. When UF rates are high, approximately half the total vol-ume depends on transport through the water-exclusive endothelial aquaporin-1 channels (ultrasmall pores); the remaining UF occurs through the small pores, leading to removal of sodium by solvent drag [7]. As a rule of thumb, 80 mmol sodium is removed per liter of ultrafiltrate. Hence, an anuric 5 kg infant with 300 mL daily UF will lose almost 5 mmol/kg Na per day, more than twice the daily urine losses of a healthy child. If the child receives 500 mL standard formula milk per day, Na intake will only be about 3–10 mmol. At normal serum Na concentrations, Na losses from UF are normally greater than the quantity ingested from infant formula. This may result in negative Na balance until a steady state is achieved at a low serum Na concentration.

3. A fall of systolic BP in the systemic circulation results in counteracting mecha-nisms that allow the infant to maintain adequate cardiac and central nervous system circulation (Fig. 5.1). Despite fluctuations in arterial BP, perfusion of the central nervous system remains constant because of the mechanism of pressure autoregula-tion, i.e., the capacity of terminal arterioles to dilate during hypotension and con-strict during hypertension. However, the physiological autoregulation operates over a range of perfusion pressures between 60–150 mmHg. With a rise or fall of perfu-sion pressure beyond this critical range, the mechanism becomes ineffective and breaks down. In chronically hypotensive PD infants, a further drop in systolic BP

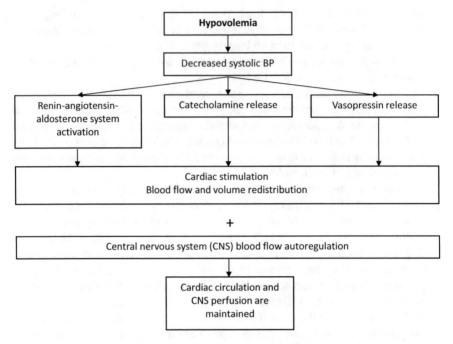

Fig. 5.1 Pathophysiologic cascade of compensatory mechanisms during arterial hypotension

caused by a "second hit" might impair the autoregulation of cerebral blood flow resulting in hypoperfusion episodes (Fig. 5.2).

Several vasoactive compounds, including endothelium-derived nitric oxide (NO), are known to modulate cerebral autoregulation. Recently, Carlström et al. reported on four infants treated with PD who developed symptomatic cerebral ischemia [8]. Blood pressure levels were low both before the event and at presentation. In two patients, the authors demonstrated that the removal of nitrate and nitrite by PD could have impaired the NO-generating systems, i.e., the classical L-arginine-dependent NO synthase or the nitrate-nitrite-NO pathway. The authors advanced the hypothesis that in infants receiving chronic PD, systolic BP persistently in the low range of normal distribution coupled with a reduction in NO bioavailability could impair the autoregulation of cerebral blood flow, thereby increasing the risk of cerebral ischemic episodes.

Posterior ciliary arteries are particularly vulnerable to a persistent drop in perfusion pressure, resulting in ischemic damage to the optic nerve head and peripapillary area [9]. The clinical picture that arises is called "nonarteritic acute ischemic optic neuropathy" (AION), which represents a cause of sudden visual loss. AION is a rare complication in patients on chronic PD, with a limited number of cases described in children to date. Recently, the Italian Registry of Pediatric Chronic Dialysis described its experience on seven children with AION among more than 700 pediatric patients treated with chronic PD over a 25-year period (1988–2013),

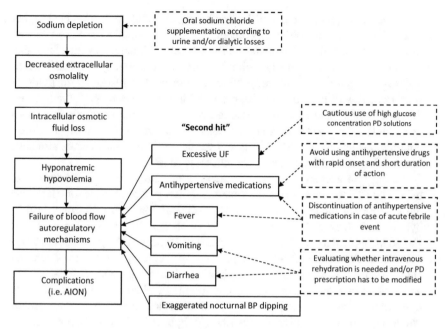

Fig. 5.2 Proposed pathophysiologic sequence of events involved in determining PD-induced hypotension and potential preventive strategies (*dashed boxes*)

corresponding to an incidence of about 1% [10]. Interestingly, the Registry included no reported cases of AION in children treated with hemodialysis during the same period. The median age of patients was 2.2 years, and most of them had some form of neurological involvement when AION developed. All patients suffered from acute-onset bilateral blindness, which was noticed at daylight after nocturnal sleep or after a nap during the day. Three patients were described as chronically hypotensive, one had undergone bilateral nephrectomy 3 months earlier, and in the remaining three patients, inappropriate use of hyperosmolar PD solution and dehydration because of gastroenteritis were considered as likely triggers of hypotension. In four out of seven cases, AION was associated with ischemic lesions in the occipital cortex: these patients did not recover visual acuity. On the contrary, those patients with absent or mild ischemic lesions on brain imaging demonstrated at least partial visual recovery.

4. The primary goal of treatment during an acute hypotensive episode is to bring BP back to normal to restore cerebral blood flow as quickly as possible, thus reducing the risk of cerebral ischemia. Another goal is to rapidly manage any underlying condition potentially leading to hypovolemia.

Dufek et al. compared 14 children on chronic PD presenting with AION with 59 non-affected patients to identify a risk profile for AION [11]. Very young age at PD initiation, autosomal recessive polycystic kidney disease as the primary cause of ESRD, anephric status, and chronic hypotension were found to be significant risk factors for AION. In this case series, five patients had a "good" visual outcome (visual acuity still quantifiable according to Snellen charts), but nine children remained blind. The outcome of AION seemed to be closely related to an aggressive and early vascular refilling therapy. All patients with a favorable outcome received fluid boluses within 12 h after the onset of symptoms, whereas patients that remained bilaterally blind did not receive resuscitation fluids or were treated with fluid boluses later than 48 h after onset of symptoms. Other therapeutic approaches, such as oral, intravenous, or intravitreal administration of steroids to accelerate resolution of disc edema, have usually shown disappointing results [10, 12]. Midodrine and various antithrombotic agents also have been attempted in a few patients without clear benefits.

Taking into account the serious outcomes of cerebral ischemic episodes in infants on PD and considering the uncertain efficacy of treatments for AION, the most important advice is to rapidly treat clinical conditions that may lead to hypovolemia (Fig. 5.2). In infants receiving chronic PD, prevention strategies should be applied to avoid those clinical events ("second hits") that could induce a further decline in blood perfusion pressure with consequent failure of cerebral autoregulation. Meticulous attention should be paid to all causes that can lead to an absolute or relative alteration in the volume of circulating blood. Absolute hypovolemia typically results from dehydration due to severe diarrhea and/or vomiting, whereas relative or distributive hypovolemia can occur with an increase in the volume of the intravascular space, e.g., during a febrile event or after exaggerated or inappropriate prescription of antihypertensive medications. In young infants, accurate calculation and frequent assessment of "dry weight" should be performed to avoid high glucose concentration PD solutions and excessive UF. In cases of acute gastroenteritis, children treated with PD should be carefully evaluated with respect to opportunities to initiate intravenous rehydration and to modify the dialysis prescription (reduced treatment time, increased dwell time, minimized dialysate glucose content, long low-glucose daytime dwell for resorption of fluid, and electrolytes on demand). The use of antihypertensive drugs with rapid onset and short duration of action should be avoided in hypertensive infants on dialysis, since these medications can cause a transient fall of BP below the critical level of autoregulation of the cerebral blood flow. In an acute febrile event, discontinuation of antihypertensive medication should also be considered.

5. Strategies for the long-term treatment and prevention of PD-induced hypotension should be used to avoid progression in the pathophysiologic cascade that leads to chronic hypotension.

In infants undergoing chronic PD, the systolic BP levels should be targeted at least at the 50th percentile adjusted for age, gender, and height. Since in infants on automated PD UF occurs exclusively at nighttime, dehydration and arterial hypotension may initially be limited to the early morning hours and thus escape detection in the outpatient setting. Regular measurements of BP and heart rate upon disconnection from the cycler are essential to diagnose subacute dehydration [13]. Moreover, small infants should receive periodic funduscopic examinations to

Table 5.2 Method for estimating sodium needs in anuric infants on PD

	Age-related dietary reference intake Ref. [14]		Losses from ultrafiltration Ref. [15]
Total daily sodium requirements (mmol) =	0–6 mol = (0.9 × kg of body weight)	+	(8 × [ml of UF/100])
	7–12 mol = (1.7 × kg of body weight)		

reveal changes potentially associated with chronic systemic arterial hypotension (optic atrophy).

To avoid chronic intravascular depletion and to promote optimal growth, infants and children with polyuric salt-wasting forms of chronic kidney disease should receive NaCl supplements. Even when anuric, infants on chronic PD are predisposed to substantial sodium losses as a result of high UF requirements. Therefore, frequent measurements of both serum and dialysate levels of sodium should be performed. Moreover, sodium balance measurements (determined from dietary and medication intake, urine, and/or dialysate losses) are suggested at least every 3 months, concurrent with measurement of dialysis adequacy [14]. Hence, the total daily sodium requirements should be calculated and eventually administered as additional oral sodium chloride (Table 5.2). If urine output is still preserved, supplemental doses of sodium as high as 5–10 mEq/kg might be required because of the combined sodium losses in urine and dialysate.

Clinical Pearls

1. Pediatric nephrologists should know the age-dependent lower BP limits and be aware of the risk of arterial hypotension in infants receiving automated PD.
2. Infants on PD are prone to become salt depleted and to develop hypovolemia. In this specific population, dietary sodium supplements represent the best therapeutic strategy to prevent a pathophysiologic cascade that eventually leads to chronic hypotension.
3. In case of acute hypotensive events, chronically hypotensive or salt-depleted infants on PD are at risk of cerebral ischemia. Posterior cerebral arteries are particularly vulnerable to a persistent drop in perfusion pressure resulting in the clinical picture of AION.
4. Administration of fluid boluses is the treatment of choice for acute hypotensive episodes. The outcome of AION also depends on rapid vascular refilling therapy, which should be provided within 12 h after the onset of symptoms.
5. Long-term management of PD-induced hypotension in infants should rest on regular BP measurements (especially in the morning, upon disconnection from the cycler), targeting systolic BP at least at the 50th percentile and on periodic fundoscopic examinations to promptly detect ischemic damage to the optic nerve.

References

1. Flynn JT. Neonatal hypertension: diagnosis and management. Pediatr Nephrol. 2000;14(4): 332–41.
2. National High Blood Pressure Education Program Working Group on High Blood Pressure in Children and Adolescents. The fourth report on the diagnosis, evaluation, and treatment of high blood pressure in children and adolescents. Pediatrics. 2004;114(2 Suppl 4th Report):555–76.
3. Kleinman ME, Chameides L, Schexnayder SM, et al. Part 14: pediatric advanced life support: 2010 American Heart Association Guidelines for Cardiopulmonary Resuscitation and Emergency Cardiovascular Care. Circulation. 2010;122(18 Suppl 3):S876–908.
4. Paulson WD, Bock GH, Nelson AP, et al. Hyponatremia in the very young chronic peritoneal dialysis patient. Am J Kidney Dis. 1989;14(3):196–9.
5. Harambat J, van Stralen KJ, Kim JJ, et al. Epidemiology of chronic kidney disease in children. Pediatr Nephrol. 2012;27:363–73.
6. Warady BA, Alexander SR, Hossli S, et al. Peritoneal membrane transport function in children receiving long term dialysis. J Am Soc Nephrol. 1996;7:2385–91.
7. Devuyst O, Goffin E. Water and solute transport in peritoneal dialysis: models and clinical applications. Nephrol Dial Transplant. 2008;23:2120–3.
8. Carlström M, Wide K, Lundvall M, et al. Plasma nitrate/nitrite removal by peritoneal dialysis might predispose infants with low blood pressure to cerebral ischaemia. Clin Kidney J. 2015;8(2):215–8.
9. Kaya S, Kolodjaschna J, Berisha F, et al. Comparison of the autoregulatory mechanisms between central retinal artery and posterior ciliary arteries after thigh cuff deflation in healthy subjects. Microvasc Res. 2011;82:269–73.
10. Di Zazzo G, Guzzo I, De Galasso L, et al. Anterior ischemic optical neuropathy in children on chronic peritoneal dialysis: report of 7 cases. Perit Dial Int. 2015;35(2):135–9.
11. Dufek S, Feldkoetter M, Vidal E, et al. Anterior ischemic optic neuropathy in pediatric peritoneal dialysis: risk factors and therapy. Pediatr Nephrol. 2014;29(7):1249–57.
12. Lee AG, Biousse V. Should steroids be offered to patients with nonarteritic anterior ischemic optic neuropathy? J Neuroophthalmol. 2010;30(2):193–8.
13. Schaefer F. Peritoneal dialysis in infants: never lose sight of-and from-arterial hypotension! Perit Dial Int. 2015;35(2):123–4.
14. National Kidney Foundation. KDOQI clinical practice guideline for nutrition in children with CKD. Am J Kidney Dis. 2009;53(Suppl 2):S1.
15. Rippe B, Venturoli D. Optimum electrolyte composition of a dialysis solution. Perit Dial Int. 2008;28(Suppl 3):S131–6.

Chapter 6
Ethical Dialysis Decisions in Infants with End-Stage Kidney Disease

Aviva M. Goldberg

Case Presentation

A 34-year-old G1P0 woman has a prenatal ultrasound at 20 weeks that shows a male fetus with severe oligohydramnios and very large kidneys without visible cysts. The suspected diagnosis is autosomal recessive polycystic kidney disease. The woman and her partner receive prenatal consultation from a pediatric nephrologist, who explains that it is likely that the baby, if born alive, will have end-stage kidney disease (ESKD) within the first few months of life. The nephrologist explains that the ESKD can be managed with dialysis, but that the mortality risk and risk of complications are higher than would be expected for an older child, and that survival may also be limited by the child's lung development. She also explains that dialysis will not cure the baby's problem, and that the baby will have lifelong kidney disease, but that kidney transplantation is a possibility within the first few years of life. The parents decide to continue the pregnancy, and the baby is born at term with moderate, but manageable, lung hypoplasia, and very poor renal function. The nephrologist on call meets with the parents to discuss the diagnosis and suggests consulting surgery for a peritoneal dialysis catheter, so that dialysis can be started in the next few days to weeks. The parents ask "Are we allowed to refuse? We didn't think this through and don't think we should do dialysis after all."

A.M. Goldberg, MD, MA, FRCPC (✉)
Section of Nephrology, Departments of Pediatric and Child Health, Max Rady College of Medicine, Winnipeg, Manitoba, Canada
e-mail: Agoldberg@exchange.hsc.mb.ca

© Springer International Publishing AG 2017
B.A. Warady et al. (eds.), *Pediatric Dialysis Case Studies*,
DOI 10.1007/978-3-319-55147-0_6

45

Clinical Questions

1. What are the outcomes for infants who have end-stage kidney disease in the first few days or weeks of life?
2. What is the role of prenatal counseling for fetuses suspected of having serious kidney disease at birth?
3. Is dialysis for newborns morally obligatory? Is this decision affected by the presence of comorbidities?

Diagnostic Discussion

1. As a high-technology intervention, there has always been the question of whether dialysis should be obligatory or optional, especially in infants, both because good data on prognosis was not available until fairly recently, and because there is a concern that subjecting young children to a life of ESKD management may promote suffering, rather that alleviate it. A 1987 paper by Cynthia Cohen argued that "in the light of the current innovative status of dialysis and transplantation for very young infants, and in view of the medical uncertainty of their short- and long-term outcomes, there are measures that physicians and parents are not required to provide to infants by either ethics or the law. Parents who refuse such treatment for their young infants, in good faith, after receiving complete information about current options, make a choice that should be respected" [1]. An article by Carl Kjellstrand at around the same time, discussing dialysis in the elderly, argued that "high-technology medicine sometimes makes dying a cruel spectacle, and patients whose lives depend on a machine want to stop" [2]. An international survey of pediatric nephrologists in the 1990s found that there was no clear standard of therapy in this group, and that many respondents were willing to defer to parental decisions, even when the respondents themselves believed that dialysis may be in the child's best interest [3].
2. Since that time, there is more evidence regarding prognosis in these infants, which could potentially inform decision making. A review of the North American Pediatric Renal Trials and Collaborative Studies (NAPRTCS) compared a historical cohort (1992–1999) to a more recent cohort (2000–2012) [4]. Another study reported recent outcomes from multiple registries, including Europe, Japan, Australia, and New Zealand [5]. These studies found that:

   (a) Survival of children starting dialysis has improved for all ages in the recent era.
   (b) Survival for infants starting dialysis in the first month of life is over 70% at 2 to 5 years post dialysis initiation.
   (c) Though survival for neonates and infants starting dialysis remains lower than that of older children, the gap has narrowed significantly compared to the previous era.

(d) Many of the children who start dialysis as neonates will receive a kidney transplant by early childhood and will have good graft outcomes.

This registry data needs to be interpreted correctly when providing pre- or postnatal counseling to parents, as only the infants who survived to the point of starting dialysis are included in these registries. Cases that have not been captured include those in which pregnancies ended with spontaneous or therapeutic abortion, infants in whom dialysis was never attempted after birth, those who were too ill to survive to dialysis initiation, and those whose renal function was better than expected prenatally and did not require neonatal dialysis. Without these caveats, there is a danger that parents receiving prenatal counseling will interpret prognosis much more optimistically than the data can justify at this time.

3. Given the better prognosis for these infants, the argument shifts from whether dialysis should ever be offered in cases of isolated ESKD (in the absence of significant comorbidities, as in the case of our patient) to whether it should be morally obligatory to provide dialysis and incumbent on parents to accept it. The Renal Physicians Association and American Society of Nephrology published joint guidelines on appropriate initiation and withdrawal from dialysis, which includes pediatric-specific recommendations. They recommend a shared decision-making model that takes into account the perspective of parents, but advocates the use of conflict resolution and child protective services when "the health care team believes that non-initiation of dialysis would constitute medical neglect" [6]. Wightman and Kett have argued that "it may not be permissible to defer to parental refusal of dialysis for a term neonate and instead that the medical team should strongly consider compelling treatment over parental objection" [7]. Warady and Lantos take a nuanced approach, pointing out that many other neonatal therapies, once considered experimental and innovative, are now considered standard care for a defined populations of infants (e.g., ECMO) [6]. While they ultimately conclude that dialysis may not yet be in the same category as these therapies, given the differences in parental burden, outcomes, costs, etc., they state "the outcomes for the infants are seen as good enough for the treatment to be strongly recommended and even considered the standard of care. But the burdens of therapy are high enough, and the chances for a bad outcome high enough, that the treatments continue to be viewed as legally and ethically optional."

When Geary and colleagues repeated their survey in 2011, they found that physicians were more likely to offer dialysis to some infants (98% vs. 93%) but less likely to offer dialysis to all (41% vs. 30%) [8]. This may be due to increased awareness of the role of comorbidities, like brain or heart disease, that can affect these decisions. Comorbidities affect 30% of children born with ESKD and can impact the benefits and burdens of dialytic therapy. Serious extrarenal disease can decrease the anticipated benefits of dialysis (e.g., life span, potential for neurocognitive development) and increase burdens (e.g., hospitalization and medicalization, pain, and suffering). Lantos and Warady have argued that future research in the field should distinguish between the two types of disease: neonatal ESKD with vs. without comorbidities in order to improve precision in reporting outcomes, prognostic counseling, and informed ethical reasoning [9].

Healthcare providers (HCPs) may find infant dialysis an especially ethically fraught area and can be expected to experience moral distress when parents make a decision that the HCP feels may deny the child a chance at life or, conversely, increase suffering in what will be a short life even with the most aggressive therapy. There has been a paucity of research into the moral distress that health-care professionals may feel when counseling a family regarding infant dialysis. In qualitative studies of HCPs regarding dialysis decisions in older adults, HCPs expressed a desire to err on the side of life, but that they worry that dialysis could prolong suffering in an individual who was close to death [10, 11]. The same may well be true for pediatric HCPs, and it is therefore prudent to ensure support for colleagues experiencing moral distress, safe spaces for staff to discuss their concerns, debriefing around difficult cases, and the use of ethics consultants, conflict-resolution teams, and other supports as required.

Clinical Pearls

1. Survival for infants started on dialysis within the first year of life has improved significantly in the last few decades, though it still lags behind survival of older children with similar disease.
2. Prenatal consultation is an essential part of the management for infants expected to have ESKD within the first few months of life. Consultation, both prenatal and after birth, should include discussion of the lifelong nature of kidney disease, the benefits and burdens of dialysis, transplantation, and conservative management/ palliative care. The recent data on prognosis should be shared, along with an acknowledgment of the limitations of this registry data and the uncertainty in the prenatal period about its relevance.
3. A parental refusal of dialysis may be genuine and well grounded or may stem from misinformation or fear. It is important to explore the reasons why the parents in the case presentation are requesting not to start dialysis and why their perspective has changed since the prenatal period. Many resources, including allied health, parent peers, and support groups, may be helpful in giving parents a realistic idea of life with end-stage kidney disease, as well as what they can expect if they do not pursue dialysis.
4. As with other pediatric decision making, the child's interests are paramount, but it is reasonable for parents to consider the benefits and burdens of the proposed therapy on both the child and the family. This is especially true for infant dialy-sis, since the dialytic therapy (usually home based), diet, and medications will require significant time, financial, and emotional investment by the parents. While it is reasonable for parents to assume some burdens in order to improve the life of their children, it must be recognized that the burdens of end-stage kidney disease are well beyond that expected of the parents of a healthy child or even a child with another chronic disease less demanding than ESKD. Forcing parents to provide a therapy which they fear might unduly burden themselves or their other children may not benefit the child in the long term.

5. Most cases involving decisions around infant dialysis can likely be resolved with a shared decision-making model that respects the viewpoints of both parents and providers, that enhances communication among the decision makers, and that involves interdisciplinary support from medical professionals, social work, clinical ethics, spiritual care, and conflict-resolution specialists. In rare cases, where it is clear that dialysis will offer a significant benefit in excess of burdens, parental refusal could constitute medical neglect and may be a reason to compel parents or involve child protection services.
6. Moral distress is an anticipated outcome for both HCPs and parents faced with this difficult decision. Support should be provided to all involved in these cases.

References

1. Cohen C. Ethical and legal considerations in the care of the infant with end-stage renal disease whose parents elect conservative therapy. An American perspective. Pediatr Nephrol. 1987;1(2):166–71.
2. Kjellstrand CM. Giving life, giving death: ethical problems of high-technology medicine. Acta Med Scand Suppl. 1988;725:1–88. Review. Erratum in: Acta Med Scand Suppl 1988; 224(2):192.
3. Geary DF. Attitudes of pediatric nephrologists to management of end-stage renal disease in infants. J Pediatr. 1998;133:154–6.
4. Carey WA, Martz KL, Warady BA. Outcome of Patients Initiating Chronic Peritoneal Dialysis During the First Year of Life. Pediatrics. 2015;136(3):e615–22.
5. van Stralen KJ. Borzych-Du_zalka D, Hataya H, et al; ESPN/ERA-EDTA registry; IPPN registry; ANZDATA registry; Japanese RRT registry. Survival and clinical outcomes of children starting renal replacement therapy in the neonatal period. Kidney Int. 2014;86(1):168–74.
6. Renal Physicians Association. Shared Decision-Making in the Appropriate Initiation of and Withdrawal from Dialysis. Rockville; 2010. Accessed online at: https://www.renalmd.org/catalogue-item.aspx?id=682.
7. Wightman A, Kett J. Has neonatal dialysis become morally obligatory? Lessons from Baby Doe. Acta Paediatr. 2015 Aug;104(8):748–50.
8. Teh JC, Frieling ML, Sienna JL, Geary DF. Attitudes of caregivers to management of end-stage renal disease in infants. Perit Dial Int. 2011;31(4):459–65.
9. Lantos JD, Warady BA. The evolving ethics of infant dialysis. Pediatr Nephrol. 2013;28(10): 1943–7.
10. Halvorsen K, Slettebø A, Nortvedt P, Pedersen R, Kirkevold M, Nordhaug M, Brinchmann BS. Priority dilemmas in dialysis: The impact of old age. J Med Ethics. 2008;34:585–9.
11. Hussain JA, Flemming K, Murtagh FE, Johnson MJ. Patient and health care professional decision-making to commence and withdraw from renal dialysis: a systematic review of qualitative research. Clin J Am Soc Nephrol. 2015;10(7):1201–15.

Chapter 7
Catheter Exit-Site and Tunnel Infections

Christine B. Sethna

Case Presentation

A 16-year-old female presents to the dialysis clinic with complaints of drainage and tenderness at her PD catheter exit site for the past 3 days. She has a history of end-stage renal disease secondary to focal segmental glomerulosclerosis and was started on continuous cycling PD 6 months ago. The patient and her mother underwent a weeklong PD training session together, but the patient primarily connects herself to PD since her mother works the evening shift. She also performs her own exit-site care. The patient was trained to perform dressing changes every 1–2 days with chlorhexidine and topical mupirocin; however, she admits that she has only been doing it every third or fourth day for the past 2 weeks since she has been busy studying for finals and running with the varsity track team after school.

The patient reports no fever, vomiting, or generalized abdominal pain; she states that the peritoneal effluent has been clear. On examination, she was afebrile with normal blood pressure and heart rate. As the patient washed her hands in preparation for removing the catheter dressing, it was noticed that she had long artificial fingernails. When asked about her nails, she said that she had them done for her junior prom. The PD nurse also noted that the patient did not perform the hand wash properly. Upon examination of the exit site, there was crusting, redness, and bluish purulent discharge surrounding the catheter. In addition, there was swelling, redness, and tenderness over the catheter tunnel. There was no abdominal tenderness beyond the subcutaneous tunnel track. Ultrasound of the tunnel demonstrated a collection of echogenic fluid surrounding the catheter throughout the tunnel track, along with

C.B. Sethna, MD, EdM (✉)
Division of Pediatric Nephrology, Cohen Children's Medical Center of New York, Queens, NY, USA

Department of Pediatrics, Hofstra Northwell School of Medicine, Hempstead, NY, USA
e-mail: csethna@northwell.edu

© Springer International Publishing AG 2017
B.A. Warady et al. (eds.), *Pediatric Dialysis Case Studies*,
DOI 10.1007/978-3-319-55147-0_7

edema of the surrounding subcutaneous tissue. The exit-site drainage was sent for culture and Gram's stain. PD fluid studies for peritonitis were also performed.

The patient was treated empirically with oral cephalexin until the Gram's stain results showed predominance of gram-negative rods. She was then switched to oral ciprofloxacin. The final culture identified *Pseudomonas aeruginosa*. There was no improvement in symptoms after 2 weeks of treatment, and she returned with generalized abdominal pain, cloudy PD effluent, and fever. She was treated for *Pseudomonas aeruginosa* peritonitis with intraperitoneal cefepime and gentamicin; however, the culture remained positive after 2 weeks and the catheter was removed. The patient transitioned to hemodialysis in the interim. The patient and her mother underwent re-training prior to returning to PD.

Clinical Questions

1. What is the incidence of exit-site infections (ESIs) and tunnel infections (TIs) in children on chronic PD?
2. How are ESIs and TIs diagnosed?
3. How can ESIs and TIs be prevented?
4. What are the treatment options?
5. Why are *Pseudomonas* infections difficult to treat?

Diagnostic Discussion

1. Exit-site infections (ESIs) and tunnel infections (TIs) are catheter-related infectious complications of chronic peritoneal dialysis (PD) in children that are associated with significant morbidity, frequent hospitalizations, and increased costs. In the North American Pediatric Renal Trials and Collaborative Studies (NAPRTCS) experience, one-third of PD patients developed an ESI/TI within the first year of dialysis. Compared to those without infection, children with ESIs/TIs had a twofold increased risk of developing peritonitis and requiring access revision and a threefold increased risk for catheter-related hospitalization [1]. From the Standardizing Care to Improve Outcomes in Pediatric End-Stage Renal Disease (SCOPE) collaborative, the incidence of ESIs/TIs was reported to be 1 in 69 patient-months among 644 children [2]. The incidence varies from 1 in 7.8 to 46.8 patient-months from other single-center reports [3, 4].

   The pathogenesis of ESIs/TIs is not entirely clear, but it is known that bacteria may colonize the catheter and exit-site soon after catheter placement. Colonization does not represent infection unless there are clinical signs present; however, with inciting exit-site trauma, colonization may predispose the area to tissue invasion and actual infection. Gram-positive organisms account for the majority of ESIs. In a Canadian series, which predated the regular use of prophylactic topical

Table 7.1 Exit-site scoring system [9]

	Scoring		
		Scoring	
Indication	0	1	2
Swelling	No	Exit only <0.5 cm	Including part of or the entire tunnel
Crust	No	<0.5 cm	>0.5 cm
Redness	No	<0.5 cm	>0.5 cm
Pain on pressure	No	Slight	Severe
Secretion	No	Serous	Purulent

Infection assumed with exit-site score ≥ 4. Presence of purulent drainage alone is sufficient for diagnosis of infection

antibiotics, *Staphylococcus aureus* was the most common pathogen for ESIs (46.2%), followed by *Staphylococcus epidermidis* (25.7%) and *Pseudomonas* (10.6%) [4]. With the implementation of the routine use of topical antibiotic prophylaxis, the incidence of ESIs/TIs has decreased, and the distribution of causative organisms has changed. In the International Pediatric Peritonitis Registry (IPPR), the use of mupirocin in the United States was associated with an eight times higher rate of *Pseudomonas* peritonitis compared to Western Europe [5]. Increases in colonization and ESIs due to atypical mycobacteria, corynebacteria, and fungi have been reported with various prophylactic antibiotic regimens in adult studies [6–8].

2. Regular monitoring of the exit site and early recognition of catheter-related infections are important because ESIs/TIs are associated with an increased risk of developing peritonitis [1]. An objective exit-site scoring system (score 0 to 10) has been proposed to aid in the diagnosis of ESIs based on the presence of peri-catheter swelling, crust, redness, tenderness, and secretions (See Table 7.1) [9]. A score of ≥2 along with the isolation of a pathogenic organism, or a score of ≥4 with or without a positive culture, is considered diagnostic. Purulent drainage alone is also sufficient for a diagnosis of ESI [10]. A positive exit-site culture in the absence of signs of inflammation is suggestive of colonization and does not require treatment, but an escalation in exit-site care is recommended. For TIs, redness, edema, or tenderness over the subcutaneous section of the catheter with or without purulent drainage defines infection. Ultrasonography of the tunnel can aid in the diagnosis of TIs and may be helpful in monitoring response to treatment [11].

3. Maintaining good chronic exit-site care is important in order to prevent ESIs/TIs and the development of peritonitis. The International Society for Peritoneal Dialysis (ISPD) recommends that PD training includes the elements of hand washing, aseptic technique and exit-site care [12]. Thorough hand washing with antibacterial soap or alcohol-based cleaning gel and complete drying of the hands prior to handling of the exit-site is essential [12]. It is widely recommended that the exit site be cleaned with a sterile antiseptic solution (e.g., chlorhexidine, povidone-iodine, hydrogen peroxide, sodium hypochlorite) and sterile gauze, but there is significant global variation in the details of exit-site

care protocols. In North America and Asia, the exit site is cleansed daily or every other day, while the frequency is less in European countries. The choice of antiseptic solutions also varies by region [5].

There is wide geographic variation in the choice of topical antibiotic prophylaxis. Topical antibiotics have been shown to reduce ESIs and are suggested as a part of exit-site care by the ISPD [12]. Daily application of mupirocin has successfully reduced ESIs, especially from *Staphylococcus aureus*, but the emergence of *Pseudomonas* infections in mupirocin-treated patients is of concern [13]. In a randomized study of adults, Bernardini et al. demonstrated that topical gentamicin at the exit site resulted in an equal reduction of ESIs due to gram-positive and gram-negative organisms, whereas topical mupirocin was more effective preventing gram-positive infections [8].

Given the wide variation in PD care practices around the globe, standardization of PD techniques and care may have the potential to reduce catheter-related infections. The SCOPE collaborative is a quality improvement initiative that aims to reduce dialysis-related infections in pediatric chronic peritoneal dialysis patients through standardizing care practices by implementation of care bundles in PD training, insertion of the catheter, and follow-up care. The collaborative has demonstrated that as compliance with the follow-up bundle (which included monthly review of hand washing, exit-site care, and aseptic technique) increased, peritonitis rates decreased [2]. Analysis of the effect of these bundles on incidence of ESI/TIs is currently underway.

When an infection occurs, PD centers are encouraged to discover the root cause of the infection episode. For example, in the case presented, possible risk factors may have included nonadherence with exit-site care, improper hand hygiene, use of artificial nails, perspiration from running (i.e., increased moisture at exit site with poor exit-site care), and self-care by an adolescent. The use of artificial nails should be discouraged, as studies have shown that they are associated with increased bacterial carriage, including *Pseudomonas*, on the hands [14, 15]. Repeated mechanical trauma to the exit site, especially during the initial post-catheter implantation period, is also a risk factor for developing an ESI; therefore, preventative measures include immobilization of the catheter, protection from trauma, and cauterization of granulation tissue [12, 16]. Interestingly, there has been no association found between infection rates and participation of adolescents in managing their own PD care [17, 18]. The ISPD recommends that training should include two family members, of which one may be the patient, if appropriate [12]. Longer time on PD has also been shown to increase the risk of ESIs/TIs in both adults and children [1]. Additionally, nasal carriage with *Staphylococcus aureus* was found to be a risk factor for ESI in adults [19]. Other factors such as age, race, disease, and catheter characteristics do not appear to affect the risk for ESIs/TIs [1, 4].

After an infection episode, it is recommended that retraining of PD care practices be provided to all caregivers [12].

4. ESIs/TIs should be promptly treated empirically with antibiotics when clinical findings meet diagnostic criteria for ESI/TI (Table 7.1), beginning with a first-

generation cephalosporin or ciprofloxacin, and then modified when culture results and sensitivities become available. When the culture is negative, a first generation cephalosporin or ciprofloxacin can be continued empirically. Empiric therapy choice should be based on local antibiotic resistance patterns and type of topical antimicrobial prophylactic agent used for exit-site care. Given the potential for resistance, vancomycin should not be used routinely unless there is a history of methicillin-resistant *Staphylococcus aureus* (MRSA). The oral treatment route is generally acceptable for ESIs, while TIs may be treated via oral, intravenous, or intraperitoneal routes. The patient in our case presentation was treated promptly with oral antibiotics but went on to develop peritonitis after only 2 weeks of treatment. It can be argued that earlier use of parenteral antibiotics might have prevented the peritonitis, but it is more likely that only very early catheter removal when *Pseudomonas* was identified as the ESI and likely TI pathogen could have favorably altered the course in this patient. Gram-positive infections are treated with a first generation cephalosporin or penicillinase-resistant penicillin with the addition of rifampin in treatment-resistant *Staphylococcus* infections. Gram-negative infections caused by *Pseudomonas* should be treated with oral ciprofloxacin plus a second antipseudomonal agent due to increased resistance with monotherapy.

The recommended treatment duration for ESIs is a minimum of 2 weeks (3 weeks for *Staphylococcus aureus* or *Pseudomonas aeruginosa*) and for at least 7 days after clinical resolution of infection [12]. TIs are treated for two to four weeks [12]. Fungal prophylaxis may be considered during prolonged antibiotic use. As an adjunct to therapy, exit-site care should be performed once to twice daily and the catheter anchored to prevent further trauma. For resistant infections, catheter-salvage techniques such as cuff shaving, re-tunneling of the catheter, and exit-site relocation have been tried [20, 21]. Indications for catheter removal include: lack of clinical improvement after 2 weeks of treatment, failure to achieve complete resolution after 4 weeks of treatment, presence of an abscess, or development of peritonitis with the same causative organism (especially if *Staphylococcus aureus* or *Pseudomonas*).

5. Catheter-related infections due to *Pseudomonas aeruginosa* are a significant complication of PD owing to associated high treatment failure rates and subsequent catheter loss. *Pseudomonas* species are gram-negative rods that have the ability to colonize PD catheters by secreting a biofilm consisting of exopolysaccharides, which protects the organisms from antimicrobial agents and promotes bacterial growth. Data from the IPPR demonstrated that *Pseudomonas* was more common in centers that performed exit-site care more than two times per week and used mupirocin for antibiotic prophylaxis [5]. *Pseudomonas aeruginosa* is increasingly recognized as an opportunistic pathogen with low antibiotic susceptibility due to intrinsic resistance genes as well as acquired resistance. Anaerobic organisms are generally sensitive to drugs such as cefepime, piperacillin, imipenem, ciprofloxacin, and aminoglycosides; however, *Pseudomonas* ESIs/TIs are often difficult to treat. Adding a second antipseudomonal agent should be considered. That said, the rate for successful treatment of *Pseudomonas* catheter-related infections with various antibiotic regimens is reported to be 38–83% [22–25].

Clinical Pearls

1. ESIs and TIs are catheter-related infections that are a significant complication of PD. ESIs and TIs should be identified early and treated aggressively, as they are associated with an increased risk for peritonitis, catheter loss, frequent hospitalization, and increased costs.
2. Optimal chronic catheter care measures such as cleansing with an antiseptic solution, proper hand washing, and topical antibiotic prophylaxis may prevent ESIs and TIs.
3. Oral antibiotic treatment of ESIs with first generation cephalosporins or ciprofloxacin (for suspected *Pseudomonas*) is recommended as empiric oral treatment pending culture results. TIs can be treated with oral, intravenous, or intraperitoneal antibiotics. Treatment duration is generally 2–4 weeks and for at least 7 days after resolution of external symptoms.
4. ESI and TIs due to *Pseudomonas aeruginosa* can be difficult to treat and often result in catheter removal.

References

1. Furth SL, et al. Peritoneal dialysis catheter infections and peritonitis in children: a report of the north American pediatric renal transplant cooperative study. Pediatr Nephrol. 2000; 15(3–4):179–82.
2. Neu A, et al. Implementation of standardized follow-up care significantly reduces peritonitis in children on chronic peritoneal dialysis. Kidney Int. 2016;89(6):1346–54.
3. Chua AN, et al. Topical mupirocin/sodium hypochlorite reduces peritonitis and exit-site infection rates in children. Clin J Am Soc Nephrol. 2009;4(12):1939–43.
4. Levy M, et al. Exit-site infection during continuous and cycling peritoneal dialysis in children. Perit Dial Int. 1990;10(1):31–5.
5. Schaefer F, et al. Worldwide variation of dialysis-associated peritonitis in children. Kidney Int. 2007;72(11):1374–9.
6. Tse KC, et al. A cluster of rapidly growing mycobacterial peritoneal dialysis catheter exit-site infections. Am J Kidney Dis. 2007;50(1):e1–5.
7. Schiffl H, Mucke C, Lang SM. Exit-site infections by non-diphtheria corynebacteria in CAPD. Perit Dial Int. 2004;24(5):454–9.
8. Bernardini J, et al. Randomized, double-blind trial of antibiotic exit site cream for prevention of exit site infection in peritoneal dialysis patients. J Am Soc Nephrol. 2005;16(2):539–45.
9. Schaefer F, et al. Intermittent versus continuous intraperitoneal glycopeptide/ceftazidime treatment in children with peritoneal dialysis-associated peritonitis. The mid-European pediatric peritoneal dialysis study group (MEPPS). J Am Soc Nephrol. 1999;10(1):136–45.
10. Li PK, et al. Peritoneal dialysis-related infections recommendations: 2010 update. Perit Dial Int. 2010;30(4):393–423.
11. Karahan OI, et al. Ultrasound evaluation of peritoneal catheter tunnel in catheter related infections in CAPD. Int Urol Nephrol. 2005;37(2):363–6.
12. Warady BA, et al. Consensus guidelines for the prevention and treatment of catheter-related infections and peritonitis in pediatric patients receiving peritoneal dialysis: 2012 update. Perit Dial Int. 2012;32(Suppl 2):S32–86.

13. Piraino B. How much peritoneal dialysis is needed for optimal outcomes? Semin Dial. 2003;16(5):367–9.
14. Pottinger J, Burns S, Manske C. Bacterial carriage by artificial versus natural nails. Am J Infect Control. 1989;17(6):340–4.
15. McNeil SA, et al. Effect of hand cleansing with antimicrobial soap or alcohol-based gel on microbial colonization of artificial fingernails worn by health care workers. Clin Infect Dis. 2001;32(3):367–72.
16. Prowant BF, Khanna R, Twardowski ZJ. Peritoneal catheter exit-site morphology and pathology: prevention, diagnosis, and treatment of exit-site infections. Case reports for independent study. Perit Dial Int. 1996;16(Suppl 3):S105–14.
17. Chua AN, Warady BA. Adherence of pediatric patients to automated peritoneal dialysis. Pediatr Nephrol. 2011;26(5):789–93.
18. Sethna C, et al. Catheter-Associated Peritonitis: risk factors and outcomes in children enrolled in the SCOPE Collaborative. CJASN. 2016;11(9):1590–6.
19. Nouwen JL, et al. Persistent (not intermittent) nasal carriage of *Staphylococcus aureus* is the determinant of CPD-related infections. Kidney Int. 2005;67(3):1084–92.
20. Yoshino A, et al. Merit of the cuff-shaving procedure in children with chronic infection. Pediatr Nephrol. 2004;19(11):1267–72.
21. Macchini F, et al. Conservative surgical management of catheter infections in children on peritoneal dialysis. Pediatr Surg Int. 2009;25(8):703–7.
22. Kazmi HR, et al. Pseudomonas exit site infections in continuous ambulatory peritoneal dialysis patients. J Am Soc Nephrol. 1992;2(10):1498–501.
23. Lo CY, et al. Pseudomonas exit-site infections in CAPD patients: evolution and outcome of treatment. Perit Dial Int. 1998;18(6):637–40.
24. Szabo T, et al. Outcome of Pseudomonas Aeruginosa exit-site and tunnel infections: a single center's experience. Adv Perit Dial. 1999;15:209–12.
25. Burkhalter F, et al. Pseudomonas exit-site infection: treatment outcomes with topical gentamicin in addition to systemic antibiotics. Clin Kidney J. 2015;8(6):781–4.

Chapter 8
Peritonitis

Enrico Eugenio Verrina

Case Presentations

Case 1

L. is a male child of 2 years of age who has been on peritoneal dialysis (PD) since his first days of life due to renal hypo-dysplasia associated with psychomotor retardation, seizures, and mild liver dysfunction. At birth, he suffered from severe perinatal asphyxia owing to placental abruption that caused a multi-organ injury, including necrotizing enterocolitis, which required surgical repair. At 1 year of age, L. had an ileal intussusception which required laparoscopic bowel resection and anastomosis in the same operating session.

His first peritoneal catheter had been replaced early in the hospital where he was born, and the second catheter was replaced on a previous admission to our unit due to obstruction that occurred during a peritonitis episode caused by a methicillin-resistant strain of *Staphylococcus aureus*. The third catheter had been functioning rather well until a few months prior to this admission when tip dislocation occurred and the catheter had to be replaced. The fourth catheter was a straight Tenckhoff catheter with two Dacron cuffs. A peritonitis episode due to a strain of coagulase-negative staphylococcus occurred at the 16th month of PD treatment (no signs of catheter exit-site or tunnel infection) and was successfully treated with a 2-week course of intraperitoneal cefazolin.

During the 6-month period prior to this admission, the peritoneal catheter was functioning well, automated PD (APD) treatment was working adequately, and

E.E. Verrina (✉)
Giannina Gaslini Children's Hospital, Dialysis Unit, Genoa, Italy
e-mail: enricoverrina@gaslini.org

© Springer International Publishing AG 2017
B.A. Warady et al. (eds.), *Pediatric Dialysis Case Studies*,
DOI 10.1007/978-3-319-55147-0_8

L. (who still had a residual diuresis) was generally doing very well. He had reached a body weight (BW) of 9.2 kg and was on the waiting list for renal transplantation.

Three months prior to this admission, an exit-site infection caused by methicillin-resistant *Staphylococcus aureus* (MRSA) had occurred (Score 4: swelling 1, redness 1, secretion 2) [1]. There were no signs of involvement of the subcutaneous catheter tunnel. The infection was treated with the local application of mupirocin cream and oral ciprofloxacin (10 mg/kg BW/day) for 14 days, followed by two intravenous administrations of vancomycin for the persistence of MRSA in the culture from the exit site. Still, there were no clinical signs of tunnel infection (ultrasonographic examination was negative). Unfortunately, on day 14 peritonitis occurred, and intra-peritoneal vancomycin was started as a 1,000 mg/L loading dose, followed by 25 mg/L as a maintenance therapy on APD. Blood vancomycin levels were in the thera-peutic range. MRSA was cultured from the peritoneal effluent sample obtained just before the start of vancomycin therapy, but by day 5 of treatment, the effluent culture had become negative. Clinical signs of peritonitis resolved rapidly. On the other hand, the exit-site infection persisted, now also showing signs of tunnel involvement (Score 7: swelling 2, redness 2, secretion 2, pain on pressure 1 [1]) (Fig. 8.1). Ultrasonographic examination showed that inflammation did not reach the inner cuff of the catheter.

At this point, according to the suggestions of the consensus guidelines for the prevention and treatment of catheter-related infections and peritonitis in pediatric patients receiving peritoneal dialysis [2], we should have removed the catheter

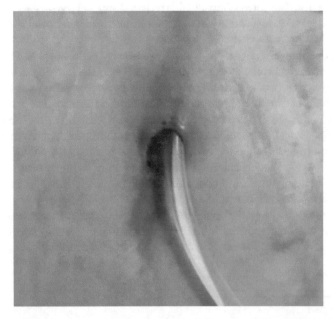

Fig. 8.1 Appearance of the peritoneal catheter exit site (Case 1) under antibiotic treatment for a methicillin-resistant *Staphylococcus aureus* infection and before surgery. Score 7: swelling 2, redness 2, secretion 2, pain on pressure 1 [1]

(see guideline 17.3) and placed another one in the same operative session (see guidelines 17.4 and 17.5). On the other hand, the child had had several abdominal interventions and four peritoneal catheter placements. During the video-laparoscopy replacement of the third catheter (the one which was dislocated), several intra-abdominal adhesions were found, and adhesiolysis was performed. The surgeons who had conducted the previous video-laparoscopic interventions were very worried about performing another abdominal intervention in this child. Moreover, he had suffered right internal jugular vein thrombosis after placement of a central venous catheter during his first months of life. Limited vascular access options, as well as L.'s small body size, made consideration of hemodialysis problematic. Lastly, the peritoneal catheter was still functioning very well.

After a thorough discussion involving the entire team of nephrologists, surgeons, infectious disease specialists, anesthesiologists, and nurses in which the *pros* and *cons* of the available therapeutic options were reviewed, it was decided to perform debridement and curettage of the exit site and unroofing of the subcutaneous tunnel, with extrusion and shaving of the superficial catheter cuff. This intervention was done on day 14 of the intraperitoneal vancomycin treatment course. An additional intravenous 20 mg/kg vancomycin dose was administered perioperatively, and a 21-day course of intraperitoneal therapy with the same antibiotic was completed. Following this intervention, the local infection healed (Fig. 8.2). As of 2 months after the completion of intraperitoneal antibiotic therapy, no recurrence of exit-site infection or peritonitis had occurred.

Fig. 8.2 Appearance of the peritoneal catheter exit site (Case 1) 1 month after conservative local surgery for a refractory methicillin-resistant *Staphylococcus aureus* infection

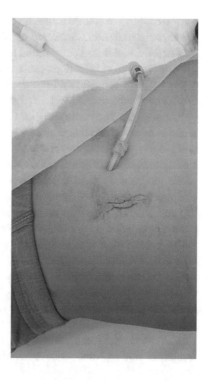

Clinical Features

1. This is the clinical case of a child on PD since the neonatal period, with several nonrenal comorbidities who had required two abdominal interventions due to intestinal necrosis and repeated peritoneal catheter replacements and who experienced an MRSA peritonitis originating from an exit-site/tunnel infection caused by the same organism.
2. As an alternative to catheter removal in a small child with a history of repeated catheter replacement and with a high operative risk, the persistence of antibiotic-resistant exit-site and tunnel infection led to a decision to perform local debridement and curettage of the infected exit site, along with unroofing of the subcutaneous tunnel and extrusion and shaving of the external Dacron cuff.

Clinical Questions

What is the optimal duration of antibiotic treatment of a peritonitis episode and/or an exit-site/tunnel infection caused by MRSA? Is there any reasonable alternative to peritoneal catheter removal for a refractory exit-site and/or tunnel infection?

Diagnostic Discussion

The currently available consensus guidelines [2] suggest that treatment for PD-associated peritonitis caused by MRSA should be based on the susceptibility of the bacteria, and the recommended length of therapy is 3 weeks. Treatment duration for exit-site/tunnel infections caused by MRSA should be 2–4 weeks, and simultaneous catheter removal and replacement are recommended for a refractory infection. The interesting aspect of this clinical case lies in the fact that treatment guidelines had been followed until the moment when the subsequent step (i.e., simultaneous peritoneal catheter removal and replacement) could have exposed the child to a risk of complications of abdominal surgery. There was a significant possibility that a new catheter would not work well in such a critical abdominal cavity, while the catheter that the child had at that moment was functioning very well. Then, it was decided to adopt a treatment solution different from that suggested by the guidelines. This decision was based on clinical judgment and on an accurate patient evaluation involving both the clinical and the surgical team. Indeed, conservative treatment of a tunnel infection, especially when caused by MRSA, can be very difficult. Because of poor blood supply to the infected area, antibiotic penetration is variable, and bacteria can adhere in clusters to the Dacron fibers of the subcutaneous cuff of the catheter which thus becomes a reservoir of bacteria [3]. Ultrasonographic examination of the tunnel may help in detecting a clinically occult infection, in evaluating its expansion and in monitoring the response to therapy [4]. Conservative surgical management of catheter infections resistant to antibiotic treatment was reported to have satisfactory results in terms of long-term catheter survival in adult as well as in pediatric PD patients [5, 6]. Conservative surgical intervention should be preoperatively planned with a surgeon experienced in PD catheter placement and revision [2]. After surgery, a shorter subcutaneous tunnel and the absence of the superficial cuff makes the catheter less stable and are associated with an increased risk of infection [7]. Therefore, it becomes even more important to securely anchor the catheter close to the exit site to minimize movement and the potential for traction injury, both of which represent risk factors for the occurrence of an exit-site infection [2]. In these cases, reevaluation of the exit-site care procedure and retraining of the patient's caretakers are strongly recommended [2].

Clinical Pearls

1. In a case of persistent and antibiotic-resistant infection of the exit site and subcutaneous tunnel, local debridement and curettage with extrusion and shaving of the external Dacron cuff can be an acceptable alternative to catheter removal in selected patients with a history of repeated catheter replacement and a high individual surgical risk.
2. Specific individual patient clinical conditions may require interventions that are not recommended in the currently available consensus treatment guidelines. In this situation, it is extremely important to conduct a thorough evaluation of each clinical case with all the members of a multidisciplinary team who are skilled in the care of patients on PD.

Case 2

R. is a 4-year-old child with end-stage renal disease due to renal dysplasia associated with congenital abnormalities of the urinary tract (bilateral vesicoureteral reflux *plus* a large urethral diverticulum) who had been on PD since his fourth day of life. Past medical history was relatively uneventful, although R. had experienced recurrent urinary tract infections likely related to his complex urinary tract abnormalities. After 26 months on PD treatment (during which he had never experienced peritonitis or a catheter exit-site infection), he was admitted to our hospital because of sudden onset of clinical signs of peritonitis (fever, abdominal pain, and cloudy peritoneal effluent). Blood and peritoneal fluid cultures were performed, and empirical intraperitoneal antibiotic therapy was started according to our internal protocol and the pediatric peritonitis treatment guidelines (cefazolin *plus* ceftazidime) [2]. By day 3, no clinical improvement had been observed (Disease Severity Score = 3 [1]). The laboratory reported yeast (subsequently identified as *Candida parapsilosis*) growing from peritoneal fluid and blood cultures. After 2 days of intravenous and intraperitoneal fluconazole administration, clinical conditions and inflammatory parameters did not improve, and cultures of peritoneal effluent remained positive for *Candida*. Fluconazole was replaced with caspofungin (50 mg/m^2 once a day). The peritoneal catheter was removed and a central venous catheter was inserted for administration of systemic antifungal therapy and to perform hemodialysis.

With this management, clinical conditions improved, and blood and peritoneal fluid cultures became negative. Antifungal treatment with caspofungin was continued for a total of 4 weeks without side effects. During treatment, serial determinations of 1-3-β-D-glucan (BDG), a fungal cell wall component, were performed on peritoneal fluid and serum (Fungitell assay, Associates of Cape Cod, Inc., Falmouth, MA, USA). The BDG test was positive at very high levels in the peritoneal fluid (>523 pg/ml that was the upper limit of detection) in the first days of fungal peritonitis, with lower but still positive levels in serum (positive cutoff, 80 pg/ml). After catheter removal the levels of serum BDG rapidly decreased, reaching <80 pg/ml after 12 days of caspofungin treatment. BDG in the peritoneal fluid and blood also became consistently negative after 3 weeks, when a new peritoneal dialysis catheter was video-laparoscopically placed.

Clinical Features

1. This clinical case started as an ordinary case of peritonitis in an apparently low-risk patient for fungal peritonitis: no previous peritonitis episodes, no catheter exit-site infection, no immunosuppression, no ostomy, and good clinical and nutritional conditions. Peritonitis then was revealed to be caused by a relatively uncommon strain of *Candida*.
2. *Candida parapsilosis* peritonitis occurred in a patient who had received only repeated, short courses of antibiotic treatment for recurrent urinary tract infections (UTIs). The most recent antibiotic course had been administered 1 month prior to the fungal peritonitis episode and, in the absence of prophylaxis, may have contributed to the development of fungal peritonitis.
3. When a few days of antifungal treatment with fluconazole did not clear the peritonitis, the peritoneal catheter was removed and fluconazole was replaced by caspofungin. This was done in order to administer a fungicidal drug that does not require dose reduction in patients with renal function impairment and that has no renal toxicity (the child still had residual renal function).

Clinical Questions

1. Should we have prescribed antifungal prophylaxis during the antibiotic treatments for UTIs (which had always been short: 7–10 days)?
2. Can BDG monitoring both in serum and peritoneal fluid be helpful to assess the response to therapy (with concomitant evaluation of clinical conditions and microbiology) and to optimize the timing of peritoneal catheter replacement after temporary catheter removal due to fungal peritonitis?

Diagnostic Discussion

1. Fungal peritonitis is relatively rare, accounting for only 2–3% of peritonitis episodes in an International Pediatric Peritonitis Registry (IPPR) report [8] and the 2011 North American Pediatric Renal Trials and Collaborative Studies (NAPRTCS) annual report [9], respectively. Case 2 can be regarded as a de novo fungal peritonitis episode: a peritonitis episode caused by a fungus, with no preceding episodes of bacterial peritonitis, the incidence of which has been reported to be 1.3–1.6% in pediatric series [10, 11]. In this child, the fungal infection could be effectively managed by following the currently available guidelines: (1) start with empirical antibiotic treatment at diagnosis for presumptive bacterial peritonitis; (2) evaluate clinical response at 72 h and change therapy based on PD effluent culture results showing the growth of *Candida parapsilosis*; (3) recognize an unsatisfactory clinical response to antifungal therapy when peritoneal effluent culture remains positive after 48 h; (4) change antifungal drug to an echinocandin agent in the presence of a nonresponding infection with a non-*albicans Candida*; (5) remove the PD catheter and transfer the child to hemodialysis; (6) continue antifungal treatment for 4 weeks; and (7) replace the peritoneal catheter and resume PD.

   Guideline 6 of the 2012 update of consensus guidelines for the prevention and treatment of catheter-related infections and peritonitis in pediatric patients receiving peritoneal dialysis [2] suggests that the use of oral nystatin or fluconazole should be considered at the time of antibiotic administration to PD patients to reduce the risk of fungal peritonitis. The rationale for this recommendation is that in two pediatric PD patient series, 56–78% of children with fungal peritonitis had received antibiotics in the preceding month, and 50–86% of them had been treated for bacterial peritonitis [10, 11]. Patients at high risk for fungal peritonitis are considered to be those who had been on prolonged courses of antibiotics, those experiencing frequent bacterial peritonitis, and those with impaired immune systems. Indeed, our patient did not belong to any of these categories, and he had received only short antibiotic courses for treatment UTIs (7–10 days). Moreover, our PD unit had experienced a very low rate of fungal peritonitis during the previous 10 years. However, the very serious consequences of an, even rare, episode of fungal peritonitis (peritoneal catheter removal, patient transfer to hemodialysis, prolonged intravenous treatments, risk of death) should prompt each PD unit to consider antifungal prophylaxis for any patient receiving antibiotics.

2. When combined with clinical, radiological, and microbiological findings, BDG can be a useful test for the diagnosis of invasive fungal infections in adults with hematologic malignancies or those admitted to intensive care units [12, 13]. It has been suggested that, when available, BDG testing should be performed in patients with secondary or tertiary peritonitis and at least one specific risk factor for intra-abdominal candidiasis [14]. Recently, the results of a pilot study of adult PD patients supported the use of BDG, in association with galactomannan, as surrogate biomarkers for the diagnosis of fungal peritonitis [15].

This clinical case represents the first report of the use of BDG monitoring during the treatment of *Candida* peritonitis in a child on PD [16]. We found a good correlation between 1-3-β-D-glucan levels in peritoneal fluid and serum and the microbiological and clinical outcome of the patient. The major problem with this kind of monitoring remains the possibility of a false-positive BDG test. While hemodialysis with cellulose membranes has been suggested as a possible cause for false-positive BDG results [17], the potential role of the peritoneal membrane is unknown. No data are available on the components of the polyurethane intravenous or silicon peritoneal catheters as a possible cause of a false-positive BDG test. Even if the difference in BDG levels found in peritoneal fluid before and after catheter removal could also be influenced by BDG release by yeast that is present in the infected catheter lumen, the clinical and microbiological course of our patient paralleled the improving BDG levels both in serum and peritoneal fluid, with reduction and normalization of the values clearly associated with successful clinical management (catheter removal and appropriate antifungal therapy). The fact that after the end of therapy samples for cultures and BDG testing taken through the peritoneal dialysis catheter were negative is consistent with a relatively low risk of false-positive test results due to catheter materials.

Finally, this case report supports early catheter removal as essential for treatment of fungal peritonitis [2]. Caspofungin may represent an effective therapy for invasive disease due to *Candida parapsilosis*, in spite of in vitro data suggesting a possible lower efficacy [18].

Clinical Pearls

1. It is important for each PD program to develop and periodically revise its own strategy of detection and management of potential risk factors in both the host and the environment for fungal peritonitis and to determine who would benefit most from antifungal prophylaxis during antibiotic therapy.
2. In PD patients with *Candida* peritonitis, BDG monitoring in serum and peritoneal fluid may be helpful to assess response to therapy, together with the concomitant evaluation of clinical conditions and microbiology.

Acknowledgments The author would like to thank Dr. Elio Castagnola for clinical consultation on infectious disease issues, Dr. Roberto Bandettini for laboratory analyses, and Dr. Alessio Pini Prato for surgical consultation.

References

1. Schaefer F, Klaus G, Mueller-Wiefel DE, Mehls O. Intermittent versus continuous intraperitoneal glycopeptide/ceftazidime treatment in children with peritoneal dialysis peritonitis. J Am Soc Nephrol. 1999;10:136–45.
2. Warady BA, Bakkaloglu S, Newland J, Cantwell M, Verrina E, Neu A, Chadha V, Yap HK, Schaefer F. Consensus guidelines for the prevention and treatment of catheter-related

infections and peritonitis in pediatric patients receiving peritoneal dialysis: 2012 update. Perit Dial Int. 2012;32(Suppl 2):S32–86.

3. Marrie TJ, Noble MA, Costerton JW. Examination of the morphology of bacteria adhering to peritoneal dialysis catheters by scanning and transmission electron microscopy. J Clin Microbiol. 1983;18(6):1388–98.

4. Stuart S, Booth TC, Cash CJ, Hameeduddin A, Goode JA, Harvey C, Malhotra A. Complications of continuous ambulatory peritoneal dialysis. Radiographics. 2009;29(2):441–60.

5. Crabtree JH, Burchette RJ. Surgical salvage of peritoneal dialysis catheters from chronic exit-site and tunnel infections. Am J Surg. 2005;190(1):4–8.

6. Macchini F, Testa S, Valadè A, Torricelli M, Leva E, Ardissino G, Edefonti A. Conservative surgical management of catheter infections in children on peritoneal dialysis. Pediatr Surg Int. 2009;25(8):703–7. Epub 2009 Jul 2.

7. Zurowska A, Feneberg R, Warady BA, Zimmering M, Monteverde M, Testa S, Calyskan S, Drozdz D, Salusky I, Kemper MJ, Ekim M, Verrina E, Misselwitz J, Schaefer F. Gram-negative peritonitis in children undergoing long-term peritoneal dialysis. Am J Kidney Dis. 2008;51:455–62.

8. Warady BA, Feneberg R, Verrina E, Flynn JT, Muller-Wiefel DE, Besbas N, Zurowska A, Aksu N, Fischbach M, Sojo E, Donmez O, Sever L, Sirin A, Alexander SR, Schaefer F. Peritonitis in children who receive long-term peritoneal dialysis: a prospective evaluation of therapeutic guidelines. J Am Soc Nephrol. 2007;18:2172–9.

9. North American Pediatric Renal Trials and Collaborative Studies (NAPRTCS) 2011 Annual Report (http://www.naprtcs.org).

10. Warady BA, Bashir M, Donaldson LA. Fungal peritonitis in children receiving peritoneal dialysis: a report of the NAPRTCS. Kidney Int. 2000;58:384–9.

11. Raaijmakers R, Schroeder C, Monnens L, Cornelissen E, Warris A. Fungal peritonitis in children on peritoneal dialysis. Pediatr Nephrol. 2007;22:288–93.

12. Lamoth F, Cruciani M, Mengoli C, Castagnola E, Lortholary O, Richardson M, Marchetti O. β-glucan antigenemia assay for the diagnosis of invasive fungal infections in patients with hematological malignancies: a systematic review and meta-analysis of cohort studies from the third European conference on infections in leukemia (ECIL-3). Clin Infect Dis. 2012;54(5):633–43.

13. Mohr JF, Sims C, Paetznick V, Rodriguez J, Finkelman MA, Rex JH, Ostrosky-Zeichner L. Prospective survey of (1-3)-β-D-glucan and its relationship to invasive candidiasis in the surgical intensive care unit setting. J Clin Microbiol. 2011;49:58–61.

14. Marchetti M, Chakrabarti A, Colizza S, Garnacho-Montero J, Kett DH, Munoz P, Cristini F, Andoniadou A, Viale P, Rocca GD, Roilides E, Sganga G, Walsh TJ, Tascini C, Tumbarello M, Menichetti F, Righi E, Eckmann C, Viscoli C, Shorr AF, Leroy O, Petrikos G, De Rosa FG. A research agenda on the management of intra-abdominal candidiasis: results from a consensus of multinational experts. Intensive Care Med. 2013;39(12):2092–106.

15. Worasilchai N, Leelahavanichkul A, Kanjanabuch T, Thongbor N, Lorvinitnun P, Sukhontasing K, Finkelman M, Chindamporn A. (1→3)-β-D-glucan and galactomannan testing for the diagnosis of fungal peritonitis in peritoneal dialysis patients, a pilot study. Med. Mycol. 2015;53(4):338–46.

16. Ginocchio F, Verrina E, Furfaro E, Cannavò R, Bandettini R, Castagnola E. Case report of the reliability 1,3-β-D-glucan monitoring during treatment of peritoneal candidiasis in a child receiving continuous peritoneal dialysis. Clin Vaccine Immunol. 2012;19(4):626-627. Epub 2012 Feb 22.

17. Kanda H, Kubo K, Hamasaki K, Kanda Y, Nakao A, Kitamura T, Fujita T, Yamamoto K, Mimura T. Influence of various hemodialysis membranes on the plasma (1/3)- β-D-glucan level. Kidney Int. 2001;60:319–23.

18. Kale-Pradhan PB, Morgan G, Wilhelm SM, Johnson LB. Comparative efficacy of echinocandins and nonechinocandis for the treatment of Candida parapsilosis infections: a meta-analysis. Pharmacotherapy. 2010;30:1207–13.

Chapter 9
Relapsing and Recurrent Peritonitis

Sevcan A. Bakkaloglu

Case Presentations

Case 1: Relapsing Peritonitis

A 17-year-old boy with end-stage kidney disease due to collapsing glomerulopathy and who had been receiving chronic peritoneal dialysis (CPD) for 5 months was admitted to the hospital with diffuse abdominal pain. He had a history of PD catheter replacement due to mechanical drainage problems 1 month after his initial catheter insertion, and he experienced minor trauma to his abdomen close to the catheter exit site 3 days ago. The exit-site was normal in appearance. The patient had diffuse abdominal tenderness on examination. Microscopic evaluation of the PD effluent showed 700 white blood cells/mm^3, with 85% neutrophils. Blood, PD effluent, and PD catheter exit-site cultures were obtained prior to initiating empiric antibiotic therapy with intraperitoneal (IP) cefepime, in accordance with published treatment guidelines [1]. The PD culture revealed coagulase-negative *Staphylococcus* (CNS) that was susceptible to cefepime, and IP cefepime was continued as monotherapy for 2 weeks. Full functional recovery was achieved at the end of treatment.

Three weeks after completion of the IP cefepime therapy, another peritonitis episode was diagnosed secondary to the same organism (CNS); therefore, this episode was labeled as relapsing peritonitis. Vancomycin was prescribed empirically and provided by the intraperitoneal route intermittently. An ultrasound examination of the PD catheter tunnel revealed a 4-mm fluid collection around the catheter. The patient's chronic catheter exit-site care did not include the use of an antibiotic ointment or cream. The exit-site score was 3 based on predefined criteria [1], and CNS was grown in the exit-site culture. In accordance with findings in the antibiotic

S.A. Bakkaloglu, MD (✉)
Division of Pediatric Nephrology, Gazi University School of Medicine, Ankara, Turkey
e-mail: sevcan@gazi.edu.tr

© Springer International Publishing AG 2017
B.A. Warady et al. (eds.), *Pediatric Dialysis Case Studies*,
DOI 10.1007/978-3-319-55147-0_9

susceptibility report, vancomycin was continued as treatment for catheter-related peritonitis and exit-site/tunnel infection. Although the results of a repeat catheter tunnel ultrasound assessment on the fifth day of antibiotic therapy demonstrated resolution of the fluid collection around the catheter, because of a refractory high cell count in the PD effluent (440/mm^3), the PD catheter was removed, and the patient underwent HD for 4 weeks. Vancomycin was provided by the intravenous (IV) route for an additional 3 weeks in preparation for PD catheter replacement.

Clinical Questions

1. What is the definition of relapsing peritonitis?
2. How common is relapsing peritonitis in children who receive chronic peritoneal dialysis?
3. What is the distribution of causative organisms in cases of relapsing peritonitis?
4. What are the risk factors for relapsing peritonitis?
5. What is the recommended approach to the treatment of relapsing peritonitis?
6. What is the indication for catheter removal in this case?
7. Is there a difference in outcome of relapsing peritonitis episodes compared to episodic peritonitis?

Diagnostic Discussion

1. A relapsing episode of peritonitis is defined as one that occurs within 4 weeks of completion of therapy of a prior episode with the same organism or one sterile episode [1, 2].
2. Relapsing peritonitis follows approximately 5–20% of primary peritonitis episodes in pediatric patients. In the Australian and New Zealand Dialysis and Transplant (ANZDATA) registry, a peritonitis relapse rate in children of only 5% was noted, in contrast to the Mid-European Pediatric Peritoneal Dialysis Study Group who reported a relapsing peritonitis rate of 20% between 1993 and 1997 [2–4]. By far the largest pediatric experience with relapsing peritonitis has come from the International Pediatric Peritonitis Registry (IPPR). The IPPR data showed that out of 490 episodes of non-fungal peritonitis, 52 were followed by a relapse, for a relapse rate of 11% [3].
3. In the IPPR experience, there was no significant difference in the distribution of causative organisms between cases of relapsing and non-relapsing peritonitis. Overall, relapsing episodes consisted of 46% Gram-positive organisms, 21% Gram-negative organisms, and 33% culture-negative cases. *Staphylococcus aureus* (*S. aureus*) and CNS were the causative organisms in 21% and 13% of episodes of relapsing peritonitis, respectively [3]. CNS and *S. aureus* combined were the most frequent causes of relapsing peritonitis episodes in the ANZDATA and Scottish registries, accounting for 48% and 76% of episodes, respectively [2]. However, more recently and in contrast to the pediatric experience, Szeto et al. described an

experience in the adult population in which the majority of organisms causing relapsing peritonitis were Gram-negative (62%); S. aureus was isolated in only 5.5% of relapsing peritonitis episodes [5]. The frequency of Gram-negative infections causing a relapsing infection (see Case 2 below) in adult PD patients was also threefold higher than the frequency noted among pediatric PD patients [5].

4. Independent risk factors for relapsing peritonitis identified by the IPPR include young age, single-cuff catheter, downward-pointing exit site, and chronic systemic antibiotic prophylaxis [3]. Adult data have also indicated that patients with repeated peritonitis had a higher risk of developing relapsing peritonitis compared to controls [5].

   To date, there is no accurate laboratory test to help predict which patient is going to develop relapsing or recurrent peritonitis after completion of antibiotic treatment. A recent study designed to further evaluate this issue by measuring the level of bacteria-derived DNA fragments in the PD effluent found that bacterial DNA fragment levels in PD effluent were significantly higher, both 5 days before and on the date of completion of antibiotic therapy, among patients who subsequently developed relapsing or recurrent peritonitis episodes than among those without these infections [6]. Although this study deserves further attention, the results remain to be validated. It is also important to note that the presence of bacterial DNA fragments in the PD effluent does not indicate the presence of living bacteria capable of causing an active infection.

5. Prompt and efficacious treatment of relapsing peritonitis episodes is critical. Since, by definition, the bacterial etiology of relapsing peritonitis is the same as that of the preceding episode of peritonitis, it is prudent to empirically start with the antibiotic regimen that would treat the first organism identified based on the previously determined antibiotic susceptibilities. If there is resistance to that antibiotic in the latest susceptibility report, antibiotic therapy has to be changed accordingly with a plan to continue therapy for at least 3 weeks [1]. For adult patients who present with relapsing or recurrent peritonitis, vancomycin is superior to cefazolin as empirical antibiotic treatment, especially in patients with a previous peritonitis episode caused by Gram-positive organisms [7]. Parallel to the adult experience, in the IPPR, switching to monotherapy with a first-generation cephalosporin on the basis of culture results was associated with a subsequent higher relapse rate (23%) compared to other final antibiotic therapies (0 to 9%) [3]. Similarly, in those who had a recent Gram-negative peritonitis episode, ceftazidime appears to be a better choice for empiric treatment than an aminoglycoside [7]. Finally, PD catheter removal should be considered if relapsing peritonitis is associated with a persistent or recurrent tunnel infection or in the setting of a second peritonitis relapse. Simultaneous removal and replacement of the catheter under antibiotic coverage has also been performed successfully as part of the treatment for relapsing bacterial peritonitis once the effluent clears with antibiotic therapy. The technique may be particularly beneficial with relapsing peritonitis secondary to CNS or S. aureus, as those infections may be a result of sequestration of bacteria in biofilm surrounding the intra-abdominal portion of the catheter [1].

6. The indication for catheter removal in this case is refractory peritonitis. Bacterial peritonitis that fails to resolve after 5 days of appropriate antibiotic treatment in PD patients is defined as refractory peritonitis and is unlikely to respond to continued medical management and most often responds to removal of the catheter.
7. Relapsing peritonitis episodes have been associated with a lower rate of full functional recovery (73 vs. 91%), a higher rate of ultrafiltration (UF) problems (14 vs. 2%) and a higher rate of permanent PD discontinuation (17 vs. 7%) in children [3], as well as higher rates of catheter removal (30 vs. 22%) and permanent HD therapy transfer (25 vs. 20%) in adult patients [8]. A concomitant exit-site infection has had very little impact on clinical outcome [7].

Clinical Pearls

1. Relapsing peritonitis follows approximately 5%–20% of primary peritonitis episodes in children and should not be counted as another peritonitis episode when peritonitis rates are calculated. Relapsing episodes secondary to Gram-positive organisms were twice as common as Gram-negative organisms in the IPPR data. However, in adult practice, Gram-negative organisms are more commonly seen in relapsing episodes compared to non-relapsing ones.
2. In patients who develop cloudy effluent within 4 weeks of completion of therapy for Gram-positive peritonitis, vancomycin is a better choice for empiric antibiotic coverage than cefazolin, at least until information about antibiotic susceptibilities is available. Similarly, in the setting of a recent Gram-negative peritonitis episode, ceftazidime appears to be a better empiric selection compared to an aminoglycoside.
3. The total duration of treatment for relapsing peritonitis should be 3 weeks to achieve a higher complete cure rate compared to a 2-week regimen. On the other hand, the source of the relapse may be the catheter through the development of either a biofilm, particularly in CNS or *S. aureus* peritonitis, or a tunnel infection. In these cases or in the case of repeated relapsing bacterial peritonitis, catheter removal may be necessary.

Case 2: Recurrent Peritonitis

A 14-year-old girl who had been undergoing CPD for 21 months was admitted to the hospital with nausea, abdominal pain, and cloudy dialysate effluent. Her renal failure was secondary to juvenile nephronophthisis. She was prescribed six exchanges nightly with a fill volume of 1,100 ml/m^2 and with a dry abdomen during the day.

Five weeks earlier she experienced a peritonitis episode secondary to *Escherichia coli (E. coli)*. That episode was treated with intermittent IP ceftazidime for 7 days, preceded by a 3-day course of empiric combination treatment with cefazolin and ceftazidime, with no associated change in her dialysis prescription. After a negative dialysate culture was obtained on the fifth day of treatment, along with clearing of the dialysate and resolution of her abdominal symptoms, the patient was discharged. Her mother continued IP antibiotic treatment at home over the subsequent 5 days.

On physical examination at the time of the most recent hospital admission, the patient had fever, abdominal distension, and diffuse abdominal tenderness. The PD catheter exit site was normal in appearance. Microscopic evaluation of the PD effluent showed 3,200 white blood cells/mm^3, with 90% neutrophils. Blood, PD effluent, and PD catheter exit-site cultures were obtained prior to initiating empiric antibiotic therapy with IP ceftazidime and vancomycin. Since the PD culture revealed *Klebsiella pneumoniae* that was susceptible to ceftazidime, vancomycin was discontinued, and this episode was labeled as a recurrent peritonitis episode. Because of persistent fever on the third day of therapy, ceftazidime was given by the IV route. The effluent gradually cleared over 5 days and the patient's fever subsided. However, the clinical course was further complicated by the patient's development of a delirium-like clinical condition characterized by agitation, bizarre behavior, and myoclonic jerks (rapid, irregular, uncoordinated, and high-amplitude movements). There were no metabolic disturbances other than the known uremic state, with no evidence of liver dysfunction or a refractory infection. A head MRI was normal, without any signs of bleeding, cerebral edema, meningeal or diffuse cerebral infection, or thrombus formation. An EEG demonstrated epileptic activity characterized by diffuse background slowing, with irregular, multifocal, polyspike discharges spreading to both cerebral hemispheres. Since there was no other obvious cause to explain the patients' clinical status, drug neurotoxicity was suspected as it was discovered that the patient was given IP ceftazidime for 6 days, in addition to the IV administration. Ceftazidime was discontinued, and ciprofloxacin treatment was given for an additional week. The patient's neurologic abnormalities completely disappeared promptly after cessation of ceftazidime, and she experienced full functional recovery from the episode of peritonitis following 3 weeks of antibiotic therapy.

Clinical Questions

1. What is the definition of recurrent peritonitis?
2. How common is recurrent peritonitis?
3. Which microorganisms are the most common causative agents for peritonitis in children on CPD, and is there any difference in the causative agents in cases of recurrent peritonitis?
4. Which antibiotics are preferred as empiric therapy in recurrent peritonitis?
5. Is there a difference in the outcome of recurrent peritonitis compared to relapsing and uncomplicated peritonitis?
6. What commonly used antibiotics may result in neurologic complications in patients on dialysis?

Diagnostic Discussion

1. An episode of peritonitis that occurs within 4 weeks of completion of therapy of a prior episode but with a different organism is defined as recurrent peritonitis [1, 2].
2. In a large adult study of 6,024 PD patients, first episodes of relapsing, recurrent, and control (uncomplicated) peritonitis occurred in 356, 165, and 2,021 patients, respectively. In other words, the frequency of recurrent peritonitis is two times and twelve times less than relapsing and uncomplicated peritonitis episodes, respectively.
3. Data from the IPPR revealed that Gram-positive bacteria were identified in 62% of peritonitis episodes in children in cases in which an organism was isolated. Despite regional differences across countries, overall, the most common organisms were CNS and *S. aureus*, occurring in 22% and 21% of all cases, respectively [4]. Whereas there is no data on the bacteriology of recurrent peritonitis in children, information is available from adults. In those studies, recurrent peritonitis episodes were much more frequently associated with fungal infections (8–13%) compared to uncomplicated and relapsing peritonitis episodes, particularly if management of the prior peritonitis episode did not include antifungal chemoprophylaxis [7, 8]. There were also a greater percentage of peritonitis episodes secondary to Gram-negative organisms (46%) and mixed bacterial growth (17%) [7]. In recurrent peritonitis, the patient's immunity may be impaired by the previous peritonitis episode leading to another episode of peritonitis from a completely different organism, implying a different root cause. This may be the case with fungal peritonitis. Additionally, recent antibiotic therapy may also disturb the gastrointestinal flora and provoke transmural migration of bowel organisms to the peritoneal cavity. Recurrent peritonitis episodes caused by Gram-negative and mixed bacterial growth may be explained by this mechanism or by an underlying and unrecognized bowel pathology [7].
4. Because relapsing and recurrent peritonitis episodes cannot be differentiated at presentation, empiric antibiotic treatment should cover Gram-negative and Gram-positive organisms. Vancomycin is superior to cefazolin as empiric antibiotic treatment, especially in patients with a previous peritonitis episode caused by Gram-positive organisms. Ceftazidime is preferred over an aminoglycoside as empiric treatment in patients with a previous peritonitis episode caused by Gram-negative organisms [7]. After culture and susceptibility results are available, therapy should be modified accordingly. In polymicrobial cases, metronidazole should be added to the treatment regimen, and the possibility of surgical pathology should be evaluated [9].
5. An adult study which evaluated 157 relapsing, 125 recurrent, and 764 control episodes (first peritonitis episode without relapse or recurrence) showed that compared with the control and relapsing groups, the recurrent group had a significantly lower primary response rate (86.4%, 88.5%, and 71.2%, respectively), lower complete cure rate (72.3%, 62.4%, and 42.4%, respectively), and higher mortality rate (7.7%, 7.0%, and 20.8%, respectively) [7]. However, a larger multicenter registry showed that recurrent and relapsing episodes had higher rates of catheter removal and transfer to hemodialysis, but similar rates of hospitalization or death compared to control peritonitis episodes [8].

6. Antibiotic-induced neurotoxicity in dialysis patients is often overlooked or misinterpreted despite the frequent administration of the offending agents. Cephalosporins are an underrecognized class of medications associated with neurotoxicity. The typical clinical picture is encephalopathy accompanied by myoclonus and sometimes seizures arising within days of administration [10]. The occurrence of seizures attributed to cefepime and ceftazidime has been 1/10,000 and 3/1,000 patients, respectively. The lag time until diagnosis is longer with cefepime than ceftazidime (5 vs. 3 days) [11, 12]. Neurotoxic symptoms occur most often when the cephalosporin dose is not adjusted for renal function, but can still occur despite those modifications which are instituted at the cost of inducing treatment failure or resistance [13]. Therapeutic drug monitoring has been advocated, but any relationship between cephalosporin levels and the occurrence of neurotoxicity remains to be proven [13].

Clinical Pearls

1. If a peritonitis episode is preceded by another episode within 4 weeks of completion of treatment, it cannot be distinguished as a relapsing or recurrent episode without having culture results. In these episodes, vancomycin and ceftazidime are preferred empiric antibiotic treatment options. Post-empiric antibiotic therapy should be guided by in vitro susceptibility data.
2. Recurrent peritonitis may sometimes result from impaired patient immunity due to a prior peritonitis episode. Recent antibiotic therapy may also disturb the gastrointestinal flora and provoke transmural migration of bowel organisms to the peritoneal cavity. In the case of recurrent fungal peritonitis cases, an additional risk factor is the lack of antifungal chemoprophylaxis during the prior peritonitis episode.
3. Although an adult study concluded that recurrent peritonitis episodes had a worse prognosis than relapsing ones, a large adult multicenter registry demonstrated that mortality and hospitalization rates are not different from control cases. Similar data has not been published in pediatrics.
4. Familiarity with cephalosporin neurotoxicity in dialysis patients can improve the timely diagnosis of antibiotic-associated encephalopathy and prompt antibiotic discontinuation.

References

1. Warady BA, Bakkaloglu S, Newland J, Cantwell M, Verrina E, Neu A, Chadha V, Yap HK, Schaefer F. Consensus guidelines for the prevention and treatment of catheter-related infections and peritonitis in pediatric patients receiving peritoneal dialysis: 2012 update. Perit Dial Int. 2012;32(Suppl 2):S32–86.
2. Bakkaloglu SA, Warady BA. Difficult peritonitis cases in children undergoing chronic peritoneal dialysis: relapsing, repeat, recurrent and zoonotic episodes. Pediatr Nephrol. 2015; 30:1397–406.

3. Lane JC, Warady BA, Feneberg R, Majkowski NL, Watson AR, Fischbach M, Kang HG, Bonzel KE, Simkova E, Stefanidis CJ, Klaus G, Alexander SR, Ekim M, Bilge I, Schaefer F, International Pediatric Peritonitis Registry. Relapsing peritonitis in children who undergo chronic peritoneal dialysis: a prospective study of the international pediatric peritonitis registry. Clin J Am Soc Nephrol. 2010;5:1041–6.
4. Schaefer F, Feneberg R, Aksu N, Donmez O, Sadikoglu B, Alexander SR, Mir S, Ha IS, Fischbach M, Simkova E, Watson AR, Möller K, von Baum H, Warady BA. Worldwide variation of dialysis associated peritonitis in children. Kidney Int. 2007;72:1374–9.
5. Szeto CC, Kwan BC, Chow KM, Law MC, Pang WF, Leung CB, Li PK. Repeat peritontis in peritoneal dialysis: retrospective review of 181 consecutive cases. Clin J Am Soc Nephrol. 2011;6:827–33.
6. Szeto CC, Lai KB, Kwan BC, Chow KM, Leung CB, Law MC, Yu V, Li PK. Bacteria-derived DNA fragment in peritoneal dialysis effluent as a predictor of relapsing peritonitis. Clin J Am Soc Nephrol. 2013;8:1935–41.
7. Szeto CC, Kwan BC, Chow KM, Law MC, Pang WF, Chung KY, Leung CB, Li PK. Recurrent and relapsing peritonitis: causative organisms and response to treatment. Am J Kidney Dis. 2009;54:702–10.
8. Burke M, Hawley CM, Badve SV, McDonald SP, Brown FG, Boudville N, Wiggins KJ, Bannister KM, Johnson DW. Relapsing and recurrent peritoneal dialysis-associated peritonitis: a multicenter registry study. Am J Kidney Dis. 2011;58:429–36.
9. Li PK, Szeto CC, Piraino B, de Arteaga J, Fan S, Figueiredo AE, Fish DN, Goffin E, Kim YL, Salzer W, Struijk DG, Teitelbaum I, Johnson DW. ISPD peritonitis recommendations: 2016 update on prevention and treatment. Perit Dial Int 2016;9:481–508.
10. Bhattacharyya S, Darby RR, Raibagkar P, Gonzalez Castro LN, Berkowitz AL. Antibiotic associated encephalopathy. Neurology. 2016;86:963–71.
11. Neu HC. Safety of cefepime: a new extended-spectrum parenteral cephalosporin. Am J Med. 1996;100(Suppl 6A):S68–75.
12. Chow KM, Szeto CC, Hui AC, Wong TY, Li PK. Retrospective review of neurotoxicity induced by cefepime and ceftazidime. Pharmacotherapy. 2003;23:369–73.
13. Honore PM, Shapen HD. Cefepime-induced neurotoxicity in critically ill patients undergoing continuous renal replacement therapy: beware of dose reduction! Crit Care. 2015;19:455.

Chapter 10
Peritoneal Dialysis-Associated Hydrothorax and Hernia

Dagmara Borzych-Duzalka and Franz Schaefer

Case Presentation

Fatih was born after 36 weeks of gestation. Prenatally, enlarged hyperechogenic kidneys and oligohydramnios had been observed, and the diagnosis of autosomal recessive polycystic kidney disease (ARPKD) was postnatally confirmed by the typical sonographic appearance.

Within the first 4 months of life, kidney volume gradually increased to more than 1.5 L per kidney. Malignant hypertension, progressive renal failure, and increasing signs of intra-abdominal space consumption with vena cava compression and impossibility to pass food necessitated emergency nephrectomy, which was performed as a two-stage procedure within 2 weeks in the fifth month of life. Removal of the grossly enlarged kidneys reduced body weight from 8.2 to 4.9 kg. A Tenckhoff catheter was placed, and peritoneal dialysis (PD) was started. The fill volume was gradually increased from 50 to 200 ml, and the patient was discharged with well-functioning automated PD. His home APD prescription was nine cycles of 650 ml/m^2 body surface area fill volume.

Nine weeks after commencement of PD, Fatih presented with acute tachypnea and hypotension while on the cycler. Physical examination revealed attenuated breathing sounds and dullness on percussion over the right chest. Chest X-ray showed massive right-sided pleural effusion (Fig. 10.1). A subsequent contrast radiography with intraperitoneal instillation of contrast agent established the diagnosis of paraesophageal leakage into the pleural space (Fig. 10.2).

D. Borzych-Duzalka (✉)
Department of Pediatrics, Nephrology and Hypertension, Medical University of Gdansk, Gdansk, Poland
e-mail: dagab@gumed.edu.pl

F. Schaefer
Division of Pediatric Nephrology, Center for Pediatrics and Adolescent Medicine, University of Heidelberg, Heidelberg, Germany

© Springer International Publishing AG 2017
B.A. Warady et al. (eds.), *Pediatric Dialysis Case Studies*,
DOI 10.1007/978-3-319-55147-0_10

Fig. 10.1 Right-sided hydrothorax

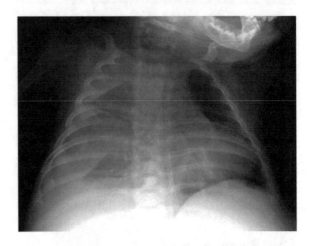

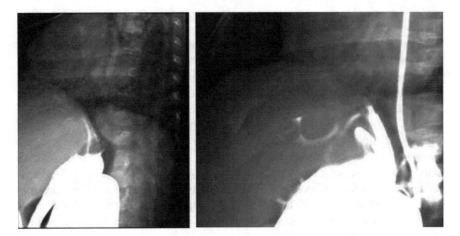

Fig. 10.2 Contrast peritoneography demonstrates peritoneopleural communication via a paraesophageal cleft

Thoracoscopy was performed, but intraperitoneal administration of methylene blue failed to detect the site of leakage. Hence, a conservative approach using dialysis with reduced fill volume was proposed. Peritoneal dialysis was resumed with 350 ml/m² fill volume. Two weeks later Fatih developed acute respiratory dysfunction while on the cycler. The diagnosis of relapsed hydrothorax was established, and the patient was admitted for open surgery. A 3 cm cleft was found in the right diaphragram, which was closed by double suture and a collagen patch. PD was resumed successfully. However, 2 weeks later when the fill volume was increased to 1,000 ml/m², Fatih developed bilateral inguinal hernias which required surgical repair.

Clinical Questions

1. What are the risk factors for developing hydrothorax and hernia?
2. How can hydrothorax and hernia be prevented?
3. What are typical symptoms of dialysis-related pleural effusion?
4. What are the diagnostic tools to confirm dialysis-associated hydrothorax?
5. What are the treatment options for a patient with pleuroperitoneal leak?

Diagnostic Discussion

1. Hydrothorax is an infrequent but potentially life-threatening complication of PD. The reported incidence is 1.6% in the adult and 2–10% in the pediatric PD population [1–4]. Hydrothorax occurs on the right side in 90% of cases. It may be caused by congenital or acquired defects of the diaphragm and manifest when a transdiaphragmatic pressure gradient builds up by instillation of peritoneal fluid. The effusion may develop shortly following PD initiation, suggesting a preexisting diaphragmatic defect, or present months to years after initiation of dialysis, commonly after physical exertion, suggesting an acquired defect in the diaphragm secondary to a sharp increase in intra-abdominal pressure. Infants and young children are predisposed to developing hernia and leakage due to their relatively thinner and more fragile peritoneal wall. Moreover, rapid increases in visceral fat mass due to enteral nutrition can lead to increased intraperitoneal pressure, increasing the risk of leakage and hernia [5–7]. The risk to develop hydrothorax appears to be increased in children with WT1 mutations (Denys-Drash and Frasier syndrome) and polycystic kidney disease (PKD). It has been speculated that since the WT1 gene plays an important role not only in kidney but also in diaphragm development, mutations in this gene might lead to dia-phragmatic defects with subsequent pleuroperitoneal leaks in dialyzed patients. In PKD intraperitoneal pressure is already high due to space consumption, mak-ing patients prone for leakage and hernia.

   The proposed explanations of the right-sided hydrothorax predominance include (i) more common tendinous defects on the right; (ii) ascending peristal-sis of the right colon, sweeping pelvic fluids into the right upper quadrant; (iii) high hydrostatic pressure in the pelvis and low in the suprahepatic region; and (iv) a piston-like action of the liver capture during diaphragm contraction, driv-ing fluid through the diaphragm pores [8].

2. According to the literature, the major factor in developing hydrothorax and her-nia is initiation of dialysis with high fill volumes or too rapidly increasing fill volumes from dialysis initiation. PD should be started with 10 ml/kg body weight for 5–7 days after catheter insertion with subsequent increase over 1 week to 1,000–1,100 ml/m^2 in children and 600–800 ml/m^2 in infants [5].

Repetitive measurements of intraperitoneal pressure may help to determine the optimal fill volume [5]. Intraperitoneal pressure should not exceed 8–10 cm H2O in infants and 12–14 cm H2O in older children [5]. Special attention is mandatory in children with organomegaly (e.g., ARPKD), WT1 mutation, obesity, or malnutrition, as these conditions increase the risk of hernia and leakage [5–7]. Among modifiable factors, constipation and abdominal pain increase the intraperitoneal pressure [7].

3. Clinical presentation may vary from an asymptomatic child to severe respiratory distress. Most children will present with cough, dyspnea, costal discomfort, chest pain and frequently with apparently inadequate ultrafiltration. Suspicion should arise in cases of dialysis-dependent respiratory symptoms, i.e., shortness of breath following dialysate infusion. Physical examination typically shows dullness on percussion and attenuated breathing signs over the affected lung.

4. The presence of a pleural effusion can be easily confirmed by radiography or sonography. However, these methods will not differentiate between dialysate leakage and a transudate caused by fluid overload, pneumonia, heart failure, or hypoalbuminemia, although one-sided appearance is highly suggestive of hydrothorax due to peritoneopleural leakage. The definitive diagnosis is established by demonstration of peritoneal fluid in the pleural space by at least one of the following procedures: (i) thoracocentesis with biochemical characteristics of dialysate (high glucose concentration), (ii) peritoneal contrast radiography, (iii) peritoneal contrast scintigraphy, (iv) peritoneal contrast MRI, or (v) contrast thoracoscopy [2].

While demonstrating high glucose concentration in the pleural space confirms the pleuroperitoneal leak, imaging studies (radiography, scintigraphy) and thoracoscopy additionally demonstrate the anatomy of the communication [2, 3]. Moreover, thoracocentesis is an invasive procedure with a potential risk of respiratory distress. In our patient contrast radiography confirmed the presence of leakage, while thoracoscopy with methylene *blue* infusion into the peritoneal cavity failed to detect the pleuroperitoneal communication.

5. The proposed treatment options depend on the severity of the symptoms and range from a conservative approach to surgical treatment. Conservative nonsurgical treatment includes (i) PD with small-volume exchanges, (ii) temporary PD cessation, or (iii) chemical pleurodesis (pleural instillation through a thoracic drain of sclerosing agents such as tetracycline, talcum powder, fibrin glue, or autologous blood) [2, 3].

The concept of temporary PD cessation or small-volume exchanges is based on the speculation that a temporary PD cessation will allow the diaphragmatic defect to heal and make resumption of regular PD feasible. Temporary PD interruption was successful in 53% of cases in ten studies including a total of 104 patients [9]. Surgical approaches range from minimally invasive video-assisted thoracoscopy to thoracotomy and is mainly indicated in patients who failed conservative management or in cases of relapsing hydrothorax [2, 3].

Clinical Pearls

1. Dialysis-associated hydrothorax is an infrequent but important complication of peritoneal dialysis and should be excluded in every patient with respiratory symptoms following PD fluid inflow and in all patients with unilateral pleural effusion.
2. Obese or malnourished patients, as well as those with organomegaly or WT1 mutation, are at increased risk of hernia and hydrothorax. PD initiation with low fill volumes, repetitive intraperitoneal pressure measurements, and constipation prophylaxis might help to prevent developing hernia, leakage, and pleural effusion.
3. Diagnosis of dialysis-related hydrothorax should be based on contrast imaging studies (scintigraphy, radiography), which are aimed to demonstrate pleuroperitoneal communication.
4. Temporary PD cessation or low fill-volume dialysis is the therapeutic option of first choice. In case of relapsing hydrothorax, surgical intervention should be considered.

References

1. Nomoto Y, Suga T, Nakajima K, Sakai H, Osawa G, Ota K, et al. Acute hydrothorax in continuous ambulatory peritoneal dialysis—a collaborative study of 161 centers. Am J Nephrol. 1989;9:363–7.
2. Szeto CC, Chow KM. Pathogenesis and management of hydrothorax complicating peritoneal dialysis. Curr Opin Pulm Med. 2004;10:315–9.
3. Chow CC, Sung JY, Cheung CK, Hamilton-Wood C, Lai KN. Massive hydrothorax in continuous ambulatory peritoneal dialysis: diagnosis, management and review of the literature. N Z Med J. 1988;101:475–7.
4. Kawaguchi AL, Dunn JC, Fonkalsrud EW. Management of peritoneal dialysis-induced hydrothorax in children. Am Surg. 1996;62:820–4.
5. Schmitt CP, Zaloszyc A, Schaefer B, Fischbach M. Peritoneal dialysis tailored to pediatric needs. Int J Nephro. 2011;2011:940267.
6. Fischbach M, Terzic J, Provot E. Itraperitoneal pressure in children: fill volume related ansd impacted by body mass index. PDI. 2003;23:391–4.
7. Fischbach M, Terzic J, Laugel V, Escande B, Dangelser C, Helmstetter A. Measurement of hydrostatic intraperitoneal pressure: a useful tool for the improvement of dialysis dose prescription. Pediatr Nephrol. 2003;18:976–80.
8. Guest S. The curious right-sided predominance dialysis-related hydrothorax. Clin Kidney J. 2015;8:212–4.
9. Chow KM, Szeto CC, Li PK. Management options for hydrothorax complicating peritoneal dialysis. Semin Dial. 2003;16:389–94.

Chapter 11
Ultrafiltration Failure in Children Undergoing Chronic PD

Franz Schaefer

Case Presentations

Case 1

Debbie developed steroid-resistant nephrotic syndrome at age 3 years. Kidney biopsy showed focal segmental glomerulosclerosis, and genetic screening revealed podocin nephropathy. While edema was reasonably well controlled with ACE inhibitor and diuretic therapy, the glomerulopathy gradually progressed to end-stage kidney disease, and peritoneal dialysis was started at age 5 years. The initial PD prescription was six cycles of 1,000 ml/m² body surface area 1.5% dextrose PD fluid dialysate with a dwell time of 90 min. A peritoneal equilibration test (PET) demonstrated a high-average transporter status. After 4 years of uneventful PD, Debbie developed peritonitis with *pseudomonas aeruginosa*, which was cultured both from the dialysis effluent and the catheter exit site. The infection was initially cleared following treatment with intraperitoneal antibiotic therapy with ceftazidime which was administered for 3 weeks, but peritonitis recurred within 1 week after discontinuation of antibiotic treatment. Antibiotic therapy was resumed and continued for another 4 weeks. At the end of this period, Debbie complained of recurrent abdominal pain and intermittently cloudy effluent. Effluent cultures were positive for *Candida albicans*. The PD catheter was explanted, intermittent hemodialysis was performed, and antifungal therapy was administered intravenously for 2 weeks. Thereafter, a new Tenckhoff catheter was placed and PD was resumed. The antifungal medication was discontinued 2 weeks later. During the subsequent 3 months, the patient's mother complained about frequent cycler alarms, decreased daily ultrafiltration, and a tendency for Debbie's blood pressure to be elevated.

F. Schaefer (✉)
Division of Pediatric Nephrology, Center for Pediatrics and Adolescent Medicine,
University of Heidelberg, Heidelberg, Germany
e-mail: Franz.Schaefer@med.uni-heidelberg.de

© Springer International Publishing AG 2017
B.A. Warady et al. (eds.), *Pediatric Dialysis Case Studies*,
DOI 10.1007/978-3-319-55147-0_11

Case 2

Tom, a 14-year-old boy, developed ESRD within 12 months of diagnosis with IgA glomerulonephritis due to a rapidly progressive course despite aggressive immunosuppressive therapy. Tom was obese due to extended high-dose glucocorticoid therapy. A Tenckhoff catheter was inserted laparoscopically, and PD was initiated electively after 7 days. After establishing the final APD prescription of 6*1,000 ml/m^2 with a good ultrafiltration rate and completion of PD training, Tom was discharged. After 2 weeks of home PD, the family reported that Tom had experienced excessive weight gain and poor ultrafiltration.

Clinical Questions

1. What is the definition and clinical significance of ultrafiltration failure in children undergoing chronic PD?
2. What is the most likely reason for ultrafiltration failure in Case 1?
3. What is the most likely reason for ultrafiltration failure in Case 2?
4. Which diagnostic procedures should be performed to explore the causes of ultrafiltration failure in both cases?
5. Which therapeutic options are available in cases of ultrafiltration failure in pediatric PD patients?

Diagnostic Discussion

1. Ultrafiltration failure (UFF) is a major cause of PD technique failure in children, second only to persistent PD associated infection [1]. In adults, UFF is defined as net ultrafiltration of less than 400 mL in 4 h on a 3.86% glucose-based dialysis solution [2]. An equivalent definition for children is given by less than 150 ml net ultrafiltration per m^2 body surface area achieved during a standard peritoneal equilibration test with 2.3% glucose-based solution. UFF usually develops gradually after 4–5 years of peritoneal dialysis [3]. Failure to produce convective ultrafiltration leads to salt and fluid overload, contributing substantially to the high prevalence of cardiovascular comorbidity in children undergoing chronic PD.
2. The two most common pathophysiological mechanisms of UFF are *membrane failure* due to long-standing exposure to PD fluid and *sequestration of PD fluid* due to intra-abdominal adhesions.

   The former phenomenon is due to a largely inevitable local inflammatory process caused mainly by exposure of the peritoneal tissue to glucose and toxic glucose degradation products (GDP) [4]. GDP are formed during heat sterilization and stimulate the local release of cytokines and growth factors such as VEGF and TGF-ß, which cause neoangiogenesis (capillary formation) and fibrosis (scar formation). "Biocompatible" PD fluids have a much reduced GDP content and show reduced tissue toxicity in experimental PD models [5]. However, they still contain glucose which per se can induce inflammatory tissue processes if administered at supraphysiological concentrations.

The formation of intraperitoneal adhesions is markedly accelerated in the case of microbial intraperitoneal infections [6]. This was likely the case in Case 1, who suffered from several episodes of bacterial and fungal peritonitis.

3. In Case 2, UFF has developed soon after implementation of PD. Membrane failure is unlikely at this early stage. UFF in this setting is more likely to be caused by a *mechanical problem*. The most common causes of mechanical dysfunction are wrapping of the catheter by omentum and catheter mislocation causing outflow obstruction and incomplete drainage. In rare cases, rupture of the peritoneal tissue layer can cause leakage into the extraperitoneal space [7].

4. The primary diagnostic procedure of choice to explore the underlying cause of UFF is the *peritoneal equilibration test* (PET) [8, 9]. For this test, the abdominal cavity is filled with 1,000–1,100 ml/m^2 2.3–2.4% PD fluid. Effluent samples are obtained after 5, 30, 60, and 120 min, and the fluid is fully drained after 4 h. A blood sample is obtained after 2 h. The peritoneal transport characteristics are assessed by determining (a) the 4-h dialysate to plasma ratio (D/P) of creatinine and (b) the ratio of effluent glucose concentration at 4 h vs. the initial concentration (D/D$_0$). The patient's peritoneal transporter status is labeled as high, high average, low average, and low if the 4-h D/P creatinine is >1 SD above, within 1 SD above, within 1 SD below, and >1 SD below the reference population, respectively. Pediatric reference values have been established in large cohorts of children undergoing chronic PD. In addition to the transporter status, the ultrafiltration volume achieved within 4 h is recorded.

The interpretation of the PET results as it pertains to UF volume is summarized in Fig. 11.1a. If adequate ultrafiltration is unexpectedly observed in the patient presumed to be experiencing UFF, and a technical issue with the PET (such as incomplete drainage prior to fill) is excluded, UFF may not actually be the cause of fluid overload. In these cases uncontrolled fluid intake or *noncompliance* with the PD prescription should be suspected.

On the other hand, poor ultrafiltration (i.e., less than 150 ml/m^2 body surface area) and the finding of a high transporter status may point to *membrane failure* (with rapid breakdown of the osmotic gradient due to increased capillarization of the peritoneal membrane) and/or *sequestration of PD fluid*. In the latter case, intra-abdominal adhesions lead to a reduced peritoneal surface area available for solute exchange. In addition, poor effluent drainage causes an increased residual dialysate volume. Mixture of the PET fill volume with a large residual volume of high creatinine and low glucose content will result in steep equilibration curves during the PET (Fig. 11.1b). The rapid solute equilibration in this condition is sometimes called "pseudo-high transporter state" since the solute exchange rate per unit of peritoneal exchange surface area may actually not be altered.

In Case 1, the PET disclosed a high transporter status with accelerated solute equilibration, pointing to membrane failure combined with extensive intra-abdominal adhesions as a consequence of long-standing PD fluid exposure and repeated severe peritonitis episodes.

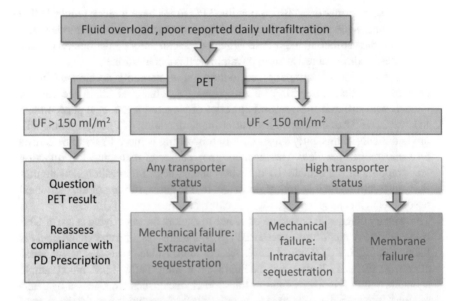

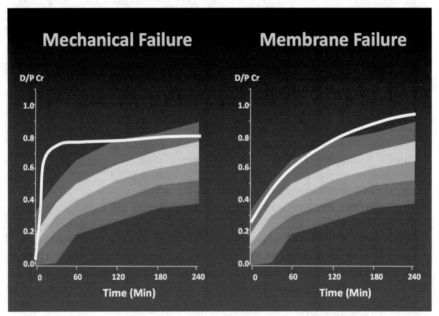

Fig. 11.1 Use of PET in patients with ultrafiltration failure. (**a**) Interpretation of PET results in patients with suspected ultrafiltration failure. (**b**) Solute equilibration curves in patients with ultrafiltration failure

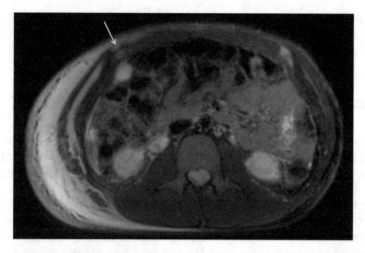

Fig. 11.2 Subcutaneous accumulation of PD fluid in Case 2. MRI was obtained after drainage of PD fluid. *Arrow* indicates site of leakage

   Low ultrafiltration in the presence of a normal transporter status may point to the rare condition of *extracavital sequestration* due to peritoneal disruption and internal leakage into the subcutaneous tissue or thoracic cavity. This was the actual cause of UFF in Case 2, who had developed a dialysate leak at the site of the instrumentation channel punched during the laparoscopic procedure for PD catheter placement. The leak was identified by a T2-weighted MRI examination without contrast agent, which revealed extensive subcutaneous fluid accumulation (Fig. 11.2). Other causes of UFF related to poor drainage include outflow obstruction due to catheter malpositioning or catheter wrapping, usually with omental tissue. Diagnostic measures to assess these mechanical causes are anterio-posterior and lateral abdominal X-ray imaging and laparoscopic inspection.

5. Early mechanical outflow obstruction can usually be corrected by surgical intervention. Late obstruction by intra-abdominal adhesions due to infection or preceding intraperitoneal surgery may be amenable to surgical adhesiolysis, but the rate of recurrence due to formation of new adhesions is high.

   UFF due to membrane failure is approached by modification of the PD prescription. Automated PD with short dwell times and use of higher PD solution dextrose concentrations will temporarily increase ultrafiltration. However, these measures are usually offset by an accelerated transformation of the peritoneal membrane due to increased glucose exposure. An alternative approach is the use of long dwells with icodextrin containing PD fluid. Icodextrin is an oligosaccharide mixture that induces slow but sustained ultrafiltration. However, the additional ultrafiltration volume obtained by a single icodextrin daytime dwell in an APD patient is small and usually insufficient to compensate for UF loss in patients with membrane failure.

It remains to be seen whether the use of biocompatible PD fluids with reduced GDP content is an effective preventative measure to attenuate membrane transformation and extend the functional integrity of the peritoneal membrane.

Clinical Pearls

1. Membrane failure usually develops after more than 5 years of PD due to chronic toxicity of PD fluid glucose and glucose degradation products which lead to hypercapillarization of the peritoneal tissue. Membrane failure is a common cause of late PD technique failure.
2. Mechanical PD failure can occur at any time in the course of PD therapy. While peritoneal disruption, catheter malpositioning, and omental obstruction typically occur soon after the start of PD, fluid sequestration due to intra-abdominal adhesions is a late complication related to repeated intraperitoneal infections.
3. The peritoneal equilibration test (with ultrafiltration assessment) is a useful tool to identify the cause and examine the extent of ultrafiltration failure. A high transporter status indicates membrane failure and/or reduced effective peritoneal surface area.
4. MRI can be useful in the detection of peritoneal rupture as a cause of ultrafiltration failure.
5. It remains to be shown whether the use of biocompatible PD fluids with reduced glucose degradation product content will attenuate the long-term risk of peritoneal membrane failure by minimizing peritoneal inflammation and neoangiogenesis.

References

1. Warady BA, Am N, Schaefer F. Optimal care of the infant, child, and adolescent on dialysis: 2014 update. Am J Kidney Dis. 2014;64:128–42.
2. Krediet RT. Ultrafiltration failure. In:Nolph and Gokal's textbook of peritoneal dialysis. 3rd ed. New York: Springer; 2009. p. 803–61.
3. Honda M, Warady BA. Long-term peritoneal dialysis and encapsulating peritoneal sclerosis in children. Pediatr Nephrol. 2010;25:75–81.
4. Saxena R. Pathogenesis and treatment of peritoneal membrane failure. Pediatr Nephrol. 2008;23:695–703.
5. Schmitt CP, Nau B, Gemulla G, Bonzel KE, Hölttä T, Testa S, Fischbach M, John U, Kemper MJ, Sander A, Arbeiter K, Schaefer F. Effect of the dialysis fluid buffer on peritoneal membrane function in children. Clin J Am Soc Nephrol. 2013;8:108–15.
6. Warady BA, Feneberg R, Verrina E, et al. Peritonitis in children who receive long-term peritoneal dialysis: a prospective evaluation of therapeutic guidelines. J Am Soc Nephrol. 2007;18:2172–9.
7. Arbeiter KM, Aufricht C, Mueller T, Balzar E, Prokesch RW. MRI in the diagnosis of a peritoneal leak in continuous ambulatory peritoneal dialysis. Pediatr Radiol. 2001;31:745–7.
8. Schaefer F, Langenbeck D, Heckert KH, Schärer K, Mehls O. Evaluation of peritoneal solute transfer by the peritoneal equilibration test in children. Adv Perit Dial. 1992;8:410–5.
9. Warady BA, Alexander SR, Hossli S, Vonesh E, Geary D, Watkins S, Salusky IB, Kohaut EC. Peritoneal membrane transport function in children receiving long-term dialysis. J Am Soc Nephrol. 1996;7:2385–91.

Chapter 12
Encapsulating Peritoneal Sclerosis

Hiroshi Hataya and Masataka Honda

Case Presentation

A 16-year-old boy was admitted with peritonitis. Several symptoms including diarrhea, abdominal distention, weakly positive C-reactive protein, and hemorrhagic effluent had been present for a few months prior to this admission.

Review of past medical history revealed that he developed anuria suddenly from an indeterminate cause at 5 years old and had been on peritoneal dialysis (PD) for 11 years due to the unavailability of a transplant donor. He suffered bacterial peritonitis several times with the last peritoneal equilibration test (PET) consistent with high peritoneal membrane transporter status (dialysate/plasma of creatinine was 0.96 and dialysate at 4 h/dialysate at 0 h of glucose 0.15).

On this admission the cell count in the dialysate was $750/mm^3$, and the culture revealed that the causative agent was coagulase-negative *Staphylococcus*. The patient also had erythropoietin-resistant anemia and a low level of albumin (2.1 g/dL). Plain radiography showed a dilated small bowel and calcification of the peritoneum (Fig 12.1). Computed tomography (CT) revealed peritoneal thickening, dilated small bowel loops, and loculated ascites (Fig 12.2). On the basis of these findings, encapsulating peritoneal sclerosis (EPS) was diagnosed, PD was discontinued, and hemodialysis (HD) was immediately started. Prednisolone 1 mg/kg/day was also administered for 1 month and then tapered every month for 6 months. One month after prednisolone administration ended, the patient experienced a recurrence of fever, abdominal pain, diarrhea, and vomiting. EPS was again diagnosed. Prednisolone 0.75 mg/kg/day was administered and tapered slowly over a period of 1 year.

H. Hataya (✉) • M. Honda
Department of Nephrology, Tokyo Metropolitan Children's Medical Center, Tokyo, Japan
e-mail: hiroshi_hataya@tmhp.jp

© Springer International Publishing AG 2017
B.A. Warady et al. (eds.), *Pediatric Dialysis Case Studies*,
DOI 10.1007/978-3-319-55147-0_12

Fig. 12.1 Plain
radiography demonstrating
a dilated small bowel and
calcifications of
peritoneum

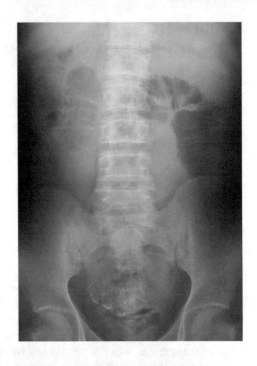

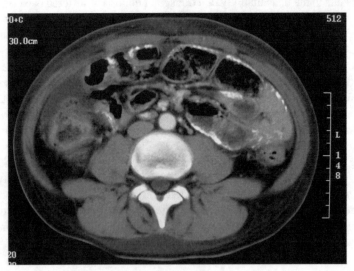

Fig. 12.2 CT demonstrating peritoneal thickening, dilated small bowel loops, and loculated
ascites

Clinical Questions

1. What is EPS and how is it diagnosed?
2. What are the risk factors for EPS?
3. What is the prognosis of EPS?
4. What are the treatment options?

Diagnostic Discussion

1. EPS is an uncommon but well-known, extremely serious, complication of long-term PD. The diagnostic criteria for EPS are based on a combination of clinical symptoms of bowel obstruction and radiological findings of features of encapsulating peritoneal fibrosis [1]. The International Society of Peritoneal Dialysis (ISPD) defines the condition as "a clinical syndrome continuously, intermittently or repeatedly presenting with symptoms of intestinal obstruction due to adhesions of a diffusely thickened peritoneum." The intestinal obstruction is partial or diffuse and is accompanied by marked sclerotic thickening of the peritoneal membrane, which exhibits cocoon-like encapsulation of the entire intestine (cocooning).

   Symptoms of bowel obstruction vary and may include vomiting, abdominal distension, abdominal pain, diarrhea or constipation, and complete intestinal obstruction. The other clinical features that may be encountered include weight loss, low-grade fever, hemorrhagic effluent, and ascites. In many patients, UF failure precedes the clinical symptoms. However, even patients with only peritoneal sclerosis experience ultrafiltration failure, making it difficult in practice to differentiate EPS from peritoneal sclerosis by ultrafiltration failure.

   A plain abdominal radiograph can reveal the bowel obstruction and peritoneal calcification. Ultrasound can detect bowel wall thickening, dilatation, and intestinal obstruction noninvasively, therefore allowing repeated examination. The CT scan can visualize signs of bowel obstruction, tethering, peritoneal calcification, and loculated ascites objectively and is recommended as the first-line modality in diagnosis due to the reproducibility of the measures obtained using this method. However, as EPS may develop within a year of a normal CT scan, this modality is not recommended when screening for EPS in asymptomatic PD patients.

   The prevalence of EPS is reportedly 1.5% to 2.0% or 8.7 per 1,000 patient-years according to three pediatric PD registries [2–4]. EPS may occur after conversion from PD to HD and transplantation.

2. The pathophysiology of EPS is mainly unknown, but several factors have been suggested as contributing to its development. The most important risk factor is long-term PD. The incidence of EPS has a strong linear association with PD duration. A Japanese registry reported its incidence as 6.6%, 12%, and 22% among children on PD longer than 5, 8, and 10 years, respectively [2]. Moreover, the median duration of PD use among those who developed EPS was 5.9 (1.6–10.2)

years, but was only 1.7 (0.7–7.7) years among those who did not develop EPS, according to a European registry [3]. The duration of PD is the key risk factor; however, not all long-term PD patients develop EPS.

The "two-hit theory" was proposed to explain the mechanism of EPS development. The first "hit" is peritoneal deterioration induced by bio-incompatible PD solutions (e.g., hyperosmolar glucose, glucose degradation products, and acid solutions) during long-term PD. The second "hit" is inflammation such as severe or recurrent peritonitis caused by bacteria or fungi. The incidence of peritonitis was higher among patients with EPS compared to those without EPS in the European EPS registry, but was nearly the same for EPS and non-EPS patients in the Japanese and Italian registries. Single episodes of severe peritonitis, however, may progress to EPS.

Recently developed biocompatible peritoneal dialysis solutions may reduce peritoneal deterioration, EPS risk, and even the severity of EPS.

3. The mortality rate is reportedly very high, ranging from 30–60% among adults. Two studies based on data from pediatric registries demonstrated a mortality rate of 30%, but a European study reported a rate of only 14% with two out of three deaths not being the result of EPS-related complications. Of the three patient registries examined, only the European registry, which showed that all patients recovered from their bowel condition, demonstrated a low mortality rate in contrast to the Italian and Japanese registries. The reasons for this discrepancy are unclear, and there is as yet little information about either adult or pediatric survivors of EPS.

4. PD should be discontinued following a diagnosis of EPS. Medical therapy at the early stages of EPS and surgical intervention at the more advanced stages are recommended. At any stage, appropriate nutritional support is essential, with parenteral nutrition being recommended for severe patients [5, 6].

Corticosteroid is the most commonly used anti-inflammatory agent, but the evidence supporting its use is still limited. Prednisolone 0.5–1.0 mg/kg/day may be administered for 1 month and then tapered and continued for at least 1 year. Combining immunosuppressants including azathioprine, cyclosporine, mycophenolate mofetil, and sirolimus with a corticosteroid is reportedly more efficacious than steroids alone.

Aside from immunosuppressants, two other drugs which may prevent peritoneal fibrosis have been reported. The first, tamoxifen, a selective estrogen receptor modulator, has been used to treat several fibrotic diseases, including retroperitoneal fibrosis. Therefore, tamoxifen may be administered to the patients with either progressive or nonprogressive EPS. The starting dose of 10–40 mg/day may be administered and continued for at least 1 year if there is clinical improvement. While several uncontrolled studies have demonstrated tamoxifen's effectiveness in combination with immunosuppressants, the evidence supporting this treatment is still inconclusive.

A second pharmacologic approach is the use of a group of renin-angiotensin-aldosterone system (RAAS) inhibitors (e.g., angiotensin converting enzyme inhibitors and angiotensin receptor blockers). The RAAS has been implicated in the pathophysiology of many harmful responses to noxious stimuli, including inflammation and fibrosis. Hence the rationale for the use of RAAS inhibitors against EPS is clear. Although the effectiveness of RAAS inhibitors against peritoneal fibrosis is poor, these agents provide another viable medical option in the treatment of PD patients who develop EPS.

Surgical treatment may enable effective removal of peritoneal adhesions without the need for an enterectomy. When performed by experienced surgical teams, surgery can result in symptom improvement and survival. The recurrence rate for EPS is about 20% after surgery [1].

Clinical Pearls

1. EPS is fatal in severe cases with intestinal obstruction. Physicians should be on the alert for EPS in its early stages based on the findings of the clinical symptoms and ultrafiltration failure.
2. The majority of long-term PD patients do not develop EPS. However, particular attention should be paid to patients who have experienced long-term PD treatment with ultrafiltration failure.
3. The mortality rate among pediatric patients may be lower than among adults. Nonetheless, EPS is a serious complication that forces patients to discontinue PD and can result in death.
4. There is no clear evidence supporting any drug intervention for EPS. Prednisolone is commonly used and may be effective in the early, inflammatory stage of EPS. Tamoxifen may contribute to preventing peritoneal fibrosis even in patients with established (nonprogressive form of) EPS.

References

1. Kawaguchi Y, Kawanishi H, Mujais S, Topley N, Oreopoulos DG. Encapsulating peritoneal sclerosis: definition, etiology, diagnosis, and treatment. International Society for Peritoneal Dialysis Ad Hoc Committee on ultrafiltration management in peritoneal dialysis. Perit Dial Int. 2000;20(Suppl 4):S43–55.
2. Hoshii S, Honda M. High incidence of encapsulating peritoneal sclerosis in pediatric patients on peritoneal dialysis longer than 10 years. Perit Dial Int. 2002;22(6):730–1.
3. Shroff R, Stefanidis CJ, Askiti V. For European paediatric dialysis working group, et al. encapsulating peritoneal sclerosis in children on chronic PD: a survey from the European paediatric dialysis working group. Nephrol Dial Transplant. 2013;28(7):1908–14.
4. Vidal E, Edefonti A, Puteo F. For Italian registry of pediatric chronic dialysis, et al. encapsulating peritoneal sclerosis in paediatric peritoneal dialysis patients: the experience of the Italian registry of pediatric chronic dialysis. Nephrol Dial Transplant. 2013;28(6):1603–9.
5. Honda M, Warady BA. Long-term peritoneal dialysis and encapsulating peritoneal sclerosis in children. Pediatr Nephrol. 2010;25(1):75–81.
6. Stefanidis CJ, Shroff R. Encapsulating peritoneal sclerosis in children. Pediatr Nephrol. 2014;29(11):2093–103.

Chapter 13
Difficult Vascular Access

Mary L. Brandt, Joseph L. Mills, and Sarah J. Swartz

Case Presentation

An 8-year-old boy presents to nephrology clinic complaining of headaches and weakness. He was diagnosed prenatally with urinary obstruction and underwent a prenatal vesiculo-aminotic shunt at 20 weeks gestation. At the time of birth, he had no urinary output. The intraperitoneal vesiculo-amniotic shunt was removed and a peritoneal dialysis catheter placed on day 2 of life.

The peritoneal dialysis catheter was removed at 2 months of age due to florid Candida peritonitis. He had a right internal jugular (RIJ) 7Fr hemodialysis (HD) catheter placed, which allowed him to be successfully dialyzed. He had multiple attempts to place a peritoneal dialysis catheter, all of which were unsuccessful due to multiple adhesions and a poorly functioning peritoneal membrane. He had placement of a 5Fr left subclavian catheter for TPN and medications during a 2-week ICU stay at age 2 for treatment of pneumonia with sepsis. He had an attempted right upper arm arteriovenous fistula (AVF) at age 4 at a different institution, which reportedly failed due to superior vena cava stenosis. He underwent successful renal transplantation at age 5, with anastomosis of the allograft renal artery to the aorta and the renal vein to the IVC. The family was lost to follow-up for the last year. He presents now with hypertension and GFR 15 ml/min/1.73m^2, BUN 80 mg/dl, and serum creatinine 3.0 mg/dl.

M.L. Brandt, MD (✉)
Division of Pediatric Surgery, Michael E. DeBakey Department of Surgery,
Baylor College of Medicine, Houston, TX, USA
e-mail: mary.brandt@bcm.edu; mlbrandt@texaschildrens.org

J.L. Mills, MD
Division of Vascular Surgery, Michael E. DeBakey Department of Surgery,
Baylor College of Medicine, Houston, TX, USA

S.J. Swartz, MD
Department of Pediatrics, Baylor College of Medicine, Houston, TX, USA

© Springer International Publishing AG 2017
B.A. Warady et al. (eds.), *Pediatric Dialysis Case Studies*,
DOI 10.1007/978-3-319-55147-0_13

95

Clinical Questions

1. What evaluation of the venous system should be done before placing a hemodialysis catheter or creating an arteriovenous fistula (AVF)?
2. Is it possible to place HD catheters or create an AV fistula in the setting of venous stenosis?
3. Should dialysis catheters be placed in the femoral vein in a patient who is being evaluated for transplant?
4. How small is too small to place an arteriovenous fistula for hemodialysis?
5. What are the "last ditch" approaches that can be used for hemodialysis in children?

Diagnostic Discussion

1. Imaging of the venous system is imperative prior to placing catheters or creating vascular access for hemodialysis [1]. Not only does imaging help identify the anatomy to plan the access, but it also prevents failure of the access from an unrecognized venous stenosis. For the upper extremity, neck, and groin, Doppler ultrasound can successfully "map" the arterial and venous systems to assess for candidate vessels for AVF creation and will usually identify issues that could affect inflow and/or outflow. For the central veins, the modality of choice is MRI/MRV without contrast or CT angiography. Because of concerns about radiation and, more importantly, the need for contrast, most pediatric renal patients undergo MRI/MRV without gadolinium to assess central venous anatomy. A history of previous subclavian catheters is associated with a markedly increased risk of subclavian stenosis. In adults, a subclavian catheter placed for TPN or chemotherapy for 2–6 weeks will result in a stenosis in approximately 30% of patients. There are no good data in children, but based on these reports, any history of prior central access – for any reason – or history of multiple prior vascular access attempts should lead to MRI/MRV evaluation of the central venous system [6]. Venography, which was previously the "gold standard," has been supplanted by MRI/MRV for children, because it is less invasive and does not expose the child to radiation or contrast. However, in select cases, venography may be the procedure of choice since anesthesia may not be needed and the duration of the procedure is shorter than an MRI/MRV.
2. Pediatric surgeons have previously been primarily responsible for obtaining access for dialysis in children. Vascular surgeons and/or interventional radiologists are now an integral part of any pediatric dialysis access team due to the rapid growth of new technologies for imaging and intervention [1, 2]. Venous stenoses can be successfully treated by percutaneous balloon angioplasty and/or stenting in a majority of patients [8]. Stenting, which is very common in adults, is rarely used in children to avoid a fixed diameter in a growing vessel but may be necessary in selected cases (Figs. 13.1 and 13.2). Options for management of complex vascular issues however continue to evolve as biodegradable stents of appropriate size are developed and approved.

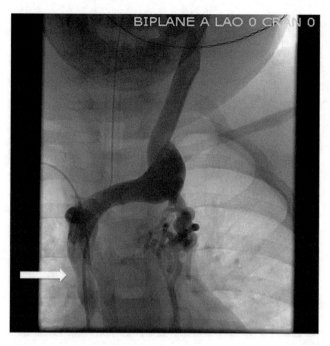

Fig. 13.1 Superior vena cavogram demonstrates severe stenosis and poor contrast opacification (*white arrow*) due to catheter-related stenosis. Residual lumen was only 2 mm by intravascular ultrasound (Courtesy of Dr. Henri Justino MD, CM, FRCPC, FACC, FSCAI, FAAP, Director, CE Mullins Cardiac Catheterization Laboratories, Texas Children's Hospital, Associate Professor of Pediatrics, Baylor College of Medicine)

3. Accessing any vein carries a risk of possible stenosis and/or occlusion. The vein that is least likely to develop clinically relevant stenosis and/or occlusion when accessed is the right internal jugular vein [5]. Although there is a slightly increased risk of central venous stenosis with use of the left internal jugular vein, it is probably the best second choice. When the internal jugular veins are not available, the debate is usually between accessing the subclavian vs. femoral veins. When considering the use of these veins for hemodialysis access, the trade-off is potential injury to, or thrombosis of, the femoral vein vs. sacrificing future permanent dialysis access options by using a subclavian vein. Femoral HD catheters are placed in the vein well proximal to the site of the venous anastomosis for a kidney transplant. Therefore, even if a stenosis develops at the site of insertion, it theoretically should not affect the outflow from the kidney. However, the catheter tip of a femoral HD catheter is positioned in the iliac vein, which can lead to endothelial damage and potential thrombosis. The relative risks and benefits of these potential sites need to be discussed by the multidisciplinary team of the nephrologists, access surgeons, and transplant surgeons caring for the child to make the best possible decision [1, 2]. In the setting of a previous transplant, it is usually wise to place the access on the side of the transplant, rather than risking the contralateral unused side.

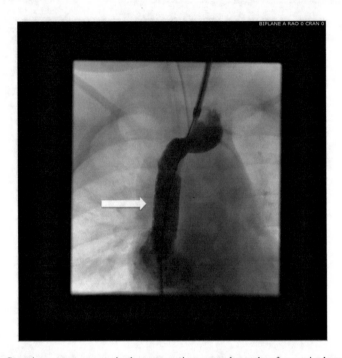

Fig. 13.2 Superior vena cavogram in the same patient several months after angioplasty and SVC stent placement (*white arrow*), demonstrating wide patency and no recurrent stenosis (Courtesy of Dr. Henri Justino MD, CM, FRCPC, FACC, FSCAI, FAAP, Director, CE Mullins Cardiac Catheterization Laboratories, Texas Children's Hospital, Associate Professor of Pediatrics, Baylor College of Medicine)

4. Small infants, even newborns, can be successfully dialyzed using hemodialysis, although this is not typically the modality of choice [7]. Hemodialysis requires placement of a catheter that is proportionally very large, which increases the risks at the time of operative placement and often results in permanent loss of the vein. AVF creation is not possible in infants and small children because of small vessel diameter and lower pressures [4, 5]. Although there are reports of successful AVF creation in children as small as 10 kg, for most vascular (or in this case, microvascular) surgeons, 20 kg is the lowest body weight at which an AVF should be considered. For all children being considered for AVF, vein mapping with ultrasound, MRV, or (rarely) venography is needed to demonstrate an adequate venous diameter and lack of any central occlusion prior to attempting AVF creation [2, 3].
5. "Last ditch" access for hemodialysis includes translumbar or transhepatic access to the inferior vena cava and access into extremely dilated collateral veins including the azygous vein. Surgical implantation of catheters directly into the superior or inferior vena cava has also been reported. In adults and more recently in pediatric patients, endoluminal recanalization and balloon angioplasty have been used to reopen chronically occluded central veins [8]. Reports of surgically bypassing a chronically occluded vein to provide additional sites for access also

exist. Autologous arteriovenous access by a femoral transposition, as described by Gradman et al., can also be considered [3].

For patients who previously failed peritoneal dialysis, diagnostic laparoscopy to evaluate the peritoneum can also be considered.

Patients with difficult access require a multidisciplinary vascular team approach with input from the pediatric nephrologist, pediatric surgeon, vascular surgeon, and interventional radiologist [1, 2].

Clinical Pearls

1. Ultrasound guided access is now standard of care for placing hemodialysis catheters. Venous access with guidance minimizes the required numbers of punctures and therefore decreases the risk of injury to the vein. For children with renal disease, their veins are truly their lifelines. Therefore, all efforts should be taken to protect the veins of these children. For example, no IV should be placed in the cephalic vein – ever – of any child with renal disease, as this is a critically important vein for the creation of arteriovenous fistulae. "Temporary" subclavian lines and PICC lines in the upper extremity should be avoided at all cost! Venous access in children with renal disease should only be undertaken, or at least supervised, by pediatric vascular access specialists and physicians with expertise and experience.

2. By far the most effective method of dealing with a venous stenosis is to prevent it. For that reason, children with renal disease should never have subclavian catheters – for any reason! For children who are not candidates for preemptive or early transplantation and are expected to require prolonged hemodialysis (longer than 1 year), early referral for AVF evaluation and creation may prevent the need for catheter placement and also help protect veins for future dialysis needs. Hence early and frequent chronic kidney disease education with discussion of renal replacement modality options is paramount and essential to reinforce this concept and achieve family assistance with preservation of vascular access [5, 9].

3. Since it is next to impossible to train all hospital personnel, the family should be taught to protect all veins in the nondominant extremity and both subclavian veins.

References

1. Baracco R, Mattoo T, Jain A, Kapur G, Valentini RP. Reducing central venous catheters in chronic hemodialysis – a commitment to arteriovenous fistula creation in children. Pediatr Nephrol. 2014;29(10):2013–20.
2. Chand DH, Geary D, Patel H, Greenbaum LA, Nailescu C, Brier ME, Valentini RP. Barriers, biases, and beliefs about arteriovenous fistula placement in children: a survey of the International Pediatric Fistula First Initiative (IPFFI) within the Midwest Pediatric Nephrology Consortium (MWPNC). Hemodial Int. 2015 Jan;19(1):100–7.

3. Gradman WS, Lerner G, Mentser M, Rodriguez H, Kamil ES. Experience with autogenous arteriovenous access in children and adolescents. Ann Vasc Surg. 2005;19(5):609–12.
4. Mak RH, Warady BA. Dialysis: vascular access in children – arteriovenous fistula or CVC? Nat Rev Nephrol. 2013 Jan;9(1):9–11.
5. Müller D, Goldstein SL. Hemodialysis in children with end-stage renal disease. Nat Rev Nephrol. 2011;7(11):650–8.
6. Rinat C, Ben-Shalom E, Becker-Cohen R, Feinstein S, Frishberg Y. Complications of central venous stenosis due to permanent central venous catheters in children on hemodialysis. Pediatr Nephrol. 2014;29(11):2235–9. 25145267
7. Tal L, Angelo JR, Akcan-Arikan A. Neonatal extracorporeal renal replacement therapy-a routine renal support modality? Pediatr Nephrol. 2016;31(11):2013–5.
8. Too CW, Sayani R, Lim EY, Leong S, Gogna A, Teo TK. REcanalisation and balloon-oriented puncture for Re-insertion of dialysis catheter in Nonpatent central veins (REBORN). Cardiovasc Intervent Radiol. 2016 Aug;39(8):1193–8.
9. Warady BA, Neu AM, Schaefer F. Optimal care of the infant, child, and adolescent on dialysis: 2014 update. Am J Kidney Dis. 2014;64(1):128–42.

Chapter 14
Hemodialysis Prescription

Klaus Arbeiter, Dagmar Csaicsich, Thomas Sacherer-Mueller, and Christoph Aufricht

Case Presentations

Case 1: Routine Hemodialysis Prescription

A 10-year-old boy (130 cm, 25 kg) is transferred to the pediatric dialysis unit for hemodialysis treatment. The primary renal disease is antenatally diagnosed posterior urethral valves with chronic obstructive nephropathy resulting in end-stage kidney failure. Renal replacement therapy by hemodialysis has been started acutely 2 years ago following deterioration of renal function because of a severe urinary tract infection. Dialysis was initiated with a central venous catheter followed by creation of an AV fistula that is successfully used for dialysis treatment since 12 months. Since 6 months the boy is anuric.

Hemodialysis was performed with a *GAMBRO AK 200 Ultra S* dialysis machine with pediatric blood lines with a priming volume of 85 mL. Treatment was delivered with the local standard prescription of three times weekly for 4 h with blood flow of 150 ml per minute using a high-flux dialyzer with 1.0 m^2 surface area. Dialysate flow was set at 500 mL/min with a temperature of 37 °C. The dialysate solution composition was as follows: potassium 3 mmol/L, Ca 1.25 mmol/L, sodium 140 mmol/L, and bicarbonate 34 mmol/L.

Anticoagulation was performed by low-molecular-weight heparin 20 mg i.v. By this prescription, dialysis dose was achieved with an average Kt/V of 1.3 and pre-dialysis blood values of 55 mmol/l BUN and inorganic phosphorus between 1.8 and 2.2 mmol/l. Growth did not improve under this dialysis prescription. About every other week, extra dialysis sessions were indicated due to volume overload and hypertension.

K. Arbeiter • D. Csaicsich • T. Sacherer-Mueller • C. Aufricht (✉)
Department of Pediatrics and Adolescent Medicine, Medical University of Vienna, Vienna, Austria
e-mail: christoph.aufricht@meduniwien.ac.at

© Springer International Publishing AG 2017
B.A. Warady et al. (eds.), *Pediatric Dialysis Case Studies*,
DOI 10.1007/978-3-319-55147-0_14

Three months ago, he was switched to hemodiafiltration. For enhanced dialysis efficacy, 2,200 mL/h substitution fluid was delivered in the predilution mode. Blood flow rate was increased to 190 ml/min, and intensive nutritional training was instituted. Volume status and blood pressure are now better controlled; repeated echocardiography has shown improvement of left ventricular hypertrophy since start of hemodiafiltration. Due to improvement of nutritional status and weight gain, dry weight is currently being reset. Quality of life is judged as acceptable by family and caretakers. The boy visits school in the morning and starts dialysis treatment in early afternoon.

Clinical Questions

1. What is the standard HD prescription for this boy?
2. What is the standard anticoagulation for this boy?
3. How can the dose of dialysis be tailored to the patient's current needs?
4. How can volume control be tailored to the patient's current needs?

Diagnostic Discussion

1. The choice of dialysis machine and the initial standard prescription of frequency and duration of dialysis sessions vary between centers and rather depend on local policies than on individual patient characteristics. The choice of the dialyzer depends on patient size and needs [1–3]. According to the patient's body surface area of 0.96 m², a dialyzer with a comparable effective surface area (1 m²) was chosen. The setting of blood flow rate depends on dialyzer characteristics and target clearance. The dialyzer chosen for the boy has a recommended flow rate of 100–300 mL/min, with a urea clearance of 180 mL/min at 200 mL/min blood flow and 500 mL/min dialysate flow. In our patient with a body weight of 25 kg, a urea clearance of 5 mL/min/kg was considered appropriate; thus, 125 mL/min should be achieved. This target urea clearance should be clearly met with a blood flow of 150 mL/min (as prescribed). In order to keep the extracorporeal blood volume (max. 8 mL/kg body weight) as low as possible, pediatric blood lines were chosen. Together with the dialyzer, the calculated extracorporeal blood volume was 138 mL, i.e., approximately 5.5 mL/kg body weight in our patient. For enhanced dialysis efficacy, hemodiafiltration was used with 2,200 mL/h substitution fluid delivered in a predilutional fashion.
2. Most standard anticoagulation regimes during hemodialysis are heparin based. Unfractionated heparin or low-molecular-weight heparin is used [4]. Dosage guidelines exist for heparin with an initial bolus dose between 10–65 IU/kg body weight and 300–1,000 IU/m² body surface area and a maintenance dose between 10–30 IU/kg/h. The smaller the child or infant, the lower the heparin dose can be when normalized to body size. To optimize the dosage, the activated clotting time (ACT) should be measured and kept around 50% over the baseline ACT

prior to anticoagulation, but should not exceed 200 s. Low-molecular-weight heparin, as used in this patient, is usually given at the beginning of the dialysis session with a dosage of about 1 mg/kg body weight. Anticoagulation dosage can be checked by measuring factor Xa activity, which should be around 0.5–0.8 U/ml 30 min after application.

Contraindications for heparin-based anticoagulation are bleeding risks, i.e., due to surgery or heparin-induced thrombocytopenia. In perioperative dialysis sessions, regional citrate anticoagulation is an alternative option [5]. Contraindications for citrate anticoagulation are insufficiency of liver function, acidosis or alkalosis, and hypernatremia. In rare cases, such as in heparin-induced thrombocytopenia, alternative medications have been used, such as glycosaminoglycan (danaparoid) and direct thrombin inhibitors like lepirudin and argatroban.

3. Hemodialysis dosing is affected by treatment time, dialyzer size, blood and dialysate flow rates, and the type of access [1, 3]. The definition of the target dialysis dose follows recommendations derived from adult guidelines. Those adult guidelines are mainly based on observed correlations of urea kinetics with patient mortality [2, 6]. The most widely used urea kinetic modeling uses the clearance of urea (K), the duration of the dialysis session (t), and the volume of urea distribution (V): Kt/V (formula by Daugirdas: $Kt/V = -\ln(Ct/Co-0{,}008\,t) + (4-3{,}5\,CtCo)\,UF/W$ where Co urea pre-dialysis, Ct urea post-dialysis, t treatment hours, UF liters of ultrafiltration, w dry weight). A minimum Kt/V level of 1.2–1.4 thrice weekly is thought to be acceptable. However, many children do not show improvement of appetite, weight gain, and statural growth despite reaching these target doses, reflecting clinical signs of underdialysis. Increasing blood flow up to 200 ml/min/m^2, using online hemodiafiltration with a high flux dialyzer, will improve not only small solute clearance but also the (not measurable) clearance of other uremic toxins. Moreover, in chronic dialysis, increasing total dialysis time via increasing the number of dialysis sessions per week should be taken into consideration (see Chap. 15 on intensified regimens).

4. Volume overload leads to hypertension and left ventricular hypertrophy, resulting in increased morbidity and mortality in pediatric and adult hemodialysis patients [7]. Volume control can be achieved by the mainstays of adequate ultrafiltration and fluid restriction. Current recommendations allow an amount of fluid removal of 1.5–2% per hour of estimated dry weight. The prescription of ultrafiltration during each hemodialysis session should have two main goals: achieving the estimated dry weight (see Chap. 26) and avoiding adverse effects of fluid removal. Aggressive fluid removal can lead to intradialytic hypotension with painful symptoms like headache, muscle cramps, abdominal pain, and vomiting. Moreover, associations between intradialytic hypotension, cardiac stunning, and poor survival have been observed, even among patients with normal coronary arteries, which is the case in most children [8]. Therefore, volume control should preferably be achieved via controlled fluid intake rather than by aggressive removal. Fluid restriction must be accompanied by a restriction of dietary salt: to maintain osmotic balance, every 8 g of salt intake prompts the intake of 1 L of free water.

Case 2: Hemodialysis Prescription in an Uncooperative Patient

A 16-year-old girl (143 cm, 40 kg) is transferred to the pediatric dialysis unit for hemodialysis treatment because of chronic transplant failure. A short trial with peritoneal dialysis had to be terminated because of relapsing peritonitis. The primary renal disease is congenital nephrotic syndrome with bilateral nephrectomy. Relevant comorbidities are inner ear deafness and severe mental retardation. Deceased donor transplantation was performed at the age of 18 months, with subsequent loss of the allograft to rejection.

Hemodialysis was started with a central venous catheter due to expected lack of cooperation and restlessness during dialysis sessions. As the catheter was repeatedly torn out by the patient, an arteriovenous fistula was created on the left upper arm and punctured with flexible cath needles. Hemodialysis sessions were performed with permanent presence of a family member. Frequently, additional sedation with diazepam was needed to allow performance of hemodialysis.

Hemodiafiltration was performed with the local standard prescription of three times weekly for 4 h with a blood flow of 250 ml/min using a high flux dialyzer with a 1.4 m^2 surface area. However, frequently interrupted sessions and flow problems led to inadequately low dialysis dose with an average weekly Kt/V of 3.6 and corresponding pre-dialysis blood values of 30 mmol/l BUN and 2.8 mmol/l phosphate. Even more importantly, excessive fluid intake at home resulted in overt chronic overhydration and high blood pressure. Repeated attempts to increase ultrafiltration or to extend the duration of the dialysis sessions were not tolerated by the patient, and additional dialysis sessions were not accepted by the stressed family. Intense and repeated training of the family aimed for strictly reduced salt intake and finally led to a tolerable level of blood pressure, although estimated dry weight was never reached.

Clinical Questions

1. How to prescribe dialysis dose in a restricted dialysis setting?
2. How to manage volume control in a restricted dialysis setting?
3. How to prescribe anticoagulation in an uncooperative patient on hemodialysis?
4. How to deal with uncooperative patients who depend on hemodialysis?

Diagnostic Discussion

1. In case of a restricted dialysis situation as exemplified by this case of a severely mentally impaired adolescent, the delivery of an optimal or even adequate dialysis dose can be challenging. In this setting with lacking cooperation and agitation during dialysis sessions, the choice of access is not necessarily guided by the optimal medical standards but needs to consider in the first place what creates the least discomfort and self-endangerment for the patient. A central venous catheter eliminates the need for repetitive puncture of an arteriovenous fistula and the risk

of needle dislocation during dialysis but subjects the patient to the risk of accidental or deliberate catheter removal. In the described patient, the sum of these factors led to a dialysis dose that remained constantly below currently suggested minimal levels.

While "conventional" dialysis aims to achieve optimal dialysis quality and is regarded as a rehabilitative treatment, in a restricted situation, it might be necessary to accept certain trade-offs. In such a situation, the approach can be to prioritize comfort and alignment with patient preferences to improve quality of life and reduce the burden of dialysis. While rigorous dialysis quality standards should be applied whenever possible, these guidelines may have less relevance for a certain subgroup of patients [9, 10]. Palliative care in ESRD has become an important issue in the "geriatric renal community," but integrating medical, social, and ethical considerations from that paradigm may be helpful to provide better individualized care for a pediatric patient with comparable needs. Such liberalizations in protocols may be regarded as medically suboptimal, yet they can make a huge difference for patients and families.

2. It was obvious that adequate fluid removal could not be performed in our patient despite increasing the prescription to the maximal tolerated ultrafiltration rate of 2% per hour of estimated dry weight.

As neither longer hemodialysis sessions nor intensified dialysis with 5–6 sessions per week were tolerated by the girl and her family, we had to focus on interdialytic fluid management. Isolated fluid restriction is often not practicable as permanent thirst will result in psychological distress to the whole family and an inacceptable reduction of quality of life. Thirst on the other hand is in most cases the result of high salt intake that subsequently has to be satisfied by water ingestion. In such patients, control of fluid status and blood pressure can only be accomplished by a substantial and sustained reduction of dietary salt intake. This approach became successful in our case when the change in dietary habits was extended to the whole family [11].

3. Anticoagulation in the extracorporeal circuit is needed to prevent clotting in the dialysis filter or tubes and inherently increases the risk of bleeding events. In patients with mental retardation, a central venous catheter includes a higher risk of bleeding if the incompliant patient pulls out the catheter. With an arteriovenous fistula, the patient may pull out the needle during dialysis, and the compliance for adequate compression after dialysis sessions may be absent.

Some patients with mental retardation have a high risk of thrombosis, i.e., if they are immobilized due to their neurological disease and therefore dependent on chronic systemic anticoagulation. These patients may benefit from heparin-based or oral anticoagulation without the need for extra medication during dialysis.

Most standard hemodialysis anticoagulation protocols are heparin based. However, if the patient is prone to auto-aggressive self-injuries or at risk of accidents due to hyperactivity, bleeding risk should be minimized with an altered anticoagulation management. In such patients, regional citrate anticoagulation may be an option [5]. For citrate dialysis, stable blood flow rates are needed, but these may be difficult to achieve in the uncooperative patient because of uncontrollable movements and arm and body position. In individual cases, even a regime without anticoagulation may be possible, with short dialysis sessions, high blood flow rates, and intermittent saline flushes.

Taken together, patients with mental retardation on hemodialysis present additional special needs and risks for bleeding or thrombotic complication that have to be taken into account when individualizing anticoagulation management. In any case, particularly close monitoring of anticoagulation to avoid over-treatment is recommended in these patients, such as frequent ACT measurements in heparinization.

4. The need to hemodialyze pediatric patients with mental retardation is increasing and presents major challenges [12]. Similar to young infants, mentally impaired patients cannot understand why they are receiving dialysis and are unable to fully cooperate with the associated procedures, in particular if these are painful or restrictive. These patients may profoundly refuse dialysis and may try to pull out dialysis needles and catheters and thereby endanger themselves, dialysis staff, and other patients. In contrast to young children, however, older children with cognitive or behavioral impairment frequently are of considerable physical strength and are able to create a hostile environment by verbal and physical acts and threats of violence.

Routine medical sedation before dialysis is risky in the chronic setting; physical restraints cause additional emotional stress and – besides violation of ethical and dignity aspects – are ineffective and will likely even exacerbate an already challenging situation. Probably the best care in patients with cognitive impairment is the introduction of strictly fixed routine protocols that allow patients to accommodate to the repeated dialysis-associated procedures, together with support of a trusted (ideally loved) contact person acting as a "sitter." This "sitter" can create an atmosphere of trust and care, while the dialysis center personnel perform their tasks, help the patients to tolerate necessary painful procedures, and distract and pacify them to remain calm during the dialysis session. In patients who are living with their families, the "sitter" is usually a family member. This represents a major advantage with regard to trust but poses additional stress on the family member who is also not used to the dialysis procedure and will need significant training and counseling to be able to see stressful conditions from the staff's point of view [13]. In contrast, nonfamily members sitting for the patient will more readily identify with the dialysis staff position but may face a greater challenge being accepted by the patient and creating a calm and trusting environment.

In any case, hemodialysis in uncooperative pediatric and adolescent patients with mental impairment causes major challenges to the patients, their families and the caregivers but are mostly feasible to handle by experienced hemodialysis staff with the support of a trusted "sitter" team. Currently, there is increasing awareness of the need for guidelines supporting the dialysis staff in these situations in adult patients due to the increasing prevalence of patients with dementia, likely resulting in valuable information for the pediatric community [14].

Clinical Pearls

1. Choice of dialysis machine, frequency, and duration of dialysis sessions depends on center policy. Choice of dialyzer, flow rates, and extracorporeal blood volume depends on patient size and treatment targets.
2. Hemodialysis dosing is determined by treatment time, dialyzer size, blood and dialysate flow rates. The definition of targets is derived from adult guidelines; therefore, individual clinical assessment of appetite, weight gain, and growth remains essential to detect underdialysis.
3. Standard anticoagulation regimes are based on unfractionated or low-molecular-weight heparin; alternate options are indicated in special situations, such as regional citrate anticoagulation in patients with increased bleeding risks or heparin-induced side effects.
4. Volume control is essential to prevent cardiovascular morbidity and mortality and should preferably be achieved via controlled fluid intake rather than by aggressive removal.
5. In restricted dialysis situations, it might be necessary to prioritize comfort and alignment with patient and family preferences to improve quality of life and reduce the burden of dialysis.

References

1. Warady BA, et al. Pediatric dialysis. New York: Springer; 2012.
2. Daugirdas JT, Blake PG, Ing TS. Handbook of dialysis. 5th ed. Philadelphia: Wolters Kluwer Health; 2014.
3. Fischbach M, et al.; The European Pediatric Dialysis Working Group. Hemodialysis in children: general practical guidelines. Pediatr Nephrol 2005;20(8):1054–66.
4. Kessler M, et al. Anticoagulation in chronic hemodialysis: progress toward an optimal approach. Semin Dial. 2015;28(5):474–89.
5. Fajardo C, et al. Inpatient citrate-based hemodialysis in pediatric patients. Pediatr Nephrol. 2016;31(10):1667–72.
6. Gotch FA, et al. A mechanistic analysis of the national cooperative dialysis study (NCDS). Kidney Int. 1985;28:526–34.
7. Paglialonga F, Consolo S, Galli MA, Testa S, Edefonti A. Interdialytic weight gain in oligoanuric children and adolescents on chronic hemodialysis. Pediatr Nephrol. 2015;30(6):999–1005.
8. Hothi DK, Rees L, McIntyre CW, Marek J. Hemodialysis-induced acute myocardial dyssynchronous impairment in children. Nephron Clin Pract. 2013;123(1–2):83–92.
9. Grubbs V, et al. A palliative approach to dialysis care: a patient-centered transition to the end of life. Clin J Am Soc Nephrol. 2014;9:2203–9.
10. Vandecasteele SJ, et al. A patient-centered vision of care for ESRD: dialysis as a bridging treatment or as a final destination? J Am Soc Nephrol. 2014;25:1647–51.
11. Lindley EJ. Reducing sodium intake in hemodialysis patients. Semin Dial. 2009;22(3):260–3.
12. Watson AR, et al. Factors influencing choice of renal replacement therapy in European paediatric nephrology units. Pediatr Nephrol. 2013;28(12):2361–8.
13. Mieto FS, et al. The mothers' experiences in the pediatrics hemodialysis unit. J Bras Nefrol. 2014;36(4):460–8.
14. Allon M, et al. The demented patient who declines to be dialyzed and the unhappy armed police officer son: what should be done? Clin J Am Soc Nephrol. 2014;9(4):804–8.

Chapter 15
Intensified Hemodialysis

Claus Peter Schmitt

Case Presentation

The 15-year-old Michel, born with hypodysplatic kidneys, underwent peritoneal dialysis (PD) from early infancy until age 4 years when his mother donated a kidney to him. Automated PD had been complicated by four episodes of peritonitis, a peritoneal leak, and frequent alarms due to outflow obstruction. The posttransplant course was stable for the first 3 years but subsequently hampered by rejection episodes treated with steroid pulses, ATG, IVIG, and rituximab. The allograft eventually failed, and the boy returned to dialysis at the age of 13 years. During the first month, 4-h hemodialysis (HD) sessions were performed twice weekly, but with residual daily urine output declining to less than 200 ml, HD was increased in a stepwise fashion to 5 h thrice weekly. The current hemodialysis dosage, achieved via a central venous catheter, is a Kt/V urea of 1.4 (according to Daugirdas single-pool equation). The 45 kg, 150 cm boy shows up with intradialytic weight gain ranging from 2 l during midweek sessions to 4.5 l after the long weekend interval. Blood pressure is elevated up to 165/95 mmHg. Echocardiography demonstrates moderate left ventricular hypertrophy. Despite repeated dietary counseling, prior to midweek dialysis sessions, serum potassium is typically around 6 mmol/l, blood urea nitrogen 75–95 mg/dl, and serum phosphorus 1.7–2.2 mmol/l. PTH is around 700 ng/ml, despite high doses of calcitriol and calcium-containing phosphate binders and treatment with 30 mg cinacalcet per day. Serum bicarbonate is below 20 mmol/l and Hb 9.2 mg/dl with erythropoietin administered twice weekly intravenously at 220 IU/kg per dose. Michel has reached Tanner stage PH2, G2; he grew 6 cm in the past year after growth hormone was started within 3 months of dialysis initiation. The boy

C.P. Schmitt (✉)
Division of Pediatric Nephrology, Center for Pediatrics and Adolescent Medicine,
University of Heidelberg, Heidelberg, Germany
e-mail: Claus.Peter.Schmitt@med.uni-heidelberg.de

© Springer International Publishing AG 2017
B.A. Warady et al. (eds.), *Pediatric Dialysis Case Studies*,
DOI 10.1007/978-3-319-55147-0_15

109

complains about fatigue, post-dialysis headache, and a lack of interest in social activities. School performance is low. The father has left the family; the mother has a full-time job and is concerned about Michel's medical condition.

Clinical Questions

1. Is dialysis treatment adequate?
2. Which alternative options of renal replacement therapy (RRT) can be offered to Michel?
3. Which modifications of hemodialysis therapy may be envisaged? What are the respective benefits and drawbacks?
4. Which complementary measures can improve treatment adequacy?

Diagnostic Discussion

1. Soon after initiation of hemodialysis, the weekly dialysis time was augmented to 15 h due to loss of residual renal function. With an average single-pool (sp) Kt/V urea of 1.4, hemodialysis is considered adequate according to current clinical practice recommendations. For adult patients, the KDOQI guidelines recommend thrice weekly hemodialysis with a target spKt/V of 1.4 and a delivered spKt/V of at least 1.2 [1]. Since no scientific evidence is available for the impact of Kt/V in children, the same targets are applied in pediatric dialysis.

   Nevertheless, this adolescent boy shows distinct clinical and biochemical signs of underdialysis. These are apparently based on the limited efficacy of dialysis and nonadherence to dietary recommendations, including a high fluid intake. Fluid status, blood pressure, anemia, and secondary hyperparathyroidism are insufficiently controlled. Growth is poor despite GH therapy, which may not be administered regularly. Physical and mental performance is poor. Thus, the overall therapy is inadequate despite a nominally adequate Kt/V urea.

2. Successful re-transplantation would be the best therapeutic option for Michel, who has been placed on the cadaveric allograft waiting list at the time of HD initiation. However, Michel is highly sensitized, so his chances to obtain a compatible donor organ within a short time period are low.

   Switching to PD is another principal option. However, PD is unlikely to function well in view of the history of drainage problems secondary to intraperitoneal adhesions following multiple peritonitis episodes. Moreover, the efficacy of PD is limited and requires good adherence to dietary restrictions and fluid intake. And the social situation is not in favor of home dialysis. Thus, intensified in-center hemodialysis currently appears as the best suited approach to improve the quality of renal replacement therapy.

3. The first measure toward a sustained increase in purification efficacy will be the replacement of the central venous catheter (CVC) by an arteriovenous fistula (AVF). Blood flow rate should be greater than 100 ml/m²/min and optimally 140–200 ml/min/m² (3–6 ml/kg/min). The latter is hardly achieved with CVC. Moreover CVC use is fraught with a much higher risk of infectious complications and significantly lower patency rates [2]. An AV fistula or AV graft should be created instead. Dialysis flow rate should be at least two times the blood flow rate, and the dialyzer surface area should equal the body surface area. In case the dialyzer allows modification of dialysate NaCl concentrations, a stepwise reduction may be aimed for in order to reduce salt load.

If available, hemodiafiltration should be established to maximize convective solute removal, ideally using online HDF with 12–15 l/m² BSA convective flow per session (predilution mode). These modifications will improve purification, in particular phosphorus removal, but also will enhance the tolerance of the dialysis sessions. The use of high-flux dialyzers and high convective-flow hemodiafiltration (HDF) presumably improves cardiovascular outcome [3].

Next to these technical modifications, the dialysis regime may be intensified by increasing the frequency and duration of dialysis sessions. Figure 15.1 gives an overview of the modifiable components of the HD prescription. The KDOQI guidelines propose to switch patients from standard hemodialysis either to frequent in-center or to long home hemodialysis. These recommendations are based on clinical trial evidence in adult HD patients, including the Frequent Hemodialysis Network (FHN) trial that compared daily in-center HD [4] and frequent home nocturnal dialysis to standard thrice weekly HD [5], and the Alberta Nocturnal trial of long home hemodialysis [6]. Altogether, intensified hemodialysis resulted in improved blood pressure control and reduced left ventricular mass [7], better anemia control, lower serum phosphorus levels and phosphate binder intake, and

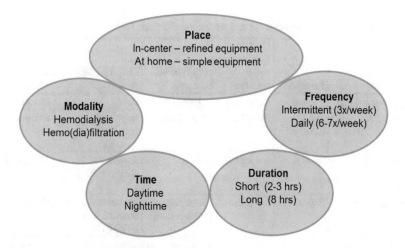

Fig. 15.1 Modifiable factors in hemodialysis

improved health-related quality of life. Twelve-month mortality was significantly lower with daily hemodialysis (hazard ratio 0.56, 95% CI 0.32–0.99) [8]. However, untoward effects were also observed on intensified dialysis schedules, including an increased rate of vascular access complications [9], an increased incidence in intradialytic hypotension [4], and a faster decline in residual function [10].

In children thrice weekly nocturnal in-center HD and HDF [11, 12], daily nocturnal home dialysis [13], and frequent in-center online HDF [14] have been performed with encouraging outcomes, including improved blood pressure control and reduced frequency of hyperphosphatemia and hyperkalemia despite little or no dietary restrictions.

Health-related quality of life and school attendance were affected favorably with nocturnal dialysis. The most convincing finding of improved dialysis adequacy in children, however, was catch-up growth observed with six times weekly online HDF [14].

Michel might benefit substantially from an intensified hemodialysis regime. The dialysis dose should be adjusted to achieve optimal fluid and salt homeostasis aiming for normal blood pressure, normophosphatemia, and a good physical performance. The preferable modality of intensified dialysis mainly depends on individual needs and the existing infrastructure of the dialysis center. Provided Michel does not live far from the dialysis center, more frequent dialysis, i.e., four times weekly or even more frequent in-center dialysis, may be envisaged. Alternatively nocturnal in-center dialysis could be carried out thrice per week if available in the dialysis center and acceptable to the patient. Home hemodialysis could be discussed but is rather unlikely to be feasible in view of the family situation.

It should be emphasized that the offer of intensified dialysis must be well balanced against the associated medical risks and the psychosocial burden of intensified treatment, which may potentially compromise quality of life (Table 15.1).

Table 15.1 Summary of conventional and intensified HD in children

HD mode	Schedule	Control of fluid status/ blood pressure	Phosphorus control	Longitudinal growth	Social rehabilitation
Conventional HD	3 × 4–5 h	Limited	Limited	Poor	Moderate
Short daily HD(F)	5–6 × 2.5–3 h	Excellent	Excellent	Improved (catch-up growth)	Acceptable
Intermittent nocturnal center HD(F)	3 × 8 h	Very good	Good	Similar to conventional HD	Very good
Daily nocturnal HD(F)	5–6 × 8 h	Excellent	Excellent – overshooting	No improvement reported with HD. HDF?	Good

The choice depends on individual patients' medical needs and available infrastructures of the dialysis center. All types of intensified HD may also be realized at home

4. A number of complementary measures are available that might help the quality of therapy in this patient beyond increasing weekly dialysis hours. First of all, dialysis adequacy should be actively monitored. Modern dialysis equipment features online measurement of small solute clearance to ensure agreement between prescribed and achieved solute removal within each dialysis session.

Bioimpedance analysis provides valuable longitudinal information on the hydration status and helps in determining the adequate dry weight, in concert with regular interdialytic ambulatory blood pressure monitoring (ABPM). The attainment of dry weight is greatly facilitated by intradialytic blood volume monitoring, which minimizes the occurrence of intradialytic hypotension.

Regular psychosocial counseling is an important cornerstone of dialysis in adolescents. Likewise, an efficient in-center schooling program is a prerequisite for frequent in-center hemodialysis programs.

The enormous "pill burden" is one of the most difficult challenges of chronic dialysis. In-center drug administration can alleviate this challenge and ensures regular intake. The administration of growth hormone can be monitored by the use of application pens with usage memory and regular measurement of serum IGF-1. If adherence is an issue, thrice weekly in-center growth hormone administration to achieve the same total weekly dose is an option.

Clinical Pearls

1. Cardiovascular disease is the leading cause of death in patients with childhood-onset end-stage renal disease. Fluid overload, high blood pressure, and hyperphosphatemia are key risk factors for long-term outcome [15–17].
2. Kt/V urea reflects small solute removal and has been associated with survival in adult dialysis patients. However, it does not mirror clearance rates of phosphate or middle-sized uremic toxins and does not correlate with fluid balance.
3. Intensified hemodialysis programs are increasingly implemented in pediatric dialysis centers in order to improve control of key pathomechanisms of dialysis-related morbidity and mortality, including fluid and salt overload, hypertension, hyperphosphatemia, and hyperparathyroidism. Clinical trial evidence in adults suggests that intensified hemodialysis improves quality of life and patient survival.
4. The apparent benefits of intensified hemodialysis must be carefully balanced in each individual patient against the potential disadvantages, such as an adverse impact on social life and schooling (Table 15.1), increased risk of access-related complications, and accelerated loss of residual renal function.
5. An arteriovenous fistula should always be preferred over a central venous catheter unless timely transplantation is envisaged. In addition to the much reduced infectious complication rates, superior patency, and lower hospitalization rates [2] achieved with arteriovenous fistulae, the preservation of central venous access options by avoidance of central venous catheterization is of utmost importance in children with end-stage renal disease who face many decades of renal replacement therapy.

References

1. KDOQI Clinical Practice Guideline for Hemodialysis Adequacy: 2015 update. National Kidney Foundation. Am J Kidney Dis. 2015;66(5):884–930. http://www.ajkd.org/article/S0272-6386(15)01019-7/fulltext#sec12.2.2.
2. Hayes WN, Watson AR, Callaghan N, Wright E, Stefanidis CJ, Ariceta G, Bakkaloglu SA, Callaghan N, Edefonti A, Me E, Ekim M, Fischbach M, Hayes W, Holtta T, Klaus G, Schmitt CP, Shroff R, Stefanidis CJ, Van de Walle J, Vondrak K, Watson AR, Wright E, Zurowska A. Vascular access: choice and complications in European paediatric haemodialysis units. Pediatr Nephrol. 2012;27(6):999–1004.
3. Nistor I, Palmer SC, Craig JC, et al. Haemodiafiltration, haemofiltration and haemodialysis for end-stage kidney disease. Cochrane Database Syst Rev. 2015;5:CD006258. doi:10.1002/14651858.CD006258.pub2.
4. The FHN Trial Group, Chertow GM, Levin NW, Beck GJ, et al. In-center hemodialysis six times per week versus three times per week. N Engl J Med. 2010;363:2287–300.
5. Culleton BF, Walsh M, Klarenbach SW, et al. Effect of frequent nocturnal hemodialysis vs. conventional hemodialysis on left ventricular mass and quality of life: a randomized controlled trial. JAMA. 2007;298:1291–9.
6. Rocco MV, Lockridge Jr RS, Beck GJ, et al. The effects of frequent nocturnal home hemodialysis: the frequent hemodialysis network nocturnal trial. Kidney Int. 2011;80(10):1080–91.
7. Susantitaphong P, Koulouridis I, Balk EM, et al. Effect of frequent or extended hemodialysis on cardiovascular parameters: a meta-analysis. Am J Kidney Dis Off J Natl Kidney Found. 2012;59:689–99.
8. Chertow GM, Levin NW, Beck GJ, Daugirdas JT, Eggers PW, Kliger AS, Larive B, Rocco MV, Greene T, Frequent Hemodialysis Network (FHN) Trials group. Long-term effects of frequent In-center hemodialysis. J Am Soc Nephrol. 2016;27(6):1830–6.
9. Suri RS, Larive B, Sherer S, et al. Risk of vascular access complications with frequent hemodialysis. J Am Soc Nephrol. 2013;24:498–505.
10. Daugirdas JT, Greene T, Rocco MV, et al. Effect of frequent hemodialysis on residual kidney function. Kidney Int. 2013;83:949–58.
11. Hoppe A, von Puttkamer C, Linke U, et al. A hospital-based intermittent nocturnal hemodialysis program for children and adolescents. J Pediatr. 2011;158:95–9.
12. Thumfart J, Hilliger T, Stiny C, et al. Is peritoneal dialysis still an equal option? Results of the Berlin pediatric nocturnal dialysis program. Pediatr Nephrol Berl Ger. 2015;30:1181–7.
13. Geary DF, Piva E, Tyrrell J, et al. Home nocturnal hemodialysis in children. J Pediatr. 2005;147:383–7.
14. Fischbach M, Terzic J, Menouer S, et al. Daily on line haemodiafiltration promotes catch-up growth in children on chronic dialysis. Nephrol Dial Transplant. 2010;25:867–73.
15. Oh J, Wunsch R, Turzer M, Bahner M, Raggi P, Querfeld U, Mehls O, Schaefer F. Advanced coronary and carotid arteriopathy in young adults with childhood-onset chronic renal failure. Circulation. 2002;106(1):100–5.
16. Chavers BM, Molony JT, Solid CA, et al. One-year mortality rates in US children with end-stage renal disease. Am J Nephrol. 2015;41:121–8. doi: 10.1159/000380828.
17. Parekh RS, Carroll CE, Wolfe RA, Port FK. Cardiovascular mortality in children and young adults with end-stage kidney disease. J Pediatr. 2002;141:191–7. doi: 10.1067/mpd.2002.125910.

Chapter 16
Home Haemodialysis

Daljit K. Hothi and Kate Sinnott

Case Presentation

An 11-year-old girl presented with steroid-resistant nephrotic syndrome at 16 months of age that was subsequently confirmed to be focal segmental glomerulosclerosis (FSGS) on renal biopsy. At 2 years of age, she underwent a living-related renal transplant from her mother, receiving plasmapheresis pre-transplantation. She developed proteinuria almost immediately after receiving the transplant. Despite escalation of her immunosuppression and further plasmapheresis, her transplant failed at 9 months and she commenced haemodialysis (HD).

Thereafter dialysis access started becoming a challenge. As a result of multiple central lines, she had developed bilateral subclavian vein stenosis and internal jugular vein stenosis with resultant superior vena cava syndrome. Consequently an arteriovenous fistula (AVF) was attempted at the right antecubital fossa. Post-operatively the arm became acutely swollen and tender with marked venous distension and obvious thrombophlebitis. Clinically as the arm deteriorated, the decision was made to ligate the fistula.

At 5 years of age, a second living non-related donor transplant was attempted. Again, she was treated with plasmapheresis pre-transplantation but proteinuria reoccurred post-transplantation. This time, the rate of decline of her renal function was much slower such that HD was not restarted until 8 years of age through a right femoral vein tunnelled catheter. This is when we first met the family after they relocated from South Africa to the UK.

On arrival to our unit, the patient was experiencing sharp pain in her leg whilst on dialysis; she was hypertensive and had markedly variable dialysis blood flows and access pressures. Subsequent imaging demonstrated migration of the femoral

D.K. Hothi (✉) • K. Sinnott
Department of Pediatric Nephrology, Great Ormond Street Hospital for Children Foundation Trust, Great Ormond Street, London, UK, WC1N 3JH
e-mail: Daljit.Hothi@gosh.nhs.uk

© Springer International Publishing AG 2017 115
B.A. Warady et al. (eds.), *Pediatric Dialysis Case Studies*,
DOI 10.1007/978-3-319-55147-0_16

line. The line was repositioned with improvement in blood flow and shortly thereafter was converted to a right external jugular vein tunnelled catheter (CVC). She subsequently developed a deep vein thrombosis and pulmonary embolus and was commenced on subcutaneous low molecular weight heparin. Treatment was complicated by a brief period of peri-vaginal bleeding.

The long-term option presented to the family at this point was another high-risk transplant or frequent, extended HD at home. The family chose the latter. Both parents trained on the mobile NxStage™ dialysis system, initially spending 2 weeks in the dialysis unit and then 2 weeks in the patient hotel to complete their training in an environment that simulated the home environment. After the family had successfully transitioned home, the patient was reassessed for an AVF and underwent a two-stage transposition surgery to create a brachio-basilic fistula. Once the fistula had matured, the parents returned to hospital to learn how to monitor, needle and dialyse through the fistula.

The patient initially dialysed at home for 5 h in the evening, 4 times per week. After 8 months she switched to nocturnal dialysis and was receiving up to 40 h of dialysis a week. The family's life changed, 'our daughter is not a dialysis patient but a young girl on dialysis'. Her energy, well-being and appetite increased. Diet restrictions were liberalised and fluid restrictions lifted. The medication burden on the whole was reduced, but with nocturnal dialysis, the patient developed hyperparathyroidism secondary to hypocalcaemia and required calcium supplementation and vitamin D. The patient was back at school full-time and the family were for the first time on dialysis able to go on holiday.

Unfortunately after 2½ years of home HD, the patient experienced access-related complications including multiple micro-thrombi in collaterals that were forming in the fistula arm and chest, worsening steal syndrome and recurrent episodes of thrombophlebitis. This resulted in frequent hospital admissions with a negative impact on the patient's health outcomes and significant disruptions to the entire family's life. This also prompted discussions about what was best for the patient in the long term: continued home HD, with the knowledge that access options are very limited, or attempt a third kidney transplant?

Clinical Questions

1. What are the benefits of home HD?
2. Which children are suitable for home HD?
3. What form of dialysis access is suitable for home HD?
4. What infrastructure is required to set up a home HD programme?
5. What dialysis systems are suitable for home HD?
6. How can you ensure the patients' safety at home?
7. What HD prescription should you use at home?
8. What are some of the disadvantages of home HD, and how can you increase treatment adherence at home?

Diagnostic Discussion

1. In the HEMO study comparing high-dose HD (urea-reduction ratio of 75%, single pool Kt/V (spKt/V) of 1.71 and equilibrated Kt/V (eKt/V) of 1.53) against standard dose HD (urea-reduction ratio of 66%, sp. Kt/V of 1.32 and eKt/V of 1.16), the relative risk of death was 0.96 [1]. On a secondary analysis, Wolfe et al. reported a 17% lower risk of mortality for every 5% increase in URR in patients with a small body mass index. This suggested a survival advantage in increasing HD dose in low BMI patients [2].

   The DOPPS review of 22,000 adult HD patients from seven countries found that a higher dialysis dose as reflected by a higher Kt/V was an independent predictor of lower mortality with a synergistic survival advantage with treatment time. Therefore survival was most pronounced by combining a higher Kt/V with longer treatment time. For every 30 min longer on HD, the relative risk of mortality was reduced by 7% [3]. An ANZDATA analysis of 4,193 patients found that the optimal dialysis dose for survival was a Kt/V greater than or equal to 1.3 and a dialysis session greater than or equal to 4.5 h. Treatment duration less than 3.5 h was associated with a higher mortality risk [4].

   Such data set the scene for 'quotidian' home dialysis, namely, more frequent and/or extended HD, or gentler and more optimal dialysis. The adult literature on quotidian dialysis practices is consistently positive and suggests clinical benefits approaching those achieved by transplantation. In a matched cohort study comparing survival between nocturnal HD and deceased and living donor kidney transplantation, there was no difference in the adjusted survival between nocturnal HD and deceased donor renal transplantation. The proportion of deaths was 14.7% for nocturnal HD, 14.3% for deceased donor transplantation and 8.5% for live donor transplantation [5].

   Literature on paediatric home HD is scarce and limited to uncontrolled single-centre experiences. Results are similar to adult data as summarised below, Table 16.1.

2. The patient criteria for a home HD programme are likely to change with time as experience grows. Programmes should start conservatively, recruiting patients with the support of 'expert' home HD families that can help to align expectations of home therapies and support new potential families in their decisions.

   Our suggested criteria for recruiting patients onto a home HD programme are listed below, but specifics may vary between programmes:

   - Commitment to dialysing at home.
   - Patient weight 10 kg and above (determined by the combined volume of the extracorporal circuit and dialyser).
   - Well-functioning vascular access.
   - Absence of psychosocial concerns that cannot be managed in the community.
   - Home of a sufficient size to accommodate the dialysis equipment and 1-month supply of dialysis consumables.

Table 16.1 Literature on paediatric home haemodialysis

Author	Cohort size	Outcomes
Tom [6]	12	Improved growth
Simonsen [7]	4	Catch up growth Freedom from dietary and fluid restrictions Improved quality of life
Geary et al. [8]	4	Improved appetite and growth Freedom from dietary and fluid restrictions Flexibility around dialysis times Improved quality of life, well-being and energy Return to full-time education and social rehabilitation Post dialysis recovery times reduced to minutes Normotension extending to hypotension with a requirement for intradialytic midodrine Reduced medication burden
Hothi [9]	4	Negative calcium balance Normal PTH Hypophosphatemia requiring dialysate phosphate
Goldstein [10]	4	Improved BP Discontinuation or reduction in antihypertensives Improved plasma phosphate and PTH levels Improved quality of life

- In consideration of the reverse osmosis dialysis systems at home, the ability to modify the water source.
- Family household hygiene that does not compromise patient risk of infection.
- Child does not live in an area with frequent and prolonged disruptions to electricity supplies. An emergency source of power must be available at all times.

The referral could be initiated for a number of reasons, including medical, social and education, or simply as a result of patients' or their families' preferences. Self-care within the HD unit often facilitates the transition to home dialysis by allowing patients and families to gradually build their confidence. We also believe that failed home PD does not preclude the possibility of home HD.

3. The quality of the dialysis access is a critical factor that influences the patient's dialysis experience. Children can be dialysed at home through a CVC or an AVF. Generally speaking CVCs are associated with a greater risk of complications, including infections, obstruction, dislodgement and central vessel stenosis. However, in our experience the complication rates with CVCs in children being dialysed at home are significantly lower than those dialysed in hospital. An AVF is undeniably the gold standard but in practice not always the easiest access solution in children. AVF placement in children requires considerable surgical expertise, and the risk of primary non-function is greater owing to the size of the blood vessels. Most children will require the help of a play therapist and/or psychologist to overcome needle phobias. However, once needling is established, most children express a preference for the fistulae due to the absence of a permanent catheter that is visible to the world and the freedom this grants, such as having the choice to swim or take a bath.

In our unit we try to encourage AVF in children that are likely to require dialysis greater than 2 years or those that have had a previous central line infection. We would not hesitate to create fistulae in children already established on a home programme if surgery is an option. Once the fistula has matured, the family returns to in-centre dialysis to allow the dialysis nurses to start needling the fistula, to establish a track for button hole needling and then to train the family.

4. Developing a home HD programme requires careful planning, resources, dedicated staff and an appreciation of the risk and governance issues arising from transitioning the patient's care home. The design of the infrastructure will affect the cost of setting up and maintaining a programme and is largely influenced by the potential size of the programme; the availability of support from a neighbouring adult programme; the choice of dialysis system; and the decision on whether patients will be trained on the HD unit or in a dedicated training facility. Finally a home HD programme is likely to impact an existing in-centre HD and peritoneal dialysis programme, and this would need monitoring.

   In our experience, staffing is key to the success of a safe, high-quality home HD programme. It is worth investing in a multidisciplinary team that can support families in their homes. At minimum the composition of the team should include a HD nurse, dialysis technician, nephrologist, dietician and social worker. The inclusion of other allied health professionals such as a pharmacist, psychologist, community nurses, local paediatricians and general practitioner is desirable for optimal support.

5. Generally speaking there are two types of dialysis systems for home HD.

   The first requires home water conversions in order to produce the large volumes of high-quality dialysate necessary for the dialysis treatment. This cost can sometimes become a barrier to delivering home HD in children where transplantation is the preferred renal replacement therapy and dialysis is viewed as a temporary interim measure. Water conversion requires the installation of a cold water outlet and a drain to allow the carbon filter, reverse osmosis unit and dialysis machine to be fitted. Families would be expected to test their water for chloride every session and bring a sample into hospital every 1–2 months to allow the dialysis technician to test for chemicals, endotoxins and microbiology.

   The alternative system, The NxStage System One™, is a portable home dialysis machine that functions with minimal home water modifications. Dialysate is prepared at home using the NxStage PureFlow™ SL integrated water purification and dialysate production system. Alternatively dialysis could be delivered using pre-prepared 5-litre, sterile, dialysate bags. The standard CAR-172-C circuit has an extracorporeal volume of 200 ml and thus would only be suitable for children weighing greater than 25 kg. We have adapted 2 CRRT circuits to lower the weight criteria. The CAR-124-C has a smaller extracorporeal volume and can house any appropriately sized dialyser, making it suitable for children weighing 20 kg and above. The CAR-125-B with an appropriately sized dialyser can treat children weighing 10 kg and above.

6. Paediatric home HD is a relatively new practice that places a high-risk clinical activity in patients' homes under the care of parents or caregivers. However, through empowering families and creating a learning environment, safety can be assured.

   Training is at the centre of our safety infrastructure. We recommend training two people at the outset, and we involve the child/young adult encouraging them to learn about the machine set-up, access and dialysis prescription. Companies often provide training material, but these have to be adapted for paediatric use. We start training on our HD unit and quickly move to a 'family step-down' training facility, co-located within hospital grounds but separate from the dialysis unit, that is set-up to simulate the home environment. This really tests the family's confidence to dialyse independently. Enhancing this we insist that three to four dialysis treatments are completed unsupervised prior to discharge, with at least one weekend treatment with no home HD staff on site within the hospital. Competencies are signed off, and both the patient and family are asked to sign a treatment adherence contract prior to discharge. Once home we offer retraining opportunities every 6 months or earlier if an adverse event has occurred at home.

   Support in the community is critical in preventing harm. Families are actively encouraged to engage with the community teams. Families have access to 24/7 telephone support with a clear communication pathway, describing who to contact for urgent medical and technical queries whilst they dialyse their children at home in the evenings, weekends and nights. To further empower them and support their decision-making, we provide them with written guidelines for normal ranges for a number of dialysis and physiological parameters, with clear instructions on how to proceed if parameters fall out of the normal range.

   Remote monitoring is not universally employed or advocated in adult or paediatric home HD programmes but, if available, may alleviate some patient or parental anxieties. Owing to concerns of central line or fistula needle dislodgement, we do mandate that families use enuresis alarms that can raise an alert over the possibility of a blood leak, and baby monitors to help amplify alarms for children on nocturnal HD.

   As part of the safety culture, it's essential to learn from adverse events and near misses. Therefore the home HD team should aim to meet at minimum quarterly to discuss problems, complications and adherence concerns, learning from these events and spreading knowledge.

7. In our experience there are many drivers for families to agree to home HD including the flexibility to dialyse around their own schedule, having the option to go on holiday and near normalisation of family and school life. The impetus for clinical teams is in improving patient outcomes. Therefore a tailored approach is required to achieve both objectives. Table 16.2 offers some guidance on different regimes, their value and expected outcomes.

8. One of the greatest concerns about home HD is the burden placed on caregivers. Geary et al. in their series described one family where the stress became so severe that a hybrid prescription was created whereby mum received respite one session per week, and the child was dialysed in centre [8]. Clearly these concerns are real; they can vary in the level of intensity and can manifest differently. These are some of the comments from some of our families:

Table 16.2 Essential considerations with different home HD prescriptions for children [11]

Prescription	Session duration, h	Sessions per week	Patient or family considerations	Prescription considerations
Short daily	2–3	6–7	Helpful for working/busy parents with a limited window for dialysing. Best for young children who cannot tolerate long sessions. Higher frequency best for children unable to tolerate aggressive UF or poorly adherent to fluid restrictions.	Most expensive due to higher dialysis consumables cost. Dialysis and blood flow typically unchanged from in-centre prescription. Seldom allows discontinuation of phosphate binders.
Extended	4.5–5.5	≥ Alternate days	Alternate-day therapy offers greater respite time for the caregiver. Teenagers become increasingly frustrated sacrificing their evenings to HD.	Dialysate and blood flow rates typically 20%–30% lower than in-centre prescription. Often allows liberalisation of dietary and fluid restrictions. Improved BP control, lower antihypertensive requirement.
Nocturnal	7–12	≥ Alternate days	Dialysing overnight can induce anxiety in caregivers and children from fear of disconnection or not hearing machine alarms. Virtually eliminates adverse intradialytic symptoms. Greatest chance of achieving complete freedom from dietary and fluid restrictions possible.	Requires additional safety considerations. Patients may develop persistently low BP. Clinicians may wish to consider prophylactic midodrine at the start of dialysis to support the BP for UF and prevent clotting. Dialyse against 1.75 mmol/L dialysate calcium to prevent negative calcium balance. Higher-frequency nocturnal HD may cause hypophosphatemia. Treat with oral supplements and/or add phosphate to the dialysate concentrate as a sodium phosphate enema. Theoretical risk of 'dialysis deficiency syndrome' (i.e. nonselective purification of essential plasma components). Some have advocated a daily dose of renal multivitamins.

These considerations are based on expert personal opinion
This table is from: Hothi et al. [11]. *Hemodial Int* is an Open Access journal and the table is used per a Creative Commons licence
BP blood pressure, *HD* haemodialysis, *UF* ultrafiltration

'Really daunting…..'
'I was quite nervy in the beginning…..'
'Massive responsibility….'
'We are parents not medical staff….'

Reassuringly, as families' confidence grows and their sense of competency and self-belief rises they build resilience, and most parents and caregivers rationalise the burden:

'We can fit dialysis around our lives……..'
'The change in our child makes it worth it……'
'The benefits outweigh the negatives…….'

Nonetheless, alone in the community, it is important that home HD families do not feel abandoned.

Clinical Pearls

1. Start with a conservative patient selection criteria until your team's confidence grows.
2. Be realistic about your budget, cohort size and local support structures when designing the infrastructure of your HHD programme.
3. Invest time and resources on your training and education programmes as they will save you time and resources later.
4. Individualise the dialysis prescription to ensure that you can achieve the right balance of meeting the needs of the 'person' and not just the clinical needs of the 'patient'.
5. Develop a robust dialysis access surveillance programme for the families, because access complications can seriously alter the experience of a home HD patient.
6. Draw up an adherence contract for your patients. This is especially important for the teenagers and young adults.
7. Monitor for signs of caregiver burden and treat seriously.

References

1. Eknoyan G, Beck GJ, Cheung AK, Daugirdas JT, Greene T, Kusek JW, Allon M, Bailey J, Delmez JA, Depner TA, Dwyer JT, Levey AS, Levin NW, Milford E, Ornt DB, Rocco MV, Schulman G, Schwab SJ, Teehan BP, Toto R, Hemodialysis (HEMO) Study Group. Effect of dialysis dose and membrane flux in maintenance hemodialysis. N Engl J Med. 2002;347:2010–9.
2. Port FK, Ashby VB, Dhingra RK, Roys EC, Wolfe RA. Dialysis dose and body mass index are strongly associated with survival in hemodialysis patients. J Am Soc Nephrol. 2002;13:1061–6.
3. Saran R, Bragg-Gresham JL, Levin NW, Twardowski ZJ, Wizemann V, Saito A, Kimata N, Gillespie BW, Combe C, Bommer J, Akiba T, Mapes DL, Young EW, Port FK. Longer treatment time and slower ultrafiltration in hemodialysis: associations with reduced mortality in the DOPPS. Kidney Int. 2006;69:1222–8.

4. Marshall MR, Byrne BG, Kerr PG, McDonald SP. Associations of hemodialysis dose and session length with mortality risk in Australian and New Zealand patients. Kidney Int. 2006;69:1229–36.

5. Pauly RP, Gill JS, Rose CL, Asad RA, Chery A, Pierratos A, Chan CT. Survival among nocturnal home haemodialysis patients compared to kidney transplant recipients. Nephrol Dial Transplant. 2009;24:2915–9.

6. Tom A, McCauley L, Bell L, Rodd C, Espinosa P, Yu G, Yu J, Girardin C, Sharma A. Growth during maintenance hemodialysis: impact of enhanced nutrition and clearance. J Pediatr. 1999;134:464–71.

7. Simonsen O. Slow nocturnal dialysis as a rescue treatment for children and young patients with end-stage renal failure. J Am Soc Nephrol. 2000;11:327A.

8. Geary DF, Piva E, Tyrrell J, Gajaria MJ, Picone G, Keating LE, Harvey EA. Home nocturnal hemodialysis in children. J Pediatr. 2005;147:383–7.

9. Hothi DK, Piva E, Keating L, Secker D, Harvey E, Geary D. Calcium and phosphate balance in children on home nocturnal hemodialysis. Pediatr Nephrol. 2006;21:835–41.

10. Goldstein SL, Silverstein DM, Leung JC, Feig DI, Soletsky B, Knight C, Warady BA. Frequent hemodialysis with NxStage system in pediatric patients receiving maintenance hemodialysis. Pediatr Nephrol. 2008;23:129–35.

11. Hothi DK, Stronach L, Sinnott K. Home hemodialysis in children. Hemodial Int. 2016;20(3):349–57.

Chapter 17
Myocardial Stunning

Daljit K. Hothi

Case Presentation

An 8-year-old boy with renal dysplasia slowly progressed to end-stage renal disease (ESRD). Owing to psychosocial concerns and the resultant lack of capacity to conduct home dialysis, he began in-center hemodialysis (HD), receiving 4 h of dialysis, three times per week through a central venous catheter. Whereas he initially had residual renal function, voiding approximately 500 ml of urine per day, within months of initiating HD, his urine output fell, and his ultrafiltration (UF) requirement had to be increased for him to achieve euvolemia at the conclusion of each dialysis session. His pre- and post-dialysis systolic BPs ranged between 110–130 mmHg and 90–115 mmHg, respectively. Almost weekly, he developed intradialytic symptoms such as cramps and headaches associated with tachycardia and a fall in blood pressure. More often than not, this resulted in interrupted UF and on occasion a requirement for a fluid bolus and premature discontinuation of his dialysis session. It was a constant struggle to achieve his dry weight at the end of each dialysis session. An echocardiogram showed good biventricular myocardial function with a left ventricular (LV) ejection fraction of 54% and with mild LV hypertrophy.

In an attempt to optimize his fluid status without precipitating further episodes of intradialytic hypotension (IDH), we adopted a number of treatment strategies, but with variable success. Specifically, we increased his dialysate calcium and bicarbonate concentrations to support his heart during dialysis; we restricted eating to the first 2 h of his dialysis session; and we increased his treatment times by incorporating a 30–60 min period of isolated UF at the end of the HD session.

D.K. Hothi (✉)
Department of Pediatric Nephrology, Great Ormond Street Hospital for Children Foundation Trust, Great Ormond Street, London, UK, WC1N 3JH
e-mail: Daljit.Hothi@gosh.nhs.uk

© Springer International Publishing AG 2017
B.A. Warady et al. (eds.), *Pediatric Dialysis Case Studies*,
DOI 10.1007/978-3-319-55147-0_17

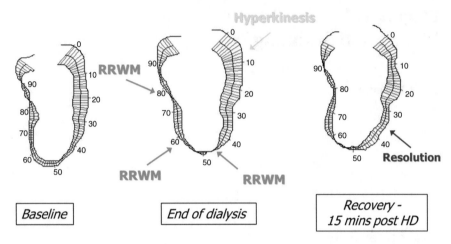

Fig. 17.1 Serial regional wall motion assessment during HD

So as to undertake a more detailed assessment of his myocardial function during his dialysis session, we conducted serial echocardiograms pre-dialysis, during the last 15 min of HD and after concluding the session. The global function, measured by ejection fraction, was normal and was preserved throughout dialysis. Using a traditional method (regional endocardial wall motion, Fig. 17.1) and a novel method (speckle tracking two-dimensional strain, Fig. 17.2), regional LV function was assessed. For both methods, the LV was divided into six segments; however, for the latter assessment, the contraction/relaxation pattern of the LV was followed in three planes: longitudinal, circumferential, and radial. Simplistically, the radial axis describes the torsional, "wringing" motion of the heart; the circumferential axis describes the circular contraction/relaxation motion; and the longitudinal axis describes the "squeezing" motion. Longitudinally directed fibers are mainly located in the subepicardium and subendocardium regions of the LV. They only form a small proportion of the total ventricular myocardial mass but play a major role in the maintenance of a normal ejection fraction. The circumferential fibers have the richest blood supply.

Our patient developed reduced regional wall motion (RRWM) in segments of the LV during dialysis, coexisting with hyperkinesis in other segments of the LV (see Fig. 17.1). This effect was transient with evidence of recovery within 15 min after completing HD. Of note, the patient's BP at the start of dialysis was 125 mmHg systolic and fell to 110 mmHg systolic at the end of the dialysis session.

The 2D speckle analysis did not demonstrate any obvious differences in the peak circumferential and radial strain, and the peak longitudinal strain fell during HD. There was also evidence of dyssynchronous LV segmental function with an obvious variation in the time taken to achieve peak strain over six segments (Fig. 17.2).

HD-induced myocardial stunning prompted us to focus our treatment strategy on preventing IDH. UF rates were limited to 10 ml/kg/hour, necessitating extended

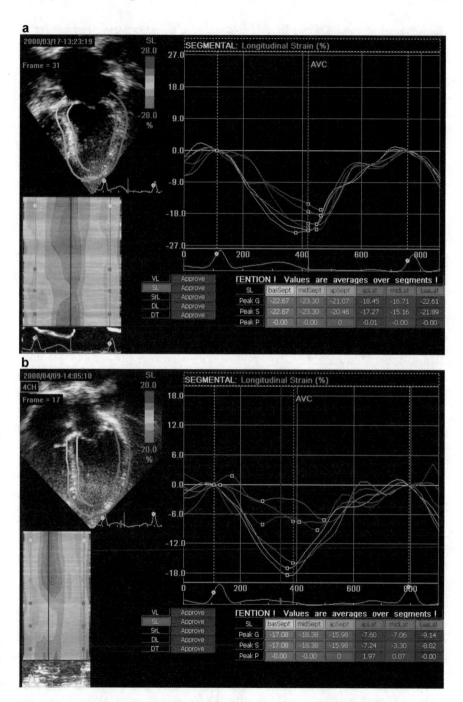

Fig. 17.2 Longitudinal strain curves. (**a**) Pre-dialysis; (**b**) at the end of dialysis

dialysis sessions or additional dialysis sessions to achieve the desired dry weight. In addition, an individualized approach to cooled dialysate was implemented by measuring the patient's tympanic temperature at the start of dialysis and then dropping the dialysate temperature by 0.5 °C from the measured tympanic temperature. After 12 months, the LV hypertrophy had resolved, and the incidence of intradialytic symptoms and hypotension significantly fell. The patient received a renal transplant 6 months later.

Clinical Questions

1. What is myocardial stunning?
2. What evidence is there that myocardial stunning occurs in dialysis patients?
3. What are the consequences of myocardial stunning?
4. Why are patients on hemodialysis prone to myocardial stunning?
5. How does one diagnose myocardial stunning?
6. How can the frequency of myocardial stunning be reduced?

Diagnostic Discussion

1. Myocardial stunning is defined as transient, postischemic LV dysfunction that can persist after the return of normal or near-normal myocardial perfusion [1]. The LV dysfunction can manifest as reduced or absent contraction globally or in discrete parts of the LV.
2. The criteria required to establish the diagnosis of myocardial stunning in the HD patient consist of (i) intradialytic myocardial ischemic injury, (ii) reduced myocardial blood flow, and (iii) segmental or global LV dysfunction. Evidence for all three criteria exists in adult HD patients and, in part, in pediatric patients.

   Conventional, intermittent HD treatments can cause significant hypovolemia and IDH. Elevated biomarkers of myocardial damage have, in turn, been demonstrated in adults and children. Acute elevation of cardiac troponin T levels during HD has been speculated to indicate subclinical myocardial cell injury [2, 3, 4]. Similarly, there are reports of silent ST segment depression during dialysis at rates that vary between 15% and 40% [5].

   The development of RRWMs is indicative of ischemia, and their onset precedes cardiac symptoms and electrocardiographic changes. In 75% of prevalent adult HD patients, RRWMs have been demonstrated, starting 2 h into dialysis, peaking at the time of maximum stress at the end of dialysis, and persisting 30 min post-dialysis in 30% of the patients. A direct correlation has been seen between both the number and intensity of RRWMs and intradialytic BP changes and UF volume [6].

A study of sequential positron emission tomography scans of adults during their HD treatments reported a 13% reduction in global myocardial blood flow 30 min into HD, a period of minimal UF. This was accompanied by a 5% fall in cardiac output, but no change in BP or heart rate. By 220 min, the global myocardial blood flow had fallen 26% on average, with a corresponding 21% drop in cardiac output. These findings were associated with a significant tachycardic response, but a nonsignificant fall in systolic and diastolic BP. The regions of the heart that demonstrated the greatest segmental decline in myocardial blood flow developed new RRWMs by the end of dialysis [7]. The duration of LV dysfunction extended beyond the period of reduced perfusion and was thus more in keeping with myocardial stunning than stress cardiomyopathy.

In children aged between 1 and 17 years and receiving conventional 4 h HD treatments, there has been evidence of transient, regional LV myocardial dysfunction in association with an elevation of plasma cardiac enzymes in 25% of patients [4]. The degree of myocardial dysfunction was associated with the size of the UF volume and the intradialytic BP change [4, 8]. The percentage decline in LV function as measured by peak strain in the longitudinal axis was also predictive of changes in systolic BP during dialysis [8].

3. Myocardial stunning is a concept traditionally associated with adult patients with coronary artery disease. Repeated episodes of ischemia and stunning are cumulative and may lead to more severe and prolonged stunning. Eventually, this scenario may progress to the phenomenon of "myocardial functional hibernation," that is, non-infarcted, scar-free myocardium with fixed myocardial dysfunction.

Myocardial hibernation is thought to represent a functional adaptation to chronic hypoperfusion that can be reversed with restoration of regional myocardial blood flow. If this fails to occur, the hibernating myocardium is highly vulnerable to increases in demand or continued reductions in oxygen supply. The subsequent stresses are cumulative and can result in eventual apoptosis or necrosis and nonviable myocardium with resultant chronic heart failure and arrhythmias.

A longitudinal study of global and regional LV performance in prevalent HD patients, 12 months apart, demonstrated a significant reduction in segmental shortening fraction in those segments that had developed RRWMs at baseline, with 32% developing a fixed reduction in segmental function. Furthermore, segments with a fixed systolic reduction of >60% showed a significant decline in ejection fraction and thus reduced global systolic function. In contrast, there was no significant change in global function in patients who did not develop fixed myocardial segmental function [9].

4. The pathophysiology of uremic cardiac disease is not fully defined, but patients with ESRD are exposed to a number of traditional and nontraditional cardiovascular risk factors.

Mechanical or hemodynamic overload and altered humoral responses are precursors for cardiac remodeling and the development of LV hypertrophy and diastolic dysfunction.

Vasculopathy is evidenced by endothelial dysfunction, increased arterial stiffness, calcification of coronary valves and carotid and coronary arteries, and increased vessel intima-media thickness. Dysregulation of blood pressure control due to abnormal baroreflex sensitivity and vasoregulatory failure translates into an imperfect relationship between blood pressure and cardiac output. UF during HD causes changes in blood volume, blood viscosity, and laminar shear stress, an environment conducive to disordered endothelial cell dynamics and function and ischemic injury.

The coronary arteries provide the blood supply to the myocardium and divide into pre-arterioles with a highly evolved autoregulation capability to ensure that the myocardial blood supply adequately meets the metabolic demand of the heart. There is a degree of reserve within the system, the coronary flow reserve, and this refers to the magnitude of the increase in coronary flow that can be achieved in going from basal coronary perfusion to maximal coronary dilatation. However, the characteristic cardiovascular phenotype in HD patients impairs coronary reserve flow. Thus, in the presence of an increased metabolic demand, such as dialysis, there is a limited ability to increase the oxygen supply to the heart with a resultant demand-supply mismatch. Ischemia prevails and this manifests as regional myocardial dysfunction. Whereas it is impossible to decipher which comes first, the hypotension or the myocardial dysfunction, it is highly probable that the two are self-perpetuating.

5. Practically, it is extremely difficult to make a definitive diagnosis of myocardial stunning in HD patients, as you need to provide evidence of myocardial ischemic injury, reduced myocardial blood flow, and segmental or global LV dysfunction while the patient is on dialysis, as described above.

A practical and reliable compromise is to seek electrocardiographic and/or biochemical evidence of myocardial injury with an ECG at the beginning and the end of dialysis looking for ST segment changes, in addition to obtaining a plasma cardiac troponin T level at the end of dialysis; these studies can be combined with serial echocardiograms throughout the dialysis and post-dialysis periods looking for evidence of regional or global LV dysfunction. Regional wall motion assessment (RWMA) is primarily an assessment in the longitudinal axis and uses the inward motion of endocardial borders as the sole marker of abnormal contraction. In contrast, 2D speckle tracking provides a multi-axis assessment of LV function and is thought to have lower inter- and intra-operator variability.

6. Myocardial stunning is preventable, as well as reversible, and the progression from stunning to myocardial hibernation and additional systemic ischemia injury can be attenuated if BP is monitored throughout dialysis and IDH is prevented. Although several prevention strategies have been deployed in children prone to IDH, the evidence to support their use is very limited. Anecdotally, using bicarbonate buffers, treating intradialytic hypocalcaemia and the avoidance of food during dialysis have positive, but limited benefits. Isolated sequential dialysis and HDF are associated with improved cardiovascular stability, but the mechanisms for this improvement remain unclear. Many believe cooling plays an important part. In fact, adult patients dialyzed against cooled dialysis have demonstrated superior BP control and a reduction in myocardial stunning [10].

There is increasing evidence that the rate of UF and not the UF volume has the greater impact on HD-related morbidity. Protocols for UF need to consider the ultrafiltration rate (UFR) in parallel with plasma refilling rates. In adult patients, an UFR greater than 10 ml/kg/hour is associated with an increased risk of hypotension and mortality [11]. In patients with high UF requirements, automated relative blood volume (RBV) biofeedback techniques or more simply RBV-driven algorithms that adjust UF rates according to RBV changes are proving to be superior in achieving equivalent or higher UF volumes with reduced cardiovascular instability [12] and myocardial stunning [13]. The alternative and technically simpler approach is maintaining a "safer" UFR by extending the dialysis time or the frequency of dialysis. This also translates to improved cardiovascular stability and attenuated myocardial stunning [13].

Clinical Pearls

1. Children who receive chronic HD commonly develop intradialytic hypotension and are at risk for the development of repetitive myocardial ischemic injury with resultant regional or global left ventricular dysfunction.
2. Myocardial stunning is reversible. However, repeated episodes are cumulative and could result in functional myocardial hibernation progressing to fixed myocardial dysfunction and myocardial cell death.
3. Ultrafiltration in the absence of intradialytic hypotension (IDH) should be a guiding principle when prescribing HD.
4. Cooled dialysis is a simple and cost-effective strategy to decrease IDH and has the potential to improve cardiovascular stability and myocardial stunning.
5. Aggressive UFR should be avoided. Euvolemia is best achieved through extended or more frequent HD sessions or RBV-driven algorithms.

References

1. Braunwald E, Kloner RA. The stunned myocardium: prolonged, postischemic ventricular dysfunction. Circulation. 1982;66(6):1146–9.
2. Tarakcioglu M, Erbagci A, Cekmen M, et al. Acute effect of haemodialysis on serum markers of myocardial damage. Int J Clin Pract. 2002;56(5):328–32.
3. Lipshultz SE, Somers MJ, Lipsitz SR, Colan SD, Jabs K, Rifai N. Serum cardiac troponin and subclinical cardiac status in pediatric chronic renal failure. Pediatrics. 2003;112(1 Pt 1):79–86.
4. Hothi DK, Rees L, Marek J, Burton J, McIntyre CW. Pediatric myocardial stunning underscores the cardiac toxicity of conventional hemodialysis treatments. Clin J Am Soc Nephrol. 2009;4(4):790–7.
5. Conlon PJ, Krucoff MW, Minda S, Schumm D, Schwab SJ. Incidence and longterm significance of transient ST segment deviation in hemodialysis patients. Clin Nephrol. 1998;49(4):236–9.

6. McIntyre CW, Burton JO, Selby NM, Leccisotti L, Korsheed S, Baker CS, Camici PG. Hemodialysis-induced cardiac dysfunction is associated with an acute reduction in global and segmental myocardial blood flow. Clin J Am Soc Nephrol. 2008;3(1):19–26.
7. Dasselaar JJ, Slart RH, Knip M, Pruim J, Tio RA, McIntyre CW, de Jong PE, Franssen CF. Haemodialysis is associated with a pronounced fall in myocardial perfusion. Nephrol Dial Transplant. 2009;24(2):604–10.
8. Hothi DK, Rees L, McIntyre CW, Marek J. Hemodialysis-induced acute myocardial dyssynchronous impairment in children. Nephron Clin Pract. 2013;123(1–2):83–92.
9. Burton JO, Jefferies H, Selby NM, McIntyre CW. Hemodialysis-induced cardiac injury: determinants and associated outcomes. Clin J Am Soc Nephrol. 2009;4:914–20.
10. Odudu A, Eldehni MT, McCann GP, McIntyre CW. Randomized controlled trial of individualized dialysate cooling for cardiac protection in hemodialysis patients. Clin J Am Soc Nephrol. 2015;10(8):1408–17.
11. Flythe JE, Brunelli SM. The risks of high ultrafiltration rate in chronic hemodialysis: implications for patient care. Semin Dial. 2011;24(3):259–65.
12. Hothi DK, Harvey E, Goia CM, Geary D. Blood-volume monitoring in paediatric haemodialysis. Pediatr Nephrol. 2008;23(5):813–20.
13. Selby NM, Lambie SH, Camici PG. Occurrence of regional left ventricular dysfunction in patients undergoing standard and biofeedback dialysis. Am J Kidney Dis. 2006;47:830–41.
14. Jefferies HJ, Virk B, Schiller B, Moran J, McIntyre CW. Frequent hemodialysis schedules are associated with reduced levels of dialysis-induced cardiac injury (myocardial stunning). Clin J Am Soc Nephrol. 2011;6(6):1326–32.

Chapter 18
Catheter-Related Bloodstream Infection

Rebecca L. Ruebner and Alicia M. Neu

Case Presentation

A 16-year-old male with end-stage kidney disease (ESRD) maintained on hemodialysis (HD) by way of a tunneled HD catheter in his right femoral vein develops fever and hypotension during his dialysis treatment. He denies a history of rhinorrhea, cough, abdominal pain, nausea, emesis, or diarrhea. He is anuric. He has had no ill contacts. Physical exam reveals no obvious source of infection, and the dialysis catheter exit site is without erythema, warmth, tenderness, or purulent drainage. Blood cultures are obtained from the HD catheter, the dialysis circuit, and a peripheral vein. He receives treatment with intravenous vancomycin and a third-generation cephalosporin in addition to intravenous fluid administration, with stabilization of his blood pressure. He is admitted to the hospital where treatment with intravenous antibiotics is continued.

The patient has ESRD due to congenital nephrotic syndrome. He required a nephrectomy and treatment with peritoneal dialysis in the neonatal period, but had recurrent peritonitis with peritoneal membrane failure prompting conversion to HD by way of a tunneled catheter at 15 months of age. He received a living-related kidney transplant at age 28 months but lost graft function secondary to acute and chronic rejection at age 12 years. He has high levels of antihuman leukocyte antigen antibodies which have thus far prevented repeat kidney transplantation. He was referred for creation of an arteriovenous fistula (AVF) or placement of an arteriovenous graft (AVG) but was felt not to be a candidate given significant central venous stenoses related to numerous prior central venous catheters. He has therefore been receiving HD by way of a central venous catheter. He has had recurrent catheter

R.L. Ruebner (✉) • A.M. Neu
Department of Pediatrics, The Johns Hopkins University School of Medicine,
Baltimore, MD, USA
e-mail: rruebne1@jhmi.edu

© Springer International Publishing AG 2017
B.A. Warady et al. (eds.), *Pediatric Dialysis Case Studies*,
DOI 10.1007/978-3-319-55147-0_18

infections and has exhausted all catheter sites except for his current site in the right femoral vein.

Within 24 h, blood cultures from both the HD catheter and dialysis circuit are positive for methicillin-resistant *Staphylococcus aureus*. Peripheral blood culture is negative. An antibiotic lock with vancomycin is initiated, in addition to ongoing treatment with intravenous vancomycin. The patient is clinically well, without fever after 36 h of antibiotic treatment, but cultures obtained from the catheter continue to grow *S. aureus*. The tunneled femoral hemodialysis catheter is exchanged over a wire and replaced with a non-tunneled catheter. Subsequent blood cultures are negative. After completion of 3 weeks of intravenous vancomycin, the non-tunneled catheter is exchanged over a wire with a tunneled hemodialysis catheter. The patient is discharged home to resume outpatient dialysis.

Clinical Questions

1. What is the definition of an HD access-related bloodstream infection (BSI) and how is it diagnosed?
2. What are the rates of HD access-related BSI in children?
3. What is the recommended treatment of an HD access-related BSI and what is the appropriate management of this child?
4. What is the most effective method to minimize the risk for HD access-related BSI?

Diagnostic Discussion

1. Although ongoing efforts seek to establish a clear and consistent definition of a catheter-related BSI, the most common definition currently used is that developed by the Centers for Disease Control and Prevention (CDC) [1]. According to the CDC, a primary BSI is a laboratory-confirmed BSI that is not secondary to an infection at another body site, and a central line-associated BSI is a laboratory-confirmed BSI where the central line was in place for >2 calendar days on the date of event [1]. The distinction between primary and catheter-associated BSI is important as the management of a positive blood culture due to an infection at another site, e.g., pneumonia, may be different than if the positive culture is reflective of infection of the catheter, particularly with regard to the management of the catheter itself [2]. Thus, diagnosis of an HD access-related BSI requires an assessment for other sites of infection, as well as careful interpretation of the blood culture results. Current guidelines from the Infectious Diseases Society of America (IDSA) suggest that if a catheter-related BSI is suspected, blood cultures should be obtained both from the catheter, after the catheter hub has been cleaned with either alcohol, tincture of iodine, or alcoholic chlorhexidine to

reduce the risk for contamination, and from a peripheral vein [2]. A definitive diagnosis of HD access-related BSI requires that the same organism grows from at least one peripheral culture and from cultures obtained from the catheter [2]. For the BSI to be attributed to the catheter, there should be a quantitative or a differential time to positivity between the cultures from the central line and peripheral vein, with at least a threefold greater colony count from blood cultures obtained from the catheter than the peripheral vein or detection of microbial growth from the catheter culture at least 2 h before the peripheral culture [2]. The IDSA guidelines recognize that there are unique aspects of managing catheters in both pediatric and HD patients, and so the guidelines specify that in HD patients in whom a peripheral venous culture cannot be obtained or is to be avoided to spare vessels for future dialysis access, a second culture may be obtained from the dialysis tubing during a dialysis session [2]. However, the IDSA guidelines recognize that it is unclear if the quantitative differential between catheter and "peripheral" cultures remains if the peripheral culture is obtained from the tubing during a dialysis session [2].

2. Given the evolving definition of an HD access-related BSI, the reported rates of these infections in children vary considerably. In addition, reports in the pediatric nephrology literature typically do not distinguish between a primary BSI and a true HD access-related BSI. Bearing this limitation in mind, previous studies have reported HD access-related BSI in pediatric patients ranging from 0.5 to 4.8 per 1,000 catheter days [3–7]. In addition, registry data have consistently demonstrated that HD access-related BSI is a leading cause of hospitalization and mortality in pediatric dialysis patients [8–10]. Gram-positive organisms account for the majority of HD access-related BSIs, with additional infections caused by gram-negative and fungal organisms [3, 6].

3. Initial management of a pediatric patient with suspected HD access-related BSI includes empiric antibiotics as well as general supportive care. Empiric antibiotic treatment should be guided by the patient's clinical status as well as the antibiogram data from the dialysis unit or hospital and should include both gram-positive and gram-negative coverage [2]. Vancomycin is recommended for empiric gram-positive coverage unless the dialysis unit has a low prevalence of methicillin-resistant *Staphylococcus aureus*, in which case cefazolin may be used [2, 11]. An aminoglycoside or third-generation cephalosporin should be used for gram-negative coverage [2, 11]. Although catheter removal is generally recommended in the setting of a catheter-associated BSI, it is recognized that in HD patients, the catheter provides access for ongoing life-sustaining dialysis, and additional vascular access sites may be limited. The potential treatment options in this setting are shown in Fig. 18.1 and include (1) intravenous antibiotics alone, (2) prompt catheter removal with placement of a new catheter after some interval of time, (3) exchange of the catheter over a guidewire, or (4) use of systemic antibiotics and an antibiotic lock [2]. Catheter removal is indicated in any clinically unstable patient and in patients who remain symptomatic for more than 36 h [2]. In patients with symptomatic improvement, catheter removal and replacement, catheter exchange, or the use of antibiotic locks should be

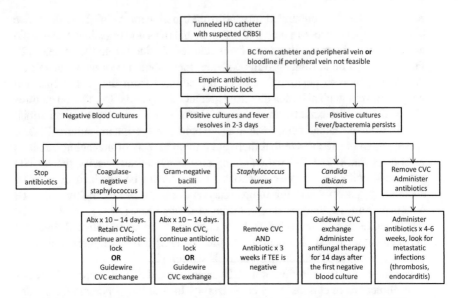

Fig. 18.1 Approach to treatment of catheter-related bloodstream infection (CRBSI) among patients who are undergoing hemodialysis (HD) with tunneled catheters. *BC* blood culture, *CVC* central venous catheter, *TEE* transesophageal echocardiograph [2] (Reprinted with permission)

considered in addition to systemic antibiotics, as data in adult HD patients demonstrate a fivefold higher rate of treatment failure with antibiotics alone compared to catheter removal [2, 11]. In particular, catheter removal with placement of a temporary catheter in another anatomical site, or catheter exchange over a wire if no alternative sites are available, is strongly recommended for HD access-related BSI due to *Staphylococcus aureus*, *Pseudomonas* species, or *Candida* species [2]. The IDSA specifically states that the indications for catheter removal for children are similar to those for adults, but acknowledge that the difficulty in obtaining alternate vascular access sites in children often necessitates antibiotic treatment without catheter removal [2]. If the decision is made to keep the existing catheter, the addition of antibiotic locks to systemic antibiotics has been shown to improve catheter survival and decrease exposure to systemic antibiotics, with some studies showing particular success in treating gram-negative infections compared to infections with *Staphylococcus aureus* [12–14]. This approach may be particularly useful for patients with limited vascular access sites in whom preservation of the existing catheter is crucial. The ultimate choice of antibiotic and duration of therapy will be based on the causative organism, the clinical course of the patient, and adjunctive therapies including removal/replacement of the catheter (Fig. 18.1) [2].

4. National and international registry data have consistently demonstrated that use of a central venous catheter rather than an AVF or AVG is associated with a significantly increased risk for infection among pediatric HD patients [10, 15–17].

Current guidelines therefore recommend the use of an AVF/AVG for HD access in children unless the patient weighs less than 20 kg, a kidney transplant is planned within 1–2 years, or HD is serving as a bridge to PD [16, 18]. Although use of an AVF/AVG is the most effective way to minimize the risk for infection, the vast majority of children continue to receive HD by way of a central venous catheter [9, 17, 19]. Given the significant morbidity and mortality associated with HD catheter-related BSI in the United States, the CDC has launched the Dialysis Bloodstream Infection Prevention Collaborative which includes recommended practices for HD catheter care, such as cleaning the catheter exit site with an antiseptic agent, preferably chlorhexidine, and use of antimicrobial ointment at the exit site with each dressing change [20]. The CDC's core interventions also include enforcing proper hand hygiene and scrubbing of the catheter hub with an antiseptic agent when it is accessed and disconnected from the dialysis tubing [20]. Studies in adult HD patients have also shown a reduction in BSI when prophylactic antibiotic locks (such as citrate with gentamicin) are used for routine catheter maintenance compared to standard heparin locks, although there are limited data on the use of prophylactic antibiotic locks in pediatric HD patients [21, 22]. While some of the current recommendations are evidence based, others reflect expert opinion. Currently, the Children's Hospital Association's Standardizing Care to Improve Outcomes in Pediatric End Stage Renal Disease (SCOPE) Collaborative is evaluating whether increased implementation of standardized catheter practices, modeled in large part after the CDC core interventions, can reduce HD access-related BSI in children maintained on chronic dialysis at participating centers located throughout the United States [23].

Clinical Pearls

1. Hemodialysis access-related BSIs are a significant source of morbidity and mortality in children with end-stage kidney disease.
2. The most effective strategy to minimize risk for HD access-related BSI is the use of an arteriovenous fistula or graft, but the majority of children continue to receive dialysis by way of a catheter.
3. Definitive diagnosis of an HD access-related BSI requires careful examination for other sites of infection and thoughtful review of blood culture results.
4. Empiric treatment of HD access-related BSI should include both gram-positive and gram-negative coverage and should be guided by the patient's clinical status and local antibiogram data.
5. Catheter removal should be considered in clinically unstable patients or in HD access-related BSI due to *Pseudomonas* species, *Staphylococcus aureus*, and *Candida* species.

References

1. O'Grady NP, Alexander M Burns LA, Dellinger EP, Garland J, Heard SO, Lipsett PA, Masur H, Mermel LA, Pearson ML, Raad II, Randolph AG, Rupp ME, Saint S. Healthcare Infection Control Practices Advisory Committee. Guidelines for the prevention of intravascular catheter-related infections. 2011. http://www.cdc.gov/hicpac/pdf/guidelines/bsi-guidelines-2011.pdf. Accessed 18 Apr 2016.
2. Mermel LA, Allon M, Bouza E, Craven DE, Flynn P, O'Grady NP, et al. Clinical practice guidelines for the diagnosis and management of intravascular catheter-related infection: 2009 update by the Infectious Diseases Society of America. Clin Infect Dis. 2009;49(1):1–45.
3. Araya CE, Fennell RS, Neiberger RE, Dharnidharka VR. Hemodialysis catheter-related bacteremia in children: increasing antibiotic resistance and changing bacteriological profile. Am J Kidney Dis. 2007;50(1):119–23.
4. Eisenstein I, Tarabeih M, Magen D, Pollack S, Kassis I, Ofer A, et al. Low infection rates and prolonged survival times of hemodialysis catheters in infants and children. Clin J Am Soc Nephrol. 2011;6(4):793–8.
5. Kovalski Y, Cleper R, Krause I, Davidovits M. Hemodialysis in children weighing less than 15 kg: a single-center experience. Pediatr Nephrol. 2007;22(12):2105–10.
6. Onder AM, Chandar J, Coakley S, Abitbol C, Montane B, Zilleruelo G. Predictors and outcome of catheter-related bacteremia in children on chronic hemodialysis. Pediatr Nephrol. 2006;21(10):1452–8.
7. Paglialonga F, Esposito S, Edefonti A, Principi N. Catheter-related infections in children treated with hemodialysis. Pediatr Nephrol. 2004;19(12):1324–33.
8. Lofaro D, Vogelzang JL, van Stralen KJ, Jager KJ, Groothoff JW. Infection-related hospitalizations over 30 years of follow-up in patients starting renal replacement therapy at pediatric age. Pediatr Nephrol. 2016;31(2):315–23.
9. NAPRTCS. 2011 annual dialysis report. http:www.emmes.com/study/ped/. Accessed 18 Apr 2016.
10. United States Renal Data System. 2015 USRDS annual data report: epidemiology of kidney disease in the United States. National Institutes of Health, National Institute of Diabetes and Digestive and Kidney Diseases, Bethesda, 2015.
11. Allon M. Treatment guidelines for dialysis catheter-related bacteremia: an update. Am J Kidney Dis. 2009;54(1):13–7.
12. Krishnasami Z, Carlton D, Bimbo L, Taylor ME, Balkovetz DF, Barker J, et al. Management of hemodialysis catheter-related bacteremia with an adjunctive antibiotic lock solution. Kidney Int. 2002;61(3):1136–42.
13. Onder AM, Billings AA, Chandar J, Nield L, Francoeur D, Simon N, et al. Antibiotic lock solutions allow less systemic antibiotic exposure and less catheter malfunction without adversely affecting antimicrobial resistance patterns. Hemodial Int. 2013;17(1):75–85.
14. Poole CV, Carlton D, Bimbo L, Allon M. Treatment of catheter-related bacteraemia with an antibiotic lock protocol: effect of bacterial pathogen. Nephrol Dial Transplant. 2004;19(5):1237–44.
15. Fadrowski JJ, Hwang W, Frankenfield DL, Fivush BA, Neu AM, Furth SL. Clinical course associated with vascular access type in a national cohort of adolescents who receive hemodialysis: findings from the clinical performance measures and US renal data system projects. Clin J Am Soc Nephrol. 2006;1(5):987–92.
16. National Kidney Foundation. KDOQI clinical practice guidelines and clinical practice recommendations for 2006 updates: hemodialysis adequacy, peritoneal dialysis adequacy and vascular access. Am J Kidney Dis. 2006;48(Suppl1):S1–S322.
17. Hayes WN, Watson AR, Callaghan N, Wright E, Stefanidis CJ, European Pediatric Dialysis Working G. Vascular access: choice and complications in European paediatric haemodialysis units. Pediatr Nephrol. 2012;27(6):999–1004.

18. Fischbach M, Edefonti A, Schroder C, Watson A, European Pediatric Dialysis Working G. Hemodialysis in children: general practical guidelines. Pediatr Nephrol. 2005;20(8):1054–66.
19. Fadrowski JJ, Hwang W, Neu AM, Fivush BA, Furth SL. Patterns of use of vascular catheters for hemodialysis in children in the United States. Am J Kidney Dis. 2009;53(1):91–8.
20. Centers for Disease Control and Prevention Dialysis Bloodstream Infection (BSI) Prevention Collaborative. http://www.cdc.gov/dialysis/collaborative. Accessed 18 Apr 2016.
21. Moore CL, Besarab A, Ajluni M, Soi V, Peterson EL, Johnson LE, et al. Comparative effectiveness of two catheter locking solutions to reduce catheter-related bloodstream infection in hemodialysis patients. Clin J Am Soc Nephrol. 2014;9(7):1232–9.
22. Moran J, Sun S, Khababa I, Pedan A, Doss S, Schiller B. A randomized trial comparing gentamicin/citrate and heparin locks for central venous catheters in maintenance hemodialysis patients. Am J Kidney Dis. 2012;59(1):102–7.
23. Children's Hospital Associations Standardizing Care to Improve Outcomes in Pediatric ESRD (SCOPE) Collaborative. https://www.childrenshospitals.org/Programs-and-Services/Quality-Improvement-and-Measurement/Collaboratives/SCOPE. Accessed 18 Apr 2016.

Chapter 19
Intradialytic Hypotension: Potential Causes and Mediating Factors

Lyndsay A. Harshman, Steven R. Alexander, and Patrick D. Brophy

Case Presentation

A 13-year-old, 50 kg male was 20 days status post second bone marrow transplant (BMT) when he developed symptoms of intradialytic hypotension, tremulousness, disorientation, and garbled speech.

The patient's past history was significant for refractory acute myelogenous leukemia (AML) secondary to juvenile myelomonocytic leukemia (JMML), for which he received his first BMT. He developed non-oliguric end-stage renal disease (ESRD) as a sequelae from several episodes of acute kidney injury, multiple nephrotoxin exposures, and tumor lysis syndrome. He was maintained on thrice-weekly hemodialysis (HD). He subsequently required a second BMT following his lack of response to re-induction chemotherapy for relapsed AML/JMML. The conditioning regimen for his second BMT included dose-reduced total body irradiation.

His clinical course leading to the second BMT was significant for the long-term use of systemic corticosteroids for chronic skin and gut graft-versus-host disease. He was malnourished but refused enteral feeding support and had received daily parenteral nutrition for 2 months prior to the second BMT. He often refused multiple prescribed medications, although he was adherent with his primary medications, such as immunosuppression.

On BMT 2 transplant day 20, while receiving routine thrice-weekly intermittent hemodialysis (IHD), he experienced an acute drop in blood pressure to 70/30 mmHg with associated dizziness and blurred vision. His weight prior to IHD had been

L.A. Harshman (✉) • P.D. Brophy
Stead Family Department of Pediatrics and Division of Pediatric Nephrology, University of Iowa Stead Family Children's Hospital, Iowa City, IA, USA
e-mail: lyndsay-harshman@uiowa.edu

S.R. Alexander
Division of Pediatric Nephrology, Department of Pediatrics, Stanford University School of Medicine, Lucile Packard Children's Hospital Stanford, Stanford, CA, USA

© Springer International Publishing AG 2017
B.A. Warady et al. (eds.), *Pediatric Dialysis Case Studies*,
DOI 10.1007/978-3-319-55147-0_19

141

50 kg which was stable and felt to be his target dry weight. Hypotension was marginally responsive to 1,500 mL normal saline fluid resuscitation. He was transferred to the pediatric intensive care unit (PICU) for further management. His laboratory evaluation included serum chemistries (sodium 134 mEq/L, potassium 5.6 mEq/L, chloride 90 mEq/L, bicarbonate 19 mEq/L), accompanied by a significant elevation in serum lactate to 9.7 mEq/L (normal = 2.2 mEq/L) with blood pH of 7.41. He was transiently febrile during the hypotensive event and received broad-spectrum antibiotic coverage; a sepsis workup was subsequently negative for fungal or bacterial infection. He required multiple pressor support including vasopressin and norepinephrine. The serum lactate continued to be elevated during the 24 h following PICU admission to 12.6 mEq/L while on pressor support. Mixed venous oxygen saturation (SVO2) remained excellent at 70–75%.

IHD was again attempted 48 h later when his blood pressure had been stabilized with inotropic support. The hemodialysis prescription utilized a saline prime and net zero ultrafiltration; however, there were still abrupt drops in blood pressure to 80–90/35–40 mmHg despite receiving continuous pressor and colloid infusions. The clinical exam in the subsequent 24 h was notable for progressive deterioration in neurological status with disorientation to place and time, intention tremor with garbled speech, and clonus on exam. He began mumbling and talking to himself, in addition to picking at unseen objects in space. With significant redirection he could follow some simple commands. He was lethargic and difficult to arouse at times. Other systemic complaints included persistent dizziness and abdominal pain with emesis.

Given the persistent elevation in lactate accompanied by a worsening neurological status, the patient was empirically administered IV thiamine due to a concern for possible Wernicke encephalopathy. Within 4 h of thiamine infusion, he had notable clinical improvement with a decrease in the serum lactate (decrease from 12.6 to 2.7 mEq/L) level and the disappearance of tremors. A thiamine level was ordered prior to the administration of thiamine, but unfortunately was not performed by the laboratory due to the presence of "interfering substances" in the blood sample. Further history revealed that the patient had been noncompliant with enteral vitamin B supplementation in the weeks leading to his onset of symptoms, and in addition, his vitamin B supplementation via the parenteral route was discontinued during the course of his hospital stay due to the perception that he was prescribed (and receiving) sufficient B vitamins orally.

Clinical Questions

1. What is the differential diagnosis for intradialytic hypotension in a pediatric HD patient?
2. What "common" diagnoses could explain the neurological symptoms exhibited by this dialysis patient? How would you approach the diagnosis of these acute neurological changes?

3. How do you explain the patient's persistent, fluid nonresponsive hypotension, especially in the setting of an elevated lactate level?
4. Describe alternative strategies for stabilizing intradialytic hypotension in the non-acute setting.

Diagnostic Discussion

1. There are many potential causes of intradialytic hypotension in a dialysis patient with more common etiologies including administration of antihypertensive medications prior to therapy, eating while on hemodialysis (with resultant splanchnic vasodilation), and/or failure to correct intradialytic hypocalcemia (see Table 19.1).

   While simultaneously evaluating for causes of hypotension, action should be taken to reduce or prevent any further acute drops in blood pressure and the development of associated complications. These actions may include suspension of the ultrafiltration rate, a 5–10 mL/kg normal saline fluid bolus, and/or discontinuation of HD in cases resistant to conservative maneuvers. Table 19.2 summarizes consequences and moderators of intradialytic hypotension in the pediatric hemodialysis patient.
2. Neurological symptoms in combination with intradialytic hypotension are cardinal features of cerebrovascular events, such as stroke or seizure. The approach to diagnosis should include head imaging (computed tomography) and/or electroencephalogram. The remainder of the investigation should take into consideration alternative etiologies, including infectious causes (with associated mental status changes) such as CNS infection, abscess, and venous sinus thrombosis.

Table 19.1 Differential diagnosis of acute intradialytic hypotension

1. Emergent medical causes
Sepsis
Cerebrovascular: stroke, seizure, venous sinus thrombosis
Cardiac: arrhythmia
Pulmonary: air/thromboembolism
New/occult hemorrhage (consider if patient receiving systemic anticoagulation)
2. Dialysis-mediated causes
Rapid ultrafiltration in excess of vascular refilling
Significant patient intradialytic weight gain (perceived need for excessive ultrafiltration rate)
Inadequate dialysis solution temperature (excessive vasodilation)
Use of antihypertensive medication (vasodilators) prior to treatment
Food ingestion on therapy
Poorly treated anemia of renal disease

Table 19.2 Consequences and moderators of intradialytic hypotension

Consequences	Moderators
Intradialytic symptoms	Withhold antihypertensive medications on dialysis days
Suspension of UF with resultant chronic hypervolemia	Avoid food intake during dialysis

Premature discontinuation of treatment and inadequate dialysis	Dialysate
	  Bicarbonate buffer
	  Higher dialysate calcium
	  Sodium profiling

Accelerated decline in residual renal function Mesenteric ischemia	UF profiling

Cerebrovascular
  Transient ischemic attacks
  Stroke
	Periods of isolated UF
	Cooled dialysate

Cardiovascular
  Regional LV dysfunction
  Ischemic cardiomyopathy progressing to heart failure
  Increased risk of arrhythmias
	Pre-dialysis or intradialytic midodrine
	Biofeedback dialysis
	RBV-driven UF algorithms
	Alternative dialysis regimens
	  Short daily dialysis
	  Hemodiafiltration
	  Prolonged/nocturnal HD

From *Pediatric Dialysis* Ed 2, Chap. 21, pp. 355

3. The differential diagnosis for persistent, fluid nonresponsive hypotension in a critically ill dialysis patient (particularly when associated with an elevated lactate level) should include:

   (a) Adrenal insufficiency
   (b) Nutritional deficiency or excess

   Adrenal insufficiency is a well-documented cause of fluid refractory hypotension in critically ill patients. Given our patient's history of total body irradiation (required for BMT conditioning), he was prone to panhypopituitarism along with secondary cortisol deficiency [1]. Similarly, he displayed evidence of glucocorticoid deficiency given euvolemic hyponatremia and hyperkalemia. Our patient's hypotension and electrolyte abnormalities improved with provision of stress-dose steroids, but serum lactate levels remained elevated.

   The most commonly considered etiologies for an elevated serum lactate level in critically ill patients are cardiac and infectious in nature; however, numerous other causes exist for an elevation of lactate, with or without acidemia (Table 19.3). Dialysis patients are at risk for nutritional deficiency, particularly water-soluble B vitamins. This risk is augmented in states of critical illness. Thiamine deficiency in the dialysis patient is a known, but rare, complication of both intermittent hemodialysis and peritoneal dialysis [2, 3]. In a thiamine-free diet, the body storage is sufficient for around 20 days in a normal adult; such a

Table 19.3 Causes of elevated serum lactate

Shock	Pharmacological agents
Distributive	Linezolid
Cardiogenic	Nucleoside reverse transcriptase inhibitors
Hypovolemic	Metformin
Obstructive	Epinephrine
Post-cardiac arrest	Propofol
Regional tissue ischemia	Acetaminophen
Mesenteric ischemia	Beta-2 agonists
Limb ischemia	Theophylline
Burns	Anaerobic muscle activity
Trauma	Seizures
Compartment syndrome	Heavy exercise
Necrotizing tissue infection	Excessive work of breathing
Diabetic ketoacidosis	Thiamine deficiency
Drugs/toxins	Malignancy
Alcohols	Liver failure
Cocaine	Mitochondrial disease
Carbon monoxide	
Cyanide	

From Andersen et al. [10]

requirement is increased in patients with a high metabolic rate or high carbohydrate intake, such as those being given a dextrose-based parenteral nutritional
formula [4, 5].

The presentation of thiamine (vitamin B1) deficiency is classically characterized by the triad of confusion, ophthalmoplegia, and ataxia – the so-called
Wernicke encephalopathy. Critical thiamine deficiency is associated with an
elevation of serum lactate without acidosis. Thiamine deficiency can directly
lead to hypotension and shock via cardiac dysfunction (also known as "wet beri-
beri"). The diagnosis can be difficult in the dialysis patient and may lead to con-
founding diagnoses associated with intradialytic hypotension such as sepsis,
seizure, and/or cerebrovascular disease (specifically stroke) [6, 7]. While the provision of IV thiamine can rapidly correct the deficient state and the associated
symptoms, it is critical to realize that magnesium is a necessary component for
the conversion of thiamine into thiamine pyrophosphate [8]. Thus, thiamine
replacement should occur together with magnesium administration. Other
sources of nutritional deficiency or excess that may lead to intradialytic hypotension include carnitine deficiency and hypermagnesemia. Hemodialysis patients
are at risk for progressive L (levo)-carnitine deficiency due to dialytic losses,
similar to that of water-soluble B vitamins [9]. Carnitine deficiency may manifest as intradialytic, poorly fluid-responsive hypotension with muscle cramping.
This amino acid derivative is essential for normal oxidative function within the

mitochondrial membrane of cardiac and endothelial cells. Supplementation with L-carnitine is typically therapeutic. Hypermagnesemia in the ESRD population (typically via inadvertent parenteral nutritional supplementation) causes profound vasodilation with fluid refractory hypotension, although this is correctable with clearance of magnesium by dialysis.

4. For the patient with persistent (chronic) intradialytic hypotension with no clear clinical or laboratory etiology for the disorder, there are alternative strategies for stabilizing the intradialytic blood pressure via the use of sodium profiling and/or ultrafiltration (UF) profiling. Sodium profiling is characterized by the use of a higher dialysate sodium concentration at dialysis initiation, with a decrease in the sodium concentration to 138 mEq/L at the end of the dialysis session, in order to allow stability of the intradialytic blood volume, along with a reduction in intradialytic cramping and fatigue [11]. Similarly, UF profiling – whereby the UF rate at the beginning of the dialysis session is high and is then progressively reduced – may yield improvement as long as the UF goal is not in excess of 10 mL/kg/h; initial, excessively high UF rates/requirements can be counterproductive in preventing hypotensive episodes [12, 13].

It is reasonable to consider a trial of midodrine to palliate symptoms associated with chronic intradialytic hypotension as well. Midodrine is a peripheral alpha-adrenergic receptor agonist that is taken ~30–60 min prior to HD, with a peak effect 60 min after medication ingestion. The standard adult oral dose of midodrine is 10 mg. There is no standard pediatric dosing. Case reports document the use of 1.25 mg in infants (unpublished experience) and 2.5–5 mg in prepubertal/adolescent patients [14].

Finally, dialysate cooling has been reported as useful therapy for symptomatic intradialytic hypotension. This approach takes account of the fact that body temperature rises during standard dialysis, likely related to a combination of factors associated with the transfer of heat to the patient from the dialysate warmer, as well as a consequence of the subtle inflammatory response of patient blood contacting the dialysis membrane [15]. Cooling of dialysate can be effectively used alone or in combination with sodium profiling and/or midodrine as described above [16]. A variety of cooling temperatures have been reported as effective, generally ranging from 35 to 36.5 °C. Data suggest that cooling of dialysate does not adversely affect dialysis adequacy, and patient-reported symptoms related to cooling of dialysate are usually well tolerated [17].

Clinical Pearls

1. There are a multitude of causes leading to intradialytic hypotension in the pediatric patient. A thorough and targeted approach should be taken to ensure that easily corrected concerns can be addressed. In cases of acute intradialytic hypotension, evaluation should first rule out emergent new medical conditions that mandate prompt intervention (see Table 19.3).

2. Thiamine deficiency and adrenal insufficiency are rare causes of intradialytic hypotension, but should be carefully considered in the differential diagnosis of intradialytic hypotension in the HD patient who shows poor fluid responsiveness, elevation of serum lactate, and/or neurological changes. Critically ill patients on HD are particularly at risk for thiamine deficiency because of preexistent malnutrition, increased consumption of thiamine in high carbohydrate nutrition, and accelerated clearance as a result of renal replacement therapy.
3. Sodium profiling, ultrafiltration profiling, midodrine therapy, and cooled dialysate have all been shown to modify or correct intradialytic hypotension in patients on HD.

References

1. Vantyghem MC, Douillard C, Balavoine AS. Hypotension from endocrine origin. Presse Med. 2012;41(11):1137–50. doi:10.1016/j.lpm.2012.03.023.
2. Ueda K, Takada D, Mii A, Tsuzuku Y, Saito SK, Kaneko T, et al. Severe thiamine deficiency resulted in Wernicke's encephalopathy in a chronic dialysis patient. Clin Exp Nephrol. 2006;10(4):290–3. doi:10.1007/s10157-006-0440-9.
3. Barbara PG, Manuel B, Elisabetta M, Giorgio S, Fabio T, Valentina C, et al. The suddenly speechless florist on chronic dialysis: the unexpected threats of a flower shop? Diagnosis: dialysis related Wernicke encephalopathy. Nephrol Dial Transplant. 2006;21(1):223–5. doi:10.1093/ndt/gfh990.
4. Sequeira Lopes da Silva JT, Almaraz Velarde R, Olgado Ferrero F, Robles Marcos M, Perez Civantos D, Ramirez Moreno JM, et al. Wernicke's encephalopathy induced by total parental nutrition. Nutr Hosp. 2010;25(6):1034–6. Epub 2011/04/27
5. Francini-Pesenti F, Brocadello F, Manara R, Santelli L, Laroni A, Caregaro L. Wernicke's syndrome during parenteral feeding: not an unusual complication. Nutrition. 2009;25(2):142–6. doi:10.1016/j.nut.2008.08.003.
6. Hung SC, Hung SH, Tarng DC, Yang WC, Chen TW, Huang TP. Thiamine deficiency and unexplained encephalopathy in hemodialysis and peritoneal dialysis patients. Am J Kidney Dis Off J Natl Kidney Found. 2001;38(5):941–7. doi:10.1053/ajkd.2001.28578.
7. Descombes E, Dessibourg CA, Fellay G. Acute encephalopathy due to thiamine deficiency (Wernicke's encephalopathy) in a chronic hemodialyzed patient: a case report. Clin Nephrol. 1991;35(4):171–5.
8. Dyckner T, Ek B, Nyhlin H, Wester PO. Aggravation of thiamine deficiency by magnesium depletion. A case report. Acta Med Scand. 1985;218(1):129–31.
9. Lynch KE, Feldman HI, Berlin JA, Flory J, Rowan CG, Brunelli SM. Effects of L-carnitine on dialysis-related hypotension and muscle cramps: a meta-analysis. Am J Kidney Dis. 2008;52(5):962–71. doi:10.1053/j.ajkd.2008.05.031. PMID: WOS:000260556000019
10. Andersen LW, Mackenhauer J, Roberts JC, Berg KM, Cocchi MN, Donnino MW. Etiology and therapeutic approach to elevated lactate levels. Mayo Clin Proc. 2013;88(10):1127–40. doi:10.1016/j.mayocp.2013.06.012. PMID: 24079682; PubMed Central PMCID: PMC3975915
11. Sadowski RH, Allred EN, Jabs K. Sodium modeling ameliorates intradialytic and interdialytic symptoms in young hemodialysis patients. J Am Soc Nephrol JASN. 1993;4(5):1192–8.
12. Hothi DK, Harvey E, Goia CM, Geary DF. Evaluating methods for improving ultrafiltration in pediatric hemodialysis. Pediatr Nephrol. 2008;23(4):631–8. doi:10.1007/s00467-007-0716-7.
13. Saran R, Bragg-Gresham JL, Levin NW, Twardowski ZJ, Wizemann V, Saito A, et al. Longer treatment time and slower ultrafiltration in hemodialysis: associations with reduced mortality in the DOPPS. Kidney Int. 2006;69(7):1222–8. doi:10.1038/sj.ki.5000186.

14. Hothi DK, Harvey E, Goia CM, Geary D. The value of sequential dialysis, mannitol and midodrine in managing children prone to dialysis failure. Pediatr Nephrol. 2009;24(8):1587–91. doi:10.1007/s00467-009-1151-8.
15. Lindholm T, Thysell H, Yamamoto Y, Forsberg B, Gullberg CA. Temperature and vascular stability in hemodialysis. Nephron. 1985;39(2):130–3.
16. Cruz DN, Mahnensmith RL, Brickel HM, Perazella MA. Midodrine and cool dialysate are effective therapies for symptomatic intradialytic hypotension. Am J Kidney Dis Off J Natl Kidney Found. 1999;33(5):920–6.
17. Selby NM, McIntyre CW. A systematic review of the clinical effects of reducing dialysate fluid temperature. Nephrol Dial Transplant. 2006;21(7):1883–98. doi:10.1093/ndt/gfl126.
18. Giacalone M, Martinelli R, Abramo A, Rubino A, Pavoni V, Iacconi P, et al. Rapid reversal of severe lactic acidosis after thiamine administration in critically ill adults: a report of 3 cases. Nutr Clin Pract. 2015;30(1):104–10. doi:10.1177/0884533614561790.

Chapter 20
Dialyzer Reaction

Elizabeth Harvey

Case Presentation

Bridget is a 15-year-old, 50 kg teenager with end-stage renal disease secondary to steroid-resistant focal segmental glomerulosclerosis (FSGS) with negative genetic workup. When she commenced hemodialysis, her medications included ramipril (for hypertension and anti-proteinuric effect), calcium carbonate, calcitriol, furosemide, cholecalciferol, iron, and darbepoetin.

Due to a precipitous decline in renal function, hemodialysis is initiated via a right internal jugular Tal Palindrome™ (Medtronic, Minneapolis, MN) double-lumen central venous catheter. Her chronic dialysis prescription is four treatments per week for 4 h each. Her initial dialysis prescription is with Dialyzer A (Table 20.1) with a total extracorporeal circuit volume of 250 ml.

The prescription for her seventh dialysis session is:

Blood flow: 250 ml/min.
Time: 4 h.
Anticoagulation: heparin.
Dialysate composition: see Table 20.2.

E. Harvey (✉)
Department of Pediatrics, Division of Nephrology, Hospital for Sick Children,
University of Toronto, Toronto, ON, Canada
e-mail: elizabeth.harvey@sickkids.ca

© Springer International Publishing AG 2017
B.A. Warady et al. (eds.), *Pediatric Dialysis Case Studies*,
DOI 10.1007/978-3-319-55147-0_20

Table 20.1 Dialyzer characteristics

	Dialyzer A	Dialyzer B
Membrane	Polysulfone	Polysulfone
Priming volume (ml)	110	112 ml
Surface area (m²)	1.8	2.0
KUF (ml/h/mmHg TMP)	55	62
Sterilization method	Ethylene oxide	Electron beam
Housing	Polycarbonate	Polycarbonate
Potting compound	Polyurethane	Polyurethane

Table 20.2 Dialysate composition

Dialysate parameter	SI units	Conventional units
Prescribed sodium	138 mmol/l	138 mEq/L
Potassium	2 mmol/l	2 mEq/L
Bicarbonate	35 mmol/l	35 mEq/L
Calcium	1.5 mmol/l	3 mEq/L
Sodium ramp	Linear: 141–136 mmol/l	Linear: 141–136 mEq/L

Part 1

Five minutes after commencing her dialysis session, Bridget becomes acutely unwell complaining of chest tightness, difficulty breathing, and headache. She is noted to be wheezing, tachycardic (HR 150 bpm), and hypotensive (BP 85/30 mmHg) and to have developed an urticarial rash over her trunk and extremities. Her oxygen saturation falls to 75%.

Clinical Questions

1. What is the appropriate course of action?
2. How are dialyzer reactions classified?
3. What are the possible causes of this type of allergic reaction?

Diagnostic Discussion

1. *Response to an anaphylactic reaction on hemodialysis:* The response to an ana-phylactic reaction on hemodialysis includes the initial response and supportive care, followed by an attempt to identify the potential allergen with stepwise removal of possible offending agents [1].

   (a) *Initial response*

   Initial management consists of immediate *cessation of dialysis without retransfusion* to avoid further exposure to presumed allergens. As there is overlap in the clinical presentation of several adverse events on dialysis (e.g., hypersensitivity reaction, hemolysis, sepsis/pyrogenic reaction, air embolism), and the cause of the patient's deterioration may not be immediately apparent, the circuit should be saved to examine later for potential causes of the reaction (e.g., kinked tubing causing hemolysis, cracked tubing or loose connections causing air embolism, expired dialyzer, sterilization method, etc.).

Blood should be taken for complete blood count, white blood cell differential, routine biochemistry (electrolytes, urea, creatinine, calcium, phosphate), blood culture, IgE levels, and C3. Bloodwork will help ascertain if dialysis is required imminently once the patient is stabilized and may give clues as to the etiology of the event.

(b) *Supportive care*

Bridget is removed from dialysis without retransfusion of the circuit and receives the following management [2]:

(i) Oxygen: high-flow oxygen via non-rebreather mask with the concentration titrated to an O2 saturation > 95%
(ii) Diphenhydramine: 1 mg/kg intravenously
(iii) Hydrocortisone: 5 mg/kg IV
(iv) Epinephrine: 1:1,000 (1 mg/ml) 0.5 ml (0.5 mg) IM
(v) Salbutamol: 1 ml (5 mg) in 3 ml saline via inhalation
(vi) Saline 10 ml/kg bolus due to hypotension

(c) *Attempt to identify the potential allergen:* Potential sources of allergy during hemodialysis include components of the dialyzer, the dialysate, the dialysis tubing, the sterilizing agent, and medications administered during the dialysis session, most notably heparin, iron, and darbepoetin [3]. Additionally, certain medications taken by the patient may precipitate severe reactions with the dialysis membrane, such as the bradykinin release reaction seen in patients taking angiotensin-converting enzyme (ACE) inhibitors during dialysis with a polyacrylonitrile AN69 membrane [4].

A dialyzer consists of a membrane, the dialyzer housing, the potting compound into which the hollow fibers are embedded, and the manufacturer's sterilizing agent, as well as any residual sterilizing chemicals for reused dialyzers. Patients may react to any component of the dialyzer, but membrane reactions are far less common with the biocompatible synthetic membranes in widespread use today. Dialysate contaminated with bacteria or endotoxin may be a source of reaction, especially with high-flux membranes. Finally, severe reactions caused by contaminated heparin have been described [5].

Recognizing the possible sources of allergy and their relative likelihood of causing symptoms allows systematic elimination of potential allergens.

2. *Classification of dialyzer reactions:* Patients may experience a wide variety of clinical symptoms during the course of a dialysis session or shortly thereafter, some of which may be due to interactions between the patient's blood and components of the dialyzer and dialysis circuit. These reactions are more common with new (non-reused) dialyzers and may be referred to as "first-use" reactions.

Table 20.3 Classification of first-use dialyzer reactions [6, 7]

Type A (anaphylaxis)		Type B (nonspecific)	Grading of severity	
Major criteria	*Minor criteria*	*Symptoms*		
Onset within 20 min of starting dialysis Dyspnea Sensation of heat/burning throughout the body or at the access Angioedema	Reproducible in subsequent dialysis treatments with the same dialysis circuit Urticaria Rhinorrhea, lacrimation Abdominal cramping Itching	Chest pain Back pain Nausea Vomiting Dyspnea Fever General malaise	Grade 1 (mild)	Not life-threatening No medications given Dialysis completed
			Grade 2 (severe)	Medications given and/or dialysis discontinued
			Grade 3 (fatal)	Death of patient
Definite (# criteria)	Probable (# criteria)			
3 major Or 2 major and 1 minor	2 major Or 1 major and 2 minor Or 3 minor			

Daugirdas and Ing [6] proposed a classification of first-use dialyzer reactions as outlined in Table 20.3, utilizing the grading system of Villarroel and Ciarkowski [7].

The incidence of dialyzer reactions is difficult to determine with accuracy in the absence of widespread, systematic reporting, but older published literature suggests a range of 3–5 per 100,000 dialysis sessions for nonfatal type A reactions to 3–5 per 100 dialysis sessions for type B reactions [6, 7]. The incidence of type A reactions is likely lower now, with more widespread use of biocompatible dialyzers, many alternative mechanisms of sterilization, and use of bicarbonate rather than acetate-containing dialysate.

3. *Causes of Bridget's type A reaction:*

Potential causes of Bridget's severe hypersensitivity reactions during HD to consider include:

Ethylene Oxide (ETO) Ethylene oxide is a bactericidal gas used as a sterilizing agent in some dialyzers. Sensitivity to ETO has been recognized since the late 1970s. Symptoms vary from full-blown anaphylactic reactions occurring within minutes of dialysis initiation, to nonspecific symptoms including fever, malaise, and myalgias. Multiple studies suggest anaphylaxis is mediated by IgE anti-ETO antibodies [8–11]. Measures to reduce the likelihood of ETO reactions include sufficient flushing of the dialysis circuit and avoidance of ETO-sterilized dialyzers and tubing [12]. The polyurethane potting compound used to secure the fibers in hollow-fiber dialyzers is a significant reservoir of ETO. Circuits which sit stagnant after the initial rinsing should be re-rinsed to remove ETO that leaches out of the potting compound. ETO may also be found as the sterilizing agent in fistula needles, dialysis tubing, and some continuous renal replacement therapy circuits. Steam sterilization, gamma irradiation, and e-beam are alternate methods of dialyzer sterilization that have not been associated with allergic reactions.

Membrane Type: Polysulfone Biocompatibility of a dialyzer relates to the propensity of the dialyzer to activate the complement, coagulation, and kallikrein systems and to cause sequestration of leukocytes [13]. A huge advance in the tolerance of dialysis has been the development of the synthetic biocompatible dialyzers.

Polysulfone dialyzers are biocompatible and are well tolerated, but all polysulfone membranes are not the same. Anaphylactic reactions to polysulfone, while rare, have been described [14, 15]. The presence of eosinophilia and elevated IgE levels has been shown in patients with recurrent anaphylactic reactions to polysulfone membranes. Polyvinylpyrrolidone (PVP), a known allergen, may be used to hydrophilize some polysulfone membranes to inhibit precipitation of platelets and plasma proteins on contact with the membrane. Reaction to PVP or the polysulfone-PVP complex may cause anaphylaxis.

Eosinophilia is not uncommon in hemodialysis patients in the absence of overt reactions, suggesting subclinical allergy to some component of the dialysis system [16]. One study of eosinophilia in patients dialyzed with polysulfone membranes showed a significant reduction in eosinophilia following a switch to a polyflux membrane [17].

Heparin Unfractionated heparin is the most common anticoagulant used during hemodialysis worldwide as it is effective, inexpensive, and readily available and has predictable kinetics. If necessary, it can be reversed with protamine. Hypersensitivity reactions directly attributable to heparin are rare but have been described [18] and may also be a manifestation of heparin-induced thrombocytopenia (HIT) as discussed below [19]. In 2008, Blossom et al. reported a widespread outbreak of adverse reactions related to heparin contamination with oversulfated chondroitin sulfate [5]. Symptoms occurred within minutes of initiation of dialysis and included facial swelling, tachycardia, hypotension, urticaria, and nausea.

Contaminated heparin as a cause of Bridget's type A reaction would be expected to affect multiple patients in the dialysis unit, rather than a single patient.

AN69/ACE Inhibitor Interaction The increased incidence of anaphylactic reactions in patients receiving treatment with ACE inhibitors while undergoing hemodialysis with an AN69 membrane was first recognized in the early 1990s [4, 20]. The presence of high bradykinin (BK) levels in affected patients implicated BK as the mediator of the allergic reaction [21]. It was shown that the negatively charged AN69 membrane generated higher levels of BK and hypothesized that ACE inhibitors blocked degradation of BK. In vitro studies and clinical experience have subsequently suggested that the "bradykinin release reaction" is a pH-dependent phenomenon occurring also in acidotic patients or those requiring a blood prime of their circuits even when not on ACE inhibitors, and which can be ameliorated by alkaline rinsing of the blood and dialysate compartments

[22] or measures to increase the pH of the circuit or the patient's blood prior to membrane contact [23]. Further investigations suggest that the propensity to develop this hypersensitivity reaction is a complex interaction between increased BK production by the negatively charged AN69 membrane, the presence of the ACE inhibitor which reduces the ability to degrade BK, and a genetic predisposition to reduced plasma levels of aminopeptidase activity [24]. Given the potential severity of this reaction, and the widespread availability of alternate biocompatible membranes, it would be prudent to avoid the use of an AN69 membrane in Bridget while she remains on the ACE inhibitor, unless she develops multiple allergic reactions to other dialyzers [25].

Endotoxins Creation of dialysate involves extensive treatment of municipal water to remove bacteria and chemical contaminants. The Association for the Advancement of Medical Instrumentation (AAMI) and other groups around the world set standards for dialysate water dictating the maximum allowable bacterial (<100 colony forming units (CFU)/ml) and endotoxin (<0.25 endotoxin unit (EU)/ml) concentrations in dialysate [26]. Endotoxins or lipopolysaccharides are large molecules found in the outer layer of gram-negative bacteria, capable of producing inflammatory reactions in humans. Water, in general, and bicarbonate dialysate in particular are good culture media for bacteria, so rigorous maintenance of dialysis water and regular testing of bacterial and endotoxin levels are essential to prevent bloodstream infections and pyrogenic reactions caused by these cytokine-inducing substances. Diffusion or backfiltration of endotoxin or other bacterial pyrogens from the dialysate across the dialyzer may cause fever, chills, rigors, and malaise during a dialysis session. The ability of bacterial endotoxins to cross the dialysis membrane appears to be more related to the nature of the membrane rather than the pore size, with polysulfone and polyamide being relatively resistant, due to adsorption on the membrane [27].

Creation of ultrapure water, defined by AAMI standards of <0.1 CFU/ml bacteria and <0.03 EU/ml endotoxin, is easily achieved by additional filtration of standard dialysate through filters which retain endotoxin and bacteria just prior to use. The benefits of ultrapure water are accumulating with evidence of reduced inflammatory markers, higher hemoglobin with lower doses of erythrocyte-stimulating agents, slower decline in residual renal function, and less dialysis-related hypotension to name a few. Ultrapure dialysate is a prerequisite for hemodiafiltration.

Endotoxin or bacterial pyrogens as a cause of Bridget's reaction should result in multiple affected patients if the central water integrity is compromised, but failure of disinfection of her specific machine could limit the reaction to Bridget alone.

Reuse Agents Few, if any, pediatric centers practice dialyzer reuse. Dialyzer reuse as a cost-saving measure and a means of reducing the incidence of "first-use" reaction with cellulosic dialyzers and ETO sterilization became a widespread practice in adult units in the 1980s and 1990s. However, with the advent of inexpensive biocompatible membranes, and improved sterilization techniques, there is a resurgence toward single-use dialyzers as the standard of care in many countries [28]. Exposure to residual sterilizing agents, particularly formaldehyde and bleach, has been associated with allergic reactions of variable severity [29]. Suboptimal concentration of germicides during reprocessing has been associated with outbreaks of bloodstream infections, and contamination with bacteria or endotoxin can cause pyrogenic reactions with fever, chills, and hypotension.

Contaminants Clusters of type A reactions, and death, have been reported related to contaminants [29] and include deaths caused by perfluorohydrocarbon contamination of dialyzers, and outbreaks of scleritis and iritis, acute loss of vision and hearing, and death associated with outdated cellulose dialyzers.

Part 2

Bridget responds well to the management provided. A decision is now required whether dialysis should be reinitiated. This must be individualized and should be based on her clinical status (blood pressure, intradialytic weight gain, pulmonary or peripheral edema) and bloodwork (potassium, urea, phosphate). Whenever possible, dialysis should be delayed at least several hours to ensure there is no rebound reaction once medication effects wane.

An assessment of the most likely cause of the reaction is essential as the starting point in stepwise elimination of potential allergens. Her next dialysis session should take place under close supervision, with anaphylaxis management readily available including medications, oxygen, and resuscitation equipment.

The timing and severity of Bridget's reaction would be most in keeping with ETO sensitivity or allergy to the polysulfone membrane and statistically less likely due to heparin. Although Bridget is not dialyzed with an AN69 membrane, this potential interaction with her ramipril medication must be considered when modifying her dialysis prescription as a result of this event.

On the basis of a presumed allergy to ethylene oxide, Bridget is switched to Dialyzer B. She tolerates this change well with no further allergic reactions or nonspecific symptoms, indicating her reaction was less likely due to the polysulfone membrane. However, her regular bloodwork 1 month later shows thrombocytopenia with a platelet count of 105,000 which is persistent on two repeated measurements over the next 2 weeks.

Clinical Question

1. What are the possible causes of Bridget's thrombocytopenia?

Diagnostic Discussion

1. **Thrombocytopenia (TCP) in Dialysis Patients** Activation of platelets is known to occur during hemodialysis, with transient drops in platelet count in the first 1–2 h of dialysis and recovery to pre-dialysis levels by the end of treatment [30]. Historically, TCP during dialysis with non-synthetic, largely cuprophane, and cellulosic membranes was one consequence of membrane bioincompatibility. Alteration in platelet function and number is far less common now, with synthetic, highly biocompatible membranes causing at most a 7–9% drop in platelet count. TCP is more likely caused by medications, immune-mediated or hematologic disorders, or sepsis. However, clinicians must be vigilant for trends occurring in response to changes in membrane configuration and sterilization techniques. For example, widespread TCP with specific pediatric-sized polymethylmethacrylate (PMMA) dialyzers lead to their discontinuation in the early 1990s (personal communication). Causes of TCP specific to dialysis include:

   (a) *Electron beam (e-beam) sterilization and polysulfone membranes:* Severe TCP in an index patient following a widespread switch to e-beam sterilized polysulfone dialyzers prompted a systematic study of pre- and post-platelet counts in 1,700 adult dialysis patients in two Canadian provinces [31]. Polysulfone e-beam sterilized dialyzers from two different manufacturers were associated with a 7% incidence of TCP as defined by an absolute platelet count of less than $100 \times 10^3/\mu l$ and/or a 15% decrease in platelet count post-dialysis. Switching to a non-e-beam sterilized polysulfone dialyzer resulted in significant improvement in the incidence of TCP in this patient population. Other authors have also reported on this phenomenon, although the mechanism of TCP has not been elucidated.

   Sterilization technique (e-beam) is likely not the only factor contributing to TCP with polysulfone membranes. Reports of improvement in significant TCP following a switch from one e-beam sterilized membrane to another suggest that the specific configuration of the polysulfone membrane itself may be implicated in the development of TCP [32], with rechallenge with the original dialyzer resulting in recurrence of TCP.

   (b) *Heparin-induced thrombocytopenia:* Heparin-induced thrombocytopenia (HIT) is an immune-mediated clinicopathological syndrome typically presenting 5–14 days after initiation of heparin and associated with the presence of HIT antibodies. The most common manifestations are TCP and thrombotic events, primarily venous, and include clotting of vascular access. Other clinical presentations include skin necrosis at heparin injection sites, ischemic limb necrosis in the absence of arterial lesions (venous gangrene), and a more recently appreciated acute systemic reaction [19]. Whether frequent clotting of the dialyzer or extracorporeal circuit is a manifestation of HIT is yet to be determined.

   The acute systemic reaction related to HIT occurs 5–30 min after intravenous injection of unfractionated heparin and may be mistaken for a dialyzer reaction. It has two presentations: an acute inflammatory reaction with fever and chills, or a cardiorespiratory event with hypotension, tachycardia, dyspnea and tachypnea, chest pain, and cardiopulmonary arrest, similar to pulmonary embolism. Symptoms are thought to result from release of interleukin 6 and von Willebrand factor as a result of endothelial injury. TCP may be transient so a platelet count should be checked following an apparent hypersensitivity reaction.

HIT is caused by the development of a heparin-platelet factor 4 (PF4) complex which binds to the platelet surface and causes platelet activation. The probability of HIT can be estimated using the "4 T's" algorithm to determine pretest probability (TCP, timing of fall in platelet count, thrombosis, or other manifestations and the presence of other causes of TCP) coupled with confirmatory laboratory measurements. These include functional tests of platelet activation which are sensitive and specific, but not readily available, and immunologic assays which detect antibodies to the heparin-PF4 complex, which are sensitive but have low specificity.

High clinical suspicion of HIT should result in prompt discontinuation of heparin, including heparin for catheter locking and low molecular weight heparins, and use of an alternate anticoagulant until tests confirm or refute the diagnosis.

HIT should be eliminated as a cause of Bridget's TCP due to the increased risk of thrombotic events and the need to alter her anticoagulation, although her pretest probability for HIT is low. Bridget should be switched to a non-e-beam sterilized polysulfone dialyzer, or a different e-beam sterilized polysulfone membrane, and the platelet response to the dialyzer substitution carefully monitored to ensure resolution of the TCP. This should not be difficult in a teenager, but may pose a challenge in tiny pediatric patients where size-appropriate dialyzers are limited.

Clinical Pearls

1. With biocompatible dialyzers and bicarbonate dialysate, severe hypersensitivity reactions have become far less common, but do occur. Patients may develop an anaphylactic reaction to any component of the dialysis circuit, including medications administered during dialysis.
2. The initial response should be to remove the patient from the circuit immediately *without retransfusion* to avoid further allergen exposure, while treating the anaphylaxis as per standard guidelines depending on the severity of the reaction.
3. A decision must be made on clinical grounds whether to resume or postpone dialysis once the patient is stabilized, with close monitoring and anaphylactic precautions during the subsequent dialysis session.
4. Stepwise elimination of potential allergens often requires a change in dialyzer to alter the dialyzer membrane or sterilization technique. Careful monitoring of the clinical response to this change is imperative.

5. Clinicians must be vigilant for clustering of unusual symptoms which may herald a problem with dialysate water integrity or a manufacturing issue resulting in a defect or contamination of one component of the dialysis circuit.

References

1. Ebo DG, Bosmans JL, Couttenye MM, Stevens WJ. Haemodialysis-associated anaphylactic and anaphylactoid reactions. Allergy. 2006;61(2):211–20.
2. Muraro A, Roberts G, Clark A, Eigenmann PA, Halken S, Lack G, et al. The management of anaphylaxis in childhood: position paper of the European academy of allergology and clinical immunology. Allergy. 2007;62(8):857–71.
3. Salem M, Ivanovich PT, Ing TS, Daugirdas JT. Adverse effects of dialyzers manifesting during the dialysis session. Nephrol Dial Transplant. 1994;9(Suppl 2):127–37.
4. Tielemans C, Madhoun P, Lenaers M, Schandene L, Goldman M, Vanherweghem JL. Anaphylactoid reactions during hemodialysis on AN69 membranes in patients receiving ACE inhibitors. Kidney Int. 1990;38(5):982–4.
5. Blossom DB, Kallen AJ, Patel PR, Elward A, Robinson L, Gao G, et al. Outbreak of adverse reactions associated with contaminated heparin. N Engl J Med. 2008;359(25):2674–84.
6. Daugirdas JT, Ing TS. First-use reactions during hemodialysis: a definition of subtypes. Kidney Int. 1988;33(Suppl 24):S37–43.
7. Villarroel F, Ciarkowski AA. A survey on hypersensitivity reactions in hemodialysis. Artif Organs. 1985;9(3):231–8.
8. Caruana RJ, Hamilton RW, Pearson FC. Dialyzer hypersensitivity syndrome: possible role of allergy to ethylene oxide. Report of 4 cases and review of one literature. Am J Nephrol. 1985;5(4):271–4.
9. Pearson F, Bruszer G, Lee W, Sagona M, Sargent H, Woods E, et al. Ethylene oxide sensitivity in hemodialysis patients. Artif Organs. 1987;11(2):100–3.
10. Nicholls A. Ethylene oxide and anaphylaxis during haemodialysis. Br Med J (Clin Res Ed). 1986;292(6530):1221–2.
11. Lemke HD. Mediation of hypersensitivity reactions during hemodialysis by IgE antibodies against ethylene oxide. Artif Organs. 1987;11(2):104–10.
12. Ansorge W, Pelger M, Dietrich W, Baurmeister U. Ethylene oxide in dialyzer rinsing fluid: effect of rinsing technique, dialyzer storage time, and potting compound. Artif Organs. 1987;11(2):118–22.
13. Kokubo K, Kurihara Y, Kobayashi K, Tsukao H, Kobayashi H. Evaluation of the biocompatibility of dialysis membranes. Blood Purif. 2015;40(4):293–7.
14. Bacelar Marques ID, Pinheiro KF, de Freitas do Carmo LP, Costa MC, Abensur H. Anaphylactic reaction induced by a polysulfone/polyvinylpyrrolidone membrane in the 10th session of hemodialysis with the same dialyzer. Hemodial Int Int Symp Home Hemodial. 2011;15(3):399–403.
15. Sayeed K, Murdakes C, Spec A, Gashti C. Anaphylactic shock at the beginning of hemodialysis. Semin Dial. 2016;29(1):81–4.
16. Hildebrand S, Corbett R, Duncan N, Ashby D. Increased prevalence of eosinophilia in a hemodialysis population: longitudinal and case control studies. Hemodial Int Int Symp Home Hemodial. 2016;20(3):414–20.
17. Li Z, Ma L, Zhao S. Effect of polyflux membranes on the improvement of hemodialysis-associated eosinophilia: a case series. Ren Fail. 2016;38(1):65–9.
18. Berkun Y, Haviv YS, Schwartz LB, Shalit M. Heparin-induced recurrent anaphylaxis. Clin Exp Allergy. 2004;34(12):1916–8.
19. Syed S, Reilly RF. Heparin-induced thrombocytopenia: a renal perspective. Nat Rev Nephrol. 2009;5(9):501–11.

20. Parnes EL, Shapiro WB. Anaphylactoid reactions in hemodialysis patients treated with the AN69 dialyzer. Kidney Int. 1991;40(6):1148–52.
21. Verresen L, Fink E, Lemke HD, Vanrenterghem Y. Bradykinin is a mediator of anaphylactoid reactions during hemodialysis with AN69 membranes. Kidney Int. 1994;45(5):1497–503.
22. Coppo R, Amore A, Cirina P, Scelfo B, Giacchino F, Comune L, et al. Bradykinin and nitric oxide generation by dialysis membranes can be blunted by alkaline rinsing solutions. Kidney Int. 2000;58(2):881–8.
23. Brophy PD, Mottes TA, Kudelka TL, McBryde KD, Gardner JJ, Maxvold NJ, et al. AN-69 membrane reactions are pH-dependent and preventable. Am J Kidney Dis Off J Natl Kidney Found. 2001;38(1):173–8.
24. Molinaro G, Duan QL, Chagnon M, Moreau ME, Simon P, Clavel P, et al. Kinin-dependent hypersensitivity reactions in hemodialysis: metabolic and genetic factors. Kidney Int. 2006;70(10):1823–31.
25. Cerqueira A, Martins PA, Carvalho BA, Vasconcelos MP. AN69-ST membrane, a useful option in two cases of severe dialysis reactions. Clin Nephrol. 2015;83(2):100–3.
26. Upadhyay A, Jaber BL. We use impure water to make dialysate for hemodialysis. Semin Dial. 2016;29(4):297–9.
27. Ward RA. Ultrapure dialysate. Semin Dial. 2004;17(6):489–97.
28. Upadhyay A, Sosa MA, Jaber BL. Single-use versus reusable dialyzers: the known unknowns. Clin J Am Soc Nephrol. 2007;2(5):1079–86.
29. Twardowski ZJ. Dialyzer reuse – part II: advantages and disadvantages. Semin Dial. 2006;19(3):41–53.
30. Daugirdas JT, Bernardo AA. Hemodialysis effect on platelet count and function and hemodialysis-associated thrombocytopenia. Kidney Int. 2012;82(2):147–57.
31. Kiaii M, Djurdjev O, Farah M, Levin A, Jung B, MacRae J. Use of electron-beam sterilized hemodialysis membranes and risk of thrombocytopenia. JAMA. 2011;306(15):1679–87.
32. De Prada L, Lee J, Gillespie A, Benjamin J. Thrombocytopenia associated with one type of polysulfone hemodialysis membrane: a report of 5 cases. Am J Kidney Dis Off J Natl Kidney Found. 2013;61(1):131–3.

Chapter 21
Nutritional Management of Infants on Dialysis

Lesley Rees and Vanessa Shaw

Case Presentation

A male foetus was found on US scan at 22 weeks gestation to have bilateral hydro-nephrosis; a distended bladder; small, bright kidneys with cysts; and a reduced amniotic fluid volume. There was spontaneous onset of labour at 37 weeks, and the baby was born by normal vaginal delivery with a birth weight of 2.1 kg, length 45 cm and head circumference 31 cm (all second centile). No respiratory support was needed. Postnatally, he was diagnosed with posterior urethral valves (PUVs) with severe bilateral cystic renal dysplasia. The baby was catheterised at birth, and the PUVs were ablated at 1 week of age. The baby was started on a standard whey-based infant formula (60:40 whey to casein ratio, electrolyte content similar to breast milk) orally and fed to meet normal neonatal nutritional requirements.

The serum creatinine, potassium, phosphate and urea subsequently increased, the serum sodium fell and the urine output was very poor. In response to poor weight gain, a nasogastric tube was passed to permit supplemental nutritional support. At 2 weeks of age, peritoneal dialysis (PD) was started. The protein content of the formula was increased, and the patient's BP was closely monitored with consideration for the provision of supplemental dietary salt.

Despite adequate dialysis with good fluid balance and BP control, accompanied by an enteral feeding plan providing adequate nutrition, growth (weight, length and head circumference) was poor. The baby was also vomiting large volumes of his feeds.

By 9 weeks of age, he weighed 4 kg (0.4th centile). A gastrostomy was inserted which resulted in decreased emesis associated with feeding, and the baby started to grow.

L. Rees (✉) • V. Shaw
Great Ormond Street Hospital for Children NHS Foundation Trust, London, WC1N3JH, UK
e-mail: Lesley.rees@gosh.nhs.uk

© Springer International Publishing AG 2017
B.A. Warady et al. (eds.), *Pediatric Dialysis Case Studies*,
DOI 10.1007/978-3-319-55147-0_21

At 3 months of age, the baby developed peritonitis. Due to increased peritoneal protein losses as a result of the infection, the serum albumin fell, which prompted a further increase in the protein content of the feedings until the baby had improved clinically. Whereas the infection was eradicated, albeit with a slow recovery, the peritonitis recurred, prompting PD catheter removal and transition to haemodialysis.

Clinical Questions

1. What factors should be considered to meet the enteral feeding requirements of the infant with CKD?
2. How can vomiting be ameliorated in the infant with CKD/ESKD?
3. When are salt supplements needed for the infant with CKD or receiving peritoneal dialysis?
4. What are the protein requirements?
5. What are the calcium and phosphate requirements?
6. What are the vitamin and mineral requirements?

Diagnostic Discussion

1. Perhaps the most challenging clinical issue in the management of infants with CKD is maintaining normal growth. This is exemplified by data from around the world showing that approximately 50% of children requiring renal replacement therapy (RRT) before their 13th birthday have a final height below the normal range [1–4]. Infants do particularly poorly. There are, thankfully, reasons for poor growth in infants with CKD that can be influenced, the most important of which is inadequate nutritional intake. Growth during infancy is predominantly dependent on nutrition, and its impact exceeds that of growth hormone, which starts to take over from nutrition as the key determinant of growth towards the end of the second year of life [5].

   Poor dietary intake may be due to anorexia, which is common in CKD, and gastro-oesophageal reflux (GER) accompanied by recurrent vomiting. Loss of height standard deviation score (Ht SDS) has been reported to be as much as 0.6 SD per month. The vulnerability of the infant due to the dependence on nutritional intake is compounded by a growth rate that is normally greater than at any other time of life, being as high as 25 cm per year at birth, 18 cm per year at 6 months of age and 12 cm per year at 12 months of age. Decreased growth rates can potentially lead to the irreversible loss of final height potential. Maintaining optimal nutrition to prevent growth failure is therefore vital, and intensive nutritional management during the infantile phase of growth can prevent or even reverse this decline [6, 7]. The daily feeding requirements at this age are shown in Table 21.1. The aim is to give, at a minimum, the Estimated Average

Table 21.1 Nutritional and fluid requirements for the term neonate/infant prior to initiating dialysis

Age	Energy (kcal/kg) estimated average requirement [8]	Protein (g/kg) reference nutrient intake [10]	Feed volume (ml/kg)
0–2 months	96–120	2.1	150–180

Table 21.2 Suggested rates for initiating and advancing tube feedings for neonates and infants with ESRD

Method	Initial infusion	Increases	Goal
Continuous feedings	1–2 ml/kg/h	1 ml/kg/h	6 ml/kg/h
Bolus feedings	10–15 ml/kg/feed	20–40 ml q 4 h	20–30 ml/kg/feed

Table adapted from KDOQI [11]

Requirement (EAR) for energy [8] and the Reference Nutrient Intake (RNI) [9] for protein for chronological age. The RNI is one of the dietary reference values (DRV) in the UK and refers to the quantity of intake of a specific nutrient which meets the needs of 95% of the population. In the mid-1990s, the Dietary Reference Intakes (DRI) replaced the Recommended Dietary Allowance (RDA) in the USA and the RNI in Canada.

Babies with CKD often cannot achieve full breast or bottle feeding spontaneously due to a poor appetite, and growth will subsequently be poor. In this situation, a nasogastric tube may be passed to provide supplemental formula in order to achieve the target volume. If a sufficient volume of formula can be delivered orally and/or per nasogastric tube, the baby will characteristically experience catch-up growth. If the mother wishes to continue breast feeding, this can be 'in addition' to the nasogastric feeds.

The formula should be offered orally first, and then the residual volume can be given via the nasogastric tube as a 'top-up' bolus feed. Alternatively, some of the formula can be delivered as an overnight continuous feed via an enteral feeding pump, with daytime oral/nasogastric boluses. Recommendations regarding the rate of infusion have been published (Table 21.2). If feeding becomes predominantly via a tube, it is important to continue to provide oral stimulation by offering the baby a dummy (pacifier) to suck. In the older child, self-feeding should be encouraged. For the child who becomes food aversive, playing with food and sitting at the table with siblings at mealtimes can help to minimise feeding problems [10].

Most centres are able to place a gastrostomy when the baby is ≥4 kg. This should be done surgically rather than percutaneously in children on PD, to reduce the infection risk [12]. There are a variety of reasons why a gastrostomy is preferable to a nasogastric or nasojejunal tube: it is less easily displaced; a gastrostomy is hidden under clothing, removing the stigma of a chronically ill child; it is not associated with abnormal development of oromotor skills; it can be safely used to feed overnight; and most importantly, gastrostomy use is associated with better growth during infancy, perhaps as a result of an accompanying decreased frequency of vomiting [12, 13].

2. Vomiting is very common in infants who receive peritoneal dialysis. When this occurs, the target formula volumes may not be achieved despite the use of a nasogastric tube [10]. The consequent energy deficit may cause a rise in potassium and urea levels and a faltering weight gain. In some cases, babies may tolerate a smaller volume of formula better. Concentrating infant formulas provides the nutritional prescription in a smaller volume; as an example, increasing the formula concentration from 13% to 15% means that the formula volume can be reduced by 20 ml/kg/day. Any extra fluid that may be needed can be provided as water, and the intake of drinking water does not seem to be affected by a loss of appetite and does not typically exacerbate vomiting (unless large volumes are taken). In fact, it is a drink that many infants enjoy and helps maintain an oral intake when all formula by mouth may be refused.

   Vomiting may also be reduced if feedings are given by slow continuous drip overnight with oral or bolus feedings offered during the day, as noted above. If the child is not under close supervision during the overnight feeding, a gastrostomy rather than a nasogastric tube is preferred because of the risk of nasogastric tube displacement. Usually half the formula volume is given overnight by an enteral feeding pump, with the remainder divided into 3–4 daytime bolus feedings. The proportion of the feeding given overnight can be increased as the baby gets older so that the burden of feeding frequently throughout the day can be reduced. In extreme cases of vomiting, it may be necessary to use the pump for the daytime feedings as well. By the time the child reaches the second year of age, some toddlers receive all of their formula intake overnight and drink only water during the day.

   Disorders of gut motility are common in infants with CKD/ESKD and may also contribute to poor intake and vomiting. There are many causes for the abnormal gut motility including a 'full abdomen' from the presence of dialysis fluid, constipation, derangements of the gastrointestinal hormones that control stomach emptying and GER. There may be a benefit from prokinetic agents such as alimemazine and erythromycin. Reduction of gastric acid secretion with H2-receptor antagonists (e.g. ranitidine) and proton pump inhibitors (e.g. lansoprazole) may also be of benefit in symptom reduction. 5HT3 receptor antagonists (e.g. ondansetron) may help with anorexia and vomiting [5, 7].

3. It is important to ensure that infants with CKD have access to adequate salt and water. Polyuria may be present in patients with CKD/ESKD because of an obligatory loss of salt and water due to abnormal renal tubular function. If fluids are inappropriately restricted (as is a common response of medical teams confronted with severe CKD in an infant), the infant can become dehydrated, and the ongoing sodium and water losses may lead to rising creatinine and potassium values. Sodium supplementation and provision of adequate fluid intake in infants with CKD can, in turn, correct declining renal function and hyperkalaemia.

   In addition to the losses of water and electrolytes in the urine, substantial losses of sodium into the PD fluid of infants frequently occurs and should be addressed at the earliest stage as hypotension is common if the losses are not repleted. Indeed, there are reports of blindness in infants on PD occurring in association with hypotension and ischaemia of the optic nerves (see Chapter 5) [14]. Poor growth may be another complication of inadequate salt management in the infant receiving PD [15]. It is therefore necessary to assess the weight and BP of the patient on PD at least daily. The sodium content of urine and spent dialysate can be measured as well. Sodium losses can be high, and long-term supplementation is often required, especially in the patient who remains polyuric despite requiring chronic dialysis. It is usual to start with sodium supplements of ≥1–2 mmol per kg per day and to increase this dose according to the patient's BP response.

4. In principle, the protein requirements for an infant with advanced CKD are not different than the requirements for a healthy infant (Table 21.1), although an amount greater than the RNI is usually given to promote growth in the poorly nourished infant. Similar recommendations have been published by KDOQI (Table 21.3).

   In the infant with CKD and high potassium and phosphorus levels, it may be necessary to substitute some of the standard whey-based infant formula with a renal-specific infant formula with a lower phosphate and potassium content until dialysis is commenced. Formula examples are shown in Table 21.4.

   With the initiation of PD, the protein content of the formula must be increased to compensate for transperitoneal losses, estimated to be 0.28 g/kg/day in the

Table 21.3 Recommended dietary protein intake in children with CKD stages 3–5 and 5D

Age	DRI (g/kg/d)	Recommended for CKD stage 3 (g/kg/d) (100–140% DRI)	Recommended for CKD stages 4–5 (g/kg/d) (100–120% DRI)	Recommended for HD (g/kg/d)[a]	Recommended for PD (g/kg/d)[b]
0–6 mos	1.5	1.5–2.1	1.5–1.8	1.6	1.8

Table modified from KDOQI [11]
[a]DRI + 0.1 g/kg/d to compensate for dialytic losses
[b]DRI + 0.15–0.3 g/kg/d depending on patient age to compensate for peritoneal losses

Table 21.4 Comparison of standard infant formula with renal infant formula

Formula concentration[a]	Energy (kcal)	Protein (g)	Potassium (mmol)	Phosphate (mg)
410 ml 13% typical standard infant formula	275 (120/kg)	5.2 (2.2/kg)	6.6 (2.9/kg)	98
410 ml 13% Renastart renal infant formula	262 (114/kg)	4.1 (1.8/kg)	2.5 (0.96/kg)	49
50:50 mixture	269 (117/kg)	4.7 (2.0/kg)	4.6 (2.0/kg)	74
Similac® PM 60:40	273 (118/kg)	6.0 (2.6/kg)	5.7 (2.5/kg)	77

180 ml/kg for 2.3 kg baby = 410 ml
[a]Normal strength standard whey-based infant formulas are prepared with an average 13 g powder in 100 ml water to provide 66 kcal/100 ml and 1.3 g protein/100 ml

Table 21.5 Concentrating feeds to meet protein requirements for peritoneal dialysis

Feed 160 ml/kg for 2.3 kg baby = 370 ml	Energy (kcal)	Protein (g)	Potassium (mmol)	Phosphate (mg)
185 ml 17% concentrated standard infant formula plus	162	3.1	3.9	58
185 ml 15% concentrated Renastart renal infant formula	136	2.1	0.8	25
Total	298	5.2	4.7	83
Per kg 50:50 mixture	129	2.26	2.0	36

first year of life [16]. KDOQI recommends an additional 0.15–0.3 g protein/kg/day to offset these losses (Table 21.3) [11]. The dietary aims remain: to enable normal growth and serum albumin and to control serum phosphorus levels. The formula can be further concentrated to increase the intake of protein, but care is needed not to provide excessive doses of potassium, phosphate, vitamins, minerals and trace elements when doing so. On occasion, the potassium concentration of the formula can also be decreased by treating the formula with a potassium resin [17]. Concern regarding the formulation of the resin and the associated risk of aluminium contamination has recently been published [18].

It is usually possible to use a combination of a concentrated infant formula and a low electrolyte formula to accomplish these nutritional goals. An example is shown in Table 21.5: if the baby is 2.3 kg, the formula volume is 160 ml/kg (370 ml) and the aim is to replace peritoneal protein losses, the protein intake will need to increase from 2.0 to 2.28 g/kg. The normal formula concentration of 13% can be increased to 17% for the standard infant formula (17 g powder in 100 ml water) and 15% (15 g powder in 100 ml water) for the renal infant formula.

Peritonitis increases protein requirements even further due to both catabolism and increased permeability of the peritoneum with a subsequent increased loss of protein. The easiest way to address this increase in protein requirement is to use a modular approach, adding a protein powder to the formula to increase the protein intake by 0.2 g/kg/day if the serum albumin falls. This formulation should be continued until the child is clinically well and the serum albumin level stabilises. The infant formula is used as the feeding base, with the addition of protein powder and glucose polymer to design a patient-specific profile for energy and protein. An example is shown in Table 21.6.

Protein requirements for haemodialysis are lower than for PD since there are no transperitoneal losses. There is, however, a requirement over and above the RNI with KDOQI recommending an additional 0.1 g/kg/day [11] due to amino acid losses in the dialysate. As before, serum potassium and phosphorus levels can typically be maintained within an acceptable range by manipulating the ratio and concentrations of standard infant formula with the renal infant formula.

5. Serum calcium and phosphorus can be manipulated by modifying the calcium and phosphate intake, in addition to the use of phosphate binders and vitamin D. In the baby on PD, the calcium in the dialysate can also be adjusted from neutral

Table 21.6 Modular approach to feeding to increase dietary protein intake

Feed	Energy (kcal)	Protein (g)	Potassium(mmol)	Phosphate (mg)
370 ml 10% standard infant formula	190	3.6	4.6	68
2 g Protifar protein powder	7	1.7	0.07	14
25 g Vitajoule glucose polymer	95	0	0	0
Per kg	127	2.3	2.0	82

(1.25 mmol/l) to a higher (1.75 mmol/l) concentration that promotes diffusion of calcium into the blood from dialysate. The recommended daily calcium balance in the first year of life is 500–600 g, which is higher than at any other age [19]. For the normal population, the RNI during the first year is 13.1 mmol (524 mg)/day. A baby on a standard whey-based infant formula may barely receive adequate calcium (e.g. 180 ml/kg standard formula for a 2 kg baby only provides an average of 190 mg calcium/day). The other important thing to remember is that the normal range for serum calcium is higher in the first year of life than at any other age [20].

The normal population safe intake for vitamin D early in the first year of life is 8.5–10 μg/day (340–400 IU/day). Standard whey-based infant formulas contain 1.2 μg (48 IU) vitamin D per 100 ml, which will require the infants to receive a vitamin D supplement until they are on a sufficient volume of formula (Scientific Advisory Committee on Nutrition. Dietary Reference Values for Energy (2011) and Vitamin D (2016), SCAN, London). However, in infants with advanced CKD/ESKD, it is also likely that activated vitamin D will be necessary to control the parathyroid hormone (PTH) level. Levels of PTH that are below 2× the upper limit of normal have been correlated with better growth and with decreased signs and symptoms of bone disease [21].

The normal serum phosphorus level is also highest during infancy [20]. It is, however, recommended that the dietary phosphorus intake of the infant with CKD/ESKD is reduced to 100% of the Dietary Reference Intake (DRI), 400 mg [9], when the serum PTH is above the target range and the serum phosphorus is within the normal reference range. This should be reduced to 80% of the DRI when the serum PTH is above the target range and the serum phosphorus exceeds the normal age-related reference range [11]. Whereas this approach to controlling serum phosphorus can typically be easily achieved with both breast milk and whey-based infant formulas which have low phosphate contents, (14 mg and an average of 27 mg per 100 ml, respectively), phosphate binders may still be required. Calcium-containing phosphate binders are prescribed with feedings and are distributed between the daytime boluses and overnight feedings so that the binder is distributed according to the intake of phosphate. What we do not know is how much of the calcium in the binders is absorbed.

In the setting of hypercalcaemia, a non-calcium-containing phosphate binder may be required. Sevelamer hydrochloride and sevelamer carbonate bind the phosphate within the formula to form an insoluble hydrogel which settles in the

Table 21.7 Suggested daily vitamin supplements for patients receiving peritoneal dialysis

	Infants	Children
Vitamin C	15 mg	60 mg
Vitamin B6	0.2 mg	1.5 mg
Folate	60 µg	400 µg

bottom of the formula bottle. This can, however, obstruct a feeding tube [22]. Ideally, the phosphate-free supernatant should be decanted and then fed, but this is not always a practical option [22]. As a compromise, sevelamer carbonate powder can be mixed with 5–10 ml of water and flushed into the feeding tube, followed by 5–10 ml of water to clean the tube. The dose can be given after a bolus feed or during a continuous feed. It is not known how effective this is in binding the phosphate.

6. Once the formula is diluted beyond its usual concentration, a vitamin, mineral and trace element supplement may be needed if sufficient quantities of these nutrients are not provided by the basic formula. The requirement for micronutrients for babies with CKD/ESKD is largely unknown, but it is recommended that they receive at least 100% of the DRI [11]. The exception to this is vitamin A; serum levels of vitamin A are elevated in children with ESKD and are associated with hypercalcaemia, anaemia and hyperlipidaemia. A vitamin A intake close to the RNI is a pragmatic approach, but is difficult to achieve when using standard infant formulas (60 µg vitamin A/100 ml). Renal infant formulas have a 30% lower vitamin A content when prepared at the same concentration.

Some water-soluble vitamins may also be needed for the infant on PD to offset transperitoneal losses. The limited literature on this subject also suggests the provision of a supplement of vitamin C, pyridoxine and folate (20) if the formula does not provide sufficient amounts (Table 21.7).

Clinical Pearls

1. Input from a paediatric renal dietitian is essential for the development of a plan for the management of nutrition for the infant with CKD and ESKD.
2. The nutrition plan should aim for a minimum EAR for energy and RNI for protein for the infant with ESKD, with the provision of additional dietary protein to account for dialysis-related losses.
3. Failure to meet the nutritional goals by the oral route alone often mandates the use of enteral feedings with either a nasogastric tube or gastrostomy.
4. Vitamin intake should meet the RNI except for vitamin A, which accumulates in children with ESKD.

References

1. Franke D, et al. Growth and maturation improvement in children on renal replacement therapy over the past 20 years. Pediatr Nephrol. 2013;28(10):2043–51.
2. Harambat J, et al. Adult height in patients with advanced CKD requiring renal replacement therapy during childhood. Clin J Am Soc Nephrol. 2014;9(1):92–9.
3. Fine RN, Martz K, Stablein D. What have 20 years of data from the North American Pediatric Renal Transplant Cooperative Study taught us about growth following renal transplantation in infants, children, and adolescents with end-stage renal disease? Pediatr Nephrol. 2010;25(4):739–46.
4. Klare B, et al. Normal adult height after steroid-withdrawal within 6 months of pediatric kidney transplantation: a 20 years single center experience. Transpl Int. 2012;25(3):276–82.
5. Rees L, Jones H. Nutritional management and growth in children with chronic kidney disease. Pediatr Nephrol. 2013;28(4):527–36.
6. Mekahli D, et al. Long-term outcome of infants with severe chronic kidney disease. Clin J Am Soc Nephrol. 2010;5(1):10–7.
7. Rees L, Mak RH. Nutrition and growth in children with chronic kidney disease. Nat Rev Nephrol. 2011;7(11):615–23.
8. Dietary reference values for energy, Scientific Advisory Committee on Nutrition, TSO, 2011: London.
9. Dietary reference values for food energy and nutrients for the United Kingdom, Report on Health and Social Subjects No 41, Department of Health, HMSO, 1991: London.
10. Ledermann SE, Shaw V, Trompeter RS. Long-term enteral nutrition in infants and young children with chronic renal failure. Pediatr Nephrol. 1999;13(9):870–5.
11. KDOQI. Clinical practice guideline for nutrition in children with CKD: 2008 update. Executive summary. Am J Kidney Dis. 2009;53(3 Suppl 2):S11–104.
12. Rees L, Brandt ML. Tube feeding in children with chronic kidney disease: technical and practical issues. Pediatr Nephrol. 2010;25(4):699–704.
13. Rees L, et al. Growth in very young children undergoing chronic peritoneal dialysis. J Am Soc Nephrol. 2011;22(12):2303–12.
14. Dufek S, et al. Anterior ischemic optic neuropathy in pediatric peritoneal dialysis: risk factors and therapy. Pediatr Nephrol. 2014;29(7):1249–57.
15. Parekh RS, et al. Improved growth in young children with severe chronic renal insufficiency who use specified nutritional therapy. J Am Soc Nephrol. 2001;12(11):2418–26.
16. Quan A, Baum M. Protein losses in children on continuous cycler peritoneal dialysis. Pediatr Nephrol. 1996;10(6):728–31.
17. Thompson K, et al. Pretreatment of formula or expressed breast milk with sodium polystyrene sulfonate (Kayexalate(R)) as a treatment for hyperkalemia in infants with acute or chronic renal insufficiency. J Ren Nutr. 2013;23(5):333–9.
18. Taylor JM, et al. Renal formulas pretreated with medications alters the nutrient profile. Pediatr Nephrol. 2015;30(10):1815–23.
19. Rees L, Shroff R. The demise of calcium-based phosphate binders-is this appropriate for children? Pediatr Nephrol. 2015;30(12):2061–71.
20. Rees L, et al. Chronic kidney disease. In:Oxford specialist handbook of paediatric nephrology. Oxford: Oxford University Press; 2011. p. 434–55.
21. Borzych D, et al. The bone and mineral disorder of children undergoing chronic peritoneal dialysis. Kidney Int. 2010;78(12):1295–304.
22. Raaijmakers R, et al. Pre-treatment of dairy and breast milk with sevelamer hydrochloride and sevelamer carbonate to reduce phosphate. Perit Dial Int. 2013;33(5):565–72.

Chapter 22
Nutritional Management of Children and Adolescents on Dialysis

Meredith Cushing and Nonnie Polderman

Case Presentation

ED is a teenage male who first presented with stage 3 chronic kidney disease at age 12 years. During his initial visits to the kidney clinic, ED's anthropometric measurements along with blood work and usual dietary intake were assessed. At that time, ED was trending along the 50% for both height and weight. Routine blood work indicated metabolic control of electrolytes and minerals, and assessment of his usual dietary intake suggested that he was consuming adequate energy and protein to promote continued growth.

Initial nutritional intervention included teaching ED and his parents about the dietary modifications that were required for his stage of chronic kidney disease (CKD). The family was instructed on a healthy diet with limited sodium, and they were provided with some preliminary information about the future need for potassium and phosphorus management.

ED was subsequently lost to follow-up for over 2 years during which time his parents conducted their own online research on dietary restrictions for CKD. Based on their findings, ED's parents were convinced that restricting dietary protein intake would help to delay the progression of their son's kidney disease, and they adopted a diet restricted in protein, as well as in overall energy. ED was no longer permitted to eat out with friends or to enjoy any of his favorite foods.

Nearly 3 years later, at the age of 15 years, ED returned to medical care presenting with end-stage kidney disease (ESKD) manifesting as seizures and tetany requiring urgent dialysis. During the period of time ED was lost to routine follow-up, his growth trends had worsened with his weight dropping, and his height dipping from the 50% to the 35% (see Figs. 22.1 and 22.2).

M. Cushing (✉) • N. Polderman (✉)
Division of Nephrology, British Columbia Children's Hospital, Vancouver, BC, Canada
e-mail: mcushing@cw.bc.ca

© Springer International Publishing AG 2017
B.A. Warady et al. (eds.), *Pediatric Dialysis Case Studies*,
DOI 10.1007/978-3-319-55147-0_22

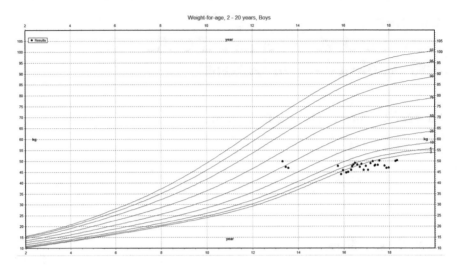

Fig. 22.1 Weight for age chart (boys 2–20 years) demonstrating significant worsening of weight with crossing of percentiles

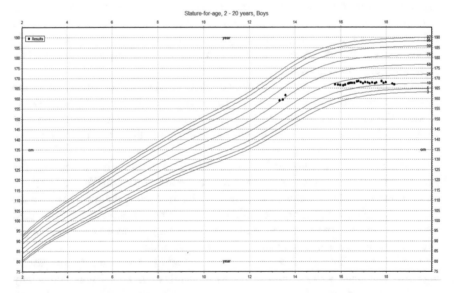

Fig. 22.2 Stature for age chart (boys 2–20 years) demonstrating significant worsening of linear growth with crossing of percentiles

Once stabilized on maintenance hemodialysis (HD), ED and his parents were reeducated about age- and dialysis-appropriate diet modifications. ED was prescribed a renal-appropriate oral nutrition supplement for additional energy and protein to help him achieve an adequate intake to stabilize his weight. ED was also prescribed an appetite stimulant; however, his adherence to this medication was not consistent. ED was provided treatment with growth hormone in an attempt to maximize his linear growth, but he was unable to commit to the daily requirement for injections. The family's financial situation had also changed, and ED was reluctant to disclose that he and his parents were experiencing food insecurity (FI) as they did not have consistent access to enough food at home to meet his recommended needs. Once the family's FI was identified, the renal team's social worker was able to assist ED's family to access some additional resources and to connect them with a local agency which helped the family gain access to a more consistent supply of groceries. Finally, as ED's urine output diminished, his diet was further restricted to a maximum of 1,000 ml of fluid per day requiring the dose of his calorie-dense nutritional supplement to be increased.

Clinical Questions

1. What are the energy and protein requirements of adolescents with progressive chronic kidney disease (CKD) or on dialysis? Is there a role for restriction of dietary protein intake in an attempt to slow the progression of CKD in pediatric patients?
2. What adjunctive therapies are available to improve appetite and increase dietary intake for children and adolescents with CKD/ESKD? What are the typical characteristics of a nutritional supplement appropriate for patients receiving dialysis?
3. How often should a child or adolescent on dialysis be evaluated for nutritional adequacy and growth?
4. How does a daily fluid restriction impact an individual's ability to meet daily caloric requirements?
5. How do food insecurity issues impact families caring for children or adolescents with chronic diseases, and how can health-care providers inquire about food insecurity?

Diagnostic Discussion

1. The ultimate goal of nutrition for the child or adolescent with CKD, on or off of dialysis, is the achievement of optimal growth and development. In clinically stable non-dialyzed pediatric CKD patients, resting energy expenditure (REE) is similar to that of age- and gender-matched healthy peers [1]. For pediatric patients being dialyzed with either hemodialysis (HD) or peritoneal dialysis (PD), REE and energy requirements are also similar to that of age- and gender-matched healthy controls [2]. Provision of 100% of the recommended nutrient intake (RNI) for protein in children with CKD is also recommended, and there is no evidence that more or less dietary protein influences the progression of CKD in children or adolescents [3]. For those patients undergoing dialysis, 100% of

the RNI for protein plus an allowance for both replacement of transperitoneal losses and daily nitrogen losses to achieve a positive nitrogen balance is recommended. Adequate energy must also be given to promote the deposition of protein.

All diet restrictions must be individualized. Overly restricted dietary prescriptions may lead to further limitations on patients' intakes resulting in poor intake and the development of malnutrition [4].

When all attempts to maximize nutritional intake and the modifiable risk factors for growth impairment (metabolic acidosis, fluid and electrolyte abnormalities, anemia, and bone disease) have been addressed and yet stature remains suboptimal, treatment with recombinant human growth hormone (rhGH) should be considered in the patient who continues to have growth potential [5–7]. The goal of treating dialysis patients with rhGH is normalization of the final adult height, defined either as the 50% of midparental height or greater than the 3% of the normal population for age and gender.

2. Multiple factors impact appetite and ultimately food intake, including uremia, dysgeusia, anemia, nausea and vomiting, time spent carrying out multiple treatments, medication intake, as well as dietary modifications and restrictions. Several appetite stimulants (Periactin® [cyproheptadine], Megace® [megestrol acetate], and Marinol® [dronabinol]) have been trialed with varying results [8]. There is also a wide array of nutritional supplements available commercially. While many contain energy and protein, not all are appropriate for the child or adolescent who is receiving dialysis. An oral nutritional supplement that contains adequate protein, while low in electrolytes and minerals, will often help meet nutritional goals while maintaining metabolic control and avoiding fluid overload. The use of protein powders or modulars containing carbohydrate and fat can be used to provide additional energy and protein for growth and development. Even small amounts of a concentrated oral nutritional supplement taken to help the patient swallow medications can add valuable nutrition on a daily basis. Much like medications, a nutrition supplement should be prescribed as part of the overall medical therapy.

When oral intake remains suboptimal, more aggressive means of nutrition support need to be considered. Offering meals while on dialysis, overnight tube feeding, as well as intradialytic parenteral nutrition (IDPN) for patients on HD should be explored.

3. Childhood and adolescence are stages of life characterized by rapid growth and development. Therefore, children and adolescents with CKD and receiving dialysis will require frequent nutritional assessment for long-term optimization of growth outcome [9]. The schedule of assessments in the NKF KDOQI Clinical Practice Guideline for Nutrition in Children with CKD offers a framework for both the parameters to be assessed, as well as the frequency of assessment at different ages and stages of CKD (Table 22.1) [10]. In centers with particular expertise, bioelectrical impedance may also be used as a component of the patient's assessment.

Table 22.1 Recommended parameters and frequency of nutritional assessment for children with CKD stages 2 to 5 and 5D

Minimum interval (mo)										
	Age 0 to <1 year			Age 1–3 years			Age > 3 years			
Measure	CKD 2–3	CKD 4–5	CKD 5D	CKD 2–3	CKD 4–5	CKD 5D	CKD 2	CKD 3	CKD 4–5	CKD 5D
Dietary intake	0.5–3	0.5–3	0.5–2	1–3	1–3	1–3	6–12	6	3–4	3–4
Height or length-for-age percentile or SDS	0.5–1.5	0.5–1.5	0.5–1	1–3	1–2	1	3–6	3–6	1–3	1–3
Height or length velocity-for-age percentile or SDS	0.5–2	0.5–2	0.5–1	1–6	1–3	1–2	6	6	6	6
Estimated dry weight and weight-for-age percentile or SDS	0.5–1.5	0.5–1.5	0.25–1	1–3	1–2	0.5–1	3–6	3–6	1–3	1–3
BMI-for-height-age percentile or SDS	0.5–1.5	0.5–1.5	0.5–1	1–3	1–2	1	3–6	3–6	1–3	1–3
Head circumference-for-age percentile or SDS	0.5–1.5	0.5–1.5	0.5–1	1–3	1–2	1–2	N/A	N/A	N/A	N/A
nPCR	N/A	N/A	N/A	N/A	N/A	N/A	N/A	N/A	N/A	1[a]

Abbreviation: *N/A* not applicable
[a]Only applies to adolescents receiving HD

4. As urine output decreases, the oral fluid intake of the dialysis patient must often be limited due to the potential of fluid overload in the oliguric/anuric patient. Having to limit daily fluid intake may inherently lead to lower dietary protein and energy consumption. Most importantly, when daily fluid intake is restricted, the nutritional value of all dietary intake is exceedingly important, and adherence to complex dietary modifications becomes even more challenging. It should be emphasized to the patient that the high sodium content of commercially processed foods also drives thirst, thus making it imperative to limit salt intake. In order to adhere to daily fluid restrictions, patients and their caregivers should also be encouraged to measure fluid intake carefully, to use smaller glassware, and to spread out fluid intake evenly throughout the day.

5. Food insecurity (FI) is defined as "the inability to acquire or consume a diet of adequate quality or sufficient quantity of food in socially acceptable ways, or the uncertainty that one will be able to do so." Food insecurity is a common problem associated with both poor health outcomes and increased health-care costs. Families living with FI will be less likely to have access to the necessary foods required by their children with chronic disease on restricted diets [11]. Early

identification of FI enables health-care providers to target services to ameliorate the health and developmental consequences associated with FI.

The food insecurity screening tool can be used in the clinic setting [12]. Answering "yes" to either of the validated two-item food insecurity screen statements quickly identifies households with young children and adolescents at risk:

(a) "within the past 12 months, we worried whether our food would run out before we got money to buy more"
(b) "within the past 12 months, the food we bought just didn't last and we didn't have enough money to get more"

Clinical Pearls

1. The protein and energy needs of the dialysis population are similar to that of the healthy population, but barriers to achieving optimal nutritional intake are numerous.
2. Nutrition supplements prescribed in the same manner and with the same importance as medications may help to improve the nutritional status of children and adolescents on dialysis.
3. Given the deterioration in nutritional intake and growth velocity that occurs as CKD progresses, regular nutritional assessment and intervention, along with consideration for treatment with rhGH, are important for both long-term survival and maximizing linear growth.
4. Limiting daily fluid intake may further compromise nutritional intake and should be addressed by careful selection and attention to food and fluid choices.
5. Health-care providers need to routinely address food insecurity with their patients and families.

References

1. Avesani CM, Kamimura MA, Cuppari L. Energy expenditure in chronic kidney disease patients. J Ren Nutr. 2011;21(1):27–30.
2. Marques de Aquino T, Avesani CM, Brasileiro RS, et al. Resting energy expenditure of children and adolescents undergoing hemodialysis. J Ren Nutr. 2008;18(3):312–9.
3. Norman LJ, Macdonald IA, Watson AR. Optimising nutrition in chronic renal insufficiency-progression of disease. Pediatr Nephrol. 2004;19(11):1253–61.
4. Kalantar-Zadeh K, Tortorici AR, Chen JL, et al. Dietary restrictions in dialysis patients: is there anything left to eat? Semin Dial. 2015;28(2):159–68.
5. Janjua HS, Mahan JD. Growth in chronic kidney disease. Adv Chronic Kidney Dis. 2011;18(5):324–31.
6. Ingulli EG, Mak RH. Growth in children with chronic kidney disease: role of nutrition, growth hormone, dialysis, and steroids. Curr Opin Pediatr. 2014;26(2):187–92.

7. Rees L. Growth hormone therapy in children with CKD after more than two decades of practice. Pediatr Nephrol. 2015;31(9):1421–35.
8. Iorember FM, Bamgbola OF. Pilot validation of objective malnutrition-inflammation scores in pediatrics and adolescent cohort on chronic maintenance dialysis. SAGE Open Med. 2014;28(2):2050312114555564.
9. Warady BA, Neu AM, Schaefer F. Optimal care of the infant, child, and adolescent on dialysis: 2014 update. Am J Kidney Dis. 2014;64(1):128–42.
10. NFK KDOQI. Clinical practice guidelines for nutrition in children with CKD: 2008 update. Am J Kidney Dis. 2009;53(Suppl 2):S1–S124.
11. Berkowitz SA, Fabreau GE. Food insecurity: what is the clinician's role? CMAJ. 2015;187(14):1031–2.
12. Hager ER, Quigg AM, Black MM, Coleman SM, et al. Development and validity of a 2-item screen to identify families at risk of food insecurity. Pediatrics. 2010;126:e26–32.

Chapter 23
Anemia Management

Bradley A. Warady

Case Presentation

A 15-year-old white male presented to his primary care physician with complaints of lethargy, poor appetite, and occasional headaches. The patient's mother also reported that her son appeared pale over the past several weeks and that his face appeared to be slightly swollen. Initial physical examination was significant for the patient's pale appearance and the presence of periorbital and pedal edema. Initial BP was 150/105 mmHg. Laboratory data were subsequently obtained and were significant for the findings of a serum creatinine of 15.5 mg/dL and blood urea nitrogen of 165 mg/dL. The patient also had evidence of hyperphosphatemia, secondary hyperparathyroidism (iPTH, 1,056 pg/ml), mild hyperkalemia, hypoalbuminemia (1.5 g/dL), and metabolic acidosis. A complete blood count revealed a normochromic, normocytic anemia with a hemoglobin value of 6.2 g/dL and a hematocrit of 19.0%. A percutaneous kidney biopsy revealed findings compatible with end-stage renal disease (ESRD) secondary to IgA nephropathy as there were <5% viable glomeruli and marked interstitial fibrosis. A right internal jugular hemodialysis catheter was inserted, and thrice weekly chronic hemodialysis was initiated soon thereafter.

Initial evaluation of the patient's anemia, in addition to the red blood cell indices, revealed a reticulocyte count of 1.0% and the absence of occult blood on stool evaluation. Iron studies revealed a serum ferritin of 865 ng/ml and a transferrin saturation of 17%. Treatment with recombinant human erythropoietin (rHuEPO) was started with an intravenous (IV) dose of 50 units/kg in association with each dialysis session, accompanied by IV sodium ferric gluconate 62.5 mg weekly. A multivitamin was

B.A. Warady (✉)
Division of Pediatric Nephrology, University of Missouri, Kansas City School of Medicine
Children's Mercy Hospital, Kansas City, MO, USA
e-mail: bwarady@cmh.edu

© Springer International Publishing AG 2017
B.A. Warady et al. (eds.), *Pediatric Dialysis Case Studies*,
DOI 10.1007/978-3-319-55147-0_23

prescribed to meet vitamin B12 and folate requirements, and both an ACE inhibitor and a calcium channel blocker were prescribed for blood pressure management.

Over the next 3 months, the patient's Hgb gradually rose to 10.6 g/dL with an adjusted IV rHuEPO dose of 3,000 units (60 units/kg) with each dialysis session. The serum ferritin was 500 ng/mL, the TSAT was 22%, and the PTH was 100 pg/ml. The patient's appetite remained somewhat poor prompting his mother to purchase and provide high doses of an over-the-counter zinc supplement (135 mg elemental zinc per day), unbeknown to the medical team. Over the subsequent 6 months, the patient developed a microcytic, hypochromic anemia as his Hgb level progressively fell to 7.2 g/dL despite a stepwise increase of the rHuEPO dose to nearly 400 units/kg/week. The reticulocyte count was only 0.8% and there was mild neutropenia. An intravenous course of replacement iron was provided over eight consecutive dialysis sessions with no improvement. There was no laboratory evidence of either lead or aluminum toxicity or inflammation. Stool evaluation for occult blood remained negative. Remarkably, a thorough review of the patient's medications by a medical student at a routine clinic visit revealed the zinc supplement, and laboratory evaluation provided evidence of zinc toxicity (serum zinc, 2.5 mcg/ml; normal, 0.60–1.2 mcg/ml). As a result of the recognized association between zinc toxicity, copper deficiency, and anemia, the copper status was assessed and revealed evidence of copper deficiency (serum copper, 15 mcg/dL; normal, 63–140 mcg/dL and serum cerruloplasmin, 1.5 mcg/dL; normal, 18–35 mcg/dL). An oral copper supplement was initiated, the zinc supplement was discontinued, and the patient experienced resolution of his anemia despite halving of his rHuEPO dose.

Clinical Questions

1. How common is anemia in association with chronic kidney disease (CKD), and what are the most common contributing factors to its development?
2. What is the etiology of the inadequate production of erythropoietin associated with impaired kidney function?
3. What factors have the greatest influence on the iron status of patients on dialysis and receiving an erythropoietic stimulating agent (ESA)?
4. How is hyporesponsiveness to ESA therapy defined, and what potentially modifiable factors can contribute to this clinical problem?
5. What factors could contribute to the development of copper deficiency and anemia in the chronic dialysis patient?

Diagnostic Discussion

1. The frequency and severity of anemia associated with CKD parallels the degree of renal impairment. The Chronic Kidney Disease in Children (CKiD) study has revealed that a fall in hemoglobin begins when the measured glomerular

filtration rate falls below 43 ml/min/1.73m^2. The North American Pediatric Renal Trials and Collaborative Studies (NAPRTCS) has reported that >93% of children with stage 5 CKD are anemic [1, 2]. The predominant causes of anemia in children and adults with CKD and ESRD are erythropoietin deficiency and lack of iron availability, as well as inflammation, blood loss, hyperparathyroidism, and vitamin deficiency (B12 and folate) [3]. A number of medications have also been associated with the development of anemia. For example, the frequently used antihypertensive agents, angiotensin-converting-enzyme inhibitors, can increase the serum level of N-acetyl-seryl-aspartyl-lysyl-proline (AcSDKP), an inhibitor of erythropoiesis [4]. In view of the factors noted above, erythropoietic-stimulating agents (ESA) and iron serve as the mainstays of therapy. The ESA can be provided as a short-acting rHuEPO formulation (e.g., epoetin alfa), or as darbepoetin alfa, an erythropoietin analogue with a 3–4 times longer half-life than rHuEPO [5, 6]. KDIGO has recommended a starting dose of 20–50 IU/kg three times weekly for epoetin and a dose of 0.45 mcg/kg once weekly or 0.75 mcg/kg every 2 weeks for darbepoetin alfa, with a target hemoglobin for children of 11–12 g/dL. Iron therapy is provided by either the oral or intravenous routes with target values of >20% for transferrin saturation and >100 ng/ml for ferritin [7].

2. Erythropoietin (EPO), the product of the erythropoietin gene on chromosome 7, acts by impairing cell apoptosis of erythroid precursor cells. EPO is a 30.4-kDa glycoprotein that is primarily derived from the liver in fetal life, but which is predominantly produced postnatally by the fibroblast-like interstitial cells of the kidney. The production of native erythropoietin involves regulation through the partial pressure of oxygen of the kidney and other organs that produce erythropoietin and the activity of hypoxia-inducible factor (HIF) [8, 9]. Three HIF-α subunits (HIF-1 α, HIF-2 α, and HIF-3 α) have been identified, and HIF-2 appears to have the greatest influence on erythropoietin synthesis. Cells continuously synthesize HIF oxygen-sensitive alpha subunits; degradation is, in turn, the manner in which HIF activity and resultant erythropoiesis is regulated.

   In the typical setting of anemia-related tissue hypoxia in the patient without CKD, the number of erythropoietin-producing cells increases in the corticomedullary region of the kidney. One of the three identified hypoxia-inducible factors (but predominantly HIF-2) stimulates erythropoietin gene transcription by binding to the hypoxia-responsive enhancer on the EPO gene. With normoxia, one of at least three prolyl hydroxylases (PHD) degrades HIF, reducing erythropoiesis.

   In the unique setting of the patient with CKD/ESRD, despite the presence of anemia, decreased renal tissue oxygen utilization and increased tissue oxygen pressure paradoxically result in decreased transcriptional activity of the HIF. Interstitial cells may also convert to myofibroblasts in the setting of severe CKD/ESRD and lose their capacity to produce EPO [10].

3. Two thirds of the body's iron resides in the red blood cells. The majority of iron required for use or storage results from the catabolism of Hgb from senescent red blood cells. Patients on dialysis require additional iron as a result of blood loss secondary to laboratory testing, gastrointestinal blood loss, and, in the hemodi-

alysis patient, blood loss in the dialyzer and tubing and at the vascular access site. In adults, the blood losses are 4–8 times that of healthy individuals [11–13]. As a result of the increased demand for iron in patients receiving therapy with an ESA, iron availability may be suboptimal as a result of absolute iron deficiency or functional iron deficiency, the latter a state in which the extraordinary demand for iron exceeds the ability of transferrin to deliver it to the bone marrow in a sufficient manner. An additional and exceedingly important influence on the iron status is the development of inflammation which may result in elevated levels of the iron-regulatory protein hepcidin [14–16]. Hepcidin, the levels of which are elevated in children and adults with CKD and ESRD following its production in the liver, binds to the cellular iron exporter ferroportin and causes its internalization and degradation. This precludes movement of iron into the circulation per the intestinal enterocytes and sequesters stored iron in macrophages. The mobilization of iron for red blood cell production, along with a decrease in the level of hepcidin, is also regulated by the release of the hormone erythroferrone by EPO-stimulated erythroblasts in the bone marrow. The production of erythroferrone is low when there are reduced numbers of erythroblasts secondary to erythropoietin deficiency and chronic inflammation [17].

4. Hyporesponsiveness to ESA therapy has historically been defined as persistence of a hemoglobin deficit (<11 g/dL) despite a weekly rHuEPO dose in excess of 400 IU/kg or 20,000 IU/week [18]. More recently, the KDIGO guidelines have defined ESA hyporesponsiveness when there have been two increases in the ESA dose up to 50% beyond the dose which had previously been stable, in an effort to maintain a stable Hgb concentration [7]. The same guidelines provide a list of modifiable (e.g., vitamin deficiency, ACEi/ARB usage) and potentially modifiable (e.g., hyperparathyroidism, bleeding) risk factors for ESA hyporesponsiveness and a recommended therapeutic approach (Table 23.1). Excessive increases in the ESA dose are to be discouraged, and doses in excess of 6,000 IU/m²/week have been associated with poorer patient survival in children receiving chronic peritoneal dialysis (Fig. 23.1) [19].

5. Copper deficiency is diagnosed by the finding of low serum copper and ceruloplasmin levels and can manifest clinically with neutropenia and an ESA-resistant anemia [20]. In cases of severe untreated deficiency, severe neurological manifestations may occur as well. The majority of dietary copper comes from vegetable sources (nuts, chocolate), and approximately 20% comes from meat, fish (particularly shellfish), and poultry. In patients with proteinuric kidney disorders, urinary copper losses can contribute to copper deficiency. In patients on peritoneal dialysis, loss of ceruloplasmin-bound copper into the dialysate can result in copper deficiency [21]. Finally, the ingestion of large quantities of zinc can result in a low copper level. Whereas the tolerable upper intake level (UL) of zinc in adolescents is 34 mg/day, an excessive intake of zinc results in the stimulation of the body's homeostatic mechanisms to limit the intestinal absorption of zinc. This consists of the synthesis of metallothionein, an intracellular ligand within the enterocytes of the small bowel which binds zinc and facilitates its excretion as enterocytes are sloughed into the gut lumen [22, 23]. When high quantities of

Table 23.1. Potentially correctable versus non-correctable factors involved in the anemia of CKD, in addition to ESA deficiency [7]

Easily correctable	Potentially correctable	Impossible to correct
Absolute iron deficiency	Infection/inflammation	Hemoglobinopathies
Vitamin B_{12}/folate deficiency	Underdialysis	Bone marrow disorders
Hypothyroidism	Hemolysis	
ACEi/ARB	Bleeding	
Nonadherence	Hyperparathyroidism	
	PRCA	
	Malignancy	
	Malnutrition	

ACEi angiotensin-converting enzyme inhibitor, *ARB* angiotensin-receptor blocker, *PRCA* pure red cell aplasia

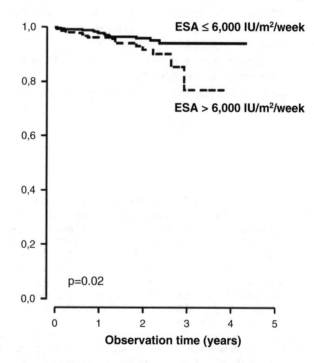

Fig. 23.1 Kaplan-Meier actuarial survival curves for patients with mean administered ESA equivalent dose ≤ or >6,000 IU/m² per week (Used with permission from *The Journal of the American Society of Nephrology* [19])

zinc are ingested, as may occur with enteral feeds or the ingestion of over-the-counter preparations, there is increased synthesis of metallothionein to which copper is competitively and preferentially bound [24]. The copper is unavailable for absorption and is excreted in the feces, contributing to the development of copper deficiency. Excessive intake of dietary iron can also limit copper absorption. Whereas the mechanism of the anemia associated with zinc-induced copper deficiency is unknown, it is likely related to the fact that copper is required for the incorporation of iron into the heme molecule, and when ceruloplasmin activity is decreased, transfer of iron from macrophages to transferrin is compromised. However, normocytic, macrocytic, and microcytic anemias have all been described in the setting of copper deficiency. Treatment of copper deficiency with oral copper supplementation is typically therapeutic with resolution of anemia and neutropenia within 6 weeks of repletion therapy. Intravenous supplementation may be necessary on occasion.

Clinical Pearls

1. Treatment with rHuEPO and iron are the key components of anemia management in children with CKD and ESRD.
2. Iron availability can be compromised by (a) the development of absolute iron deficiency, (b) the presence of functional iron deficiency as a result of ESA-stimulated erythropoiesis, or (c) inflammation-related sequestration of iron associated with elevated levels of hepcidin.
3. Hyporesponsiveness to ESA therapy can occur secondary to a variety of modifiable or potentially modifiable factors.
4. Copper deficiency can occur secondary to excessive zinc intake and can result in ESA-resistant anemia.

References

1. Fadrowski JJ, Pierce CB, Cole SR, Moxey-Mims M, Warady BA, Furth SL. Hemoglobin decline in children with chronic kidney disease: baseline results from the chronic kidney disease in children prospective cohort study. Clin J Am Soc Nephrol CJASN. 2008;3(2):457–62. PubMed PMID: 18235140. Pubmed Central PMCID: PMC2390950. Epub 2008/02/01. eng
2. Atkinson MA, Martz K, Warady BA, Neu AM. Risk for anemia in pediatric chronic kidney disease patients: a report of NAPRTCS. Pediatr Nephrol (Berlin, Germany). 2010;25(9):1699–706. PubMed PMID: 20464428. Epub 2010/05/14. eng
3. Warady BA, Silverstein DM. Management of anemia with erythropoietic-stimulating agents in children with chronic kidney disease. Pediatr Nephrol (Berlin, Germany). 2014;29(9):1493–505. PubMed PMID: 24005791
4. Kuriyama R, Kogure H, Itoh S, Kikuchi K, Ichikawa N, Nomura Y, et al. Angiotensin converting enzyme inhibitor induced anemia in a kidney transplant recipient. Transplant Proc. 1996;28(3):1635. PubMed PMID: 8658817. Epub 1996/06/01. eng
5. Warady BA, Arar MY, Lerner G, Nakanishi AM, Stehman-Breen C. Darbepoetin alfa for the treatment of anemia in pediatric patients with chronic kidney disease. Pediatr Nephrol (Berlin, Germany). 2006;21(8):1144–52. PubMed PMID: 16724235. Epub 2006/05/26. eng
6. Schaefer F, Hoppe B, Jungraithmayr T, Klaus G, Pape L, Farouk M, et al. Safety and usage of darbepoetin alfa in children with chronic kidney disease: prospective registry study. Pediatr Nephrol (Berlin, Germany). 2015;31(3):443–53. PubMed PMID: 26482252. Epub 2015/10/21. Eng
7. KDIGO. Clinical practice guideline for anemia in chronic kidney disease. Kidney Int Suppl. 2012;2(Suppl August):270–335.
8. Koury MJ, Haase VH. Anaemia in kidney disease: harnessing hypoxia responses for therapy. Nat Rev Nephrol. 2015;11(7):394–410.
9. Nangaku M, Eckardt KU. Hypoxia and the HIF system in kidney disease. J Mol Med (Berlin, Germany). 2007;85(12):1325–30. PubMed PMID: 18026918. Epub 2007/11/21. eng

10. Falke LL, Gholizadeh S, Goldschmeding R, Kok RJ, Nguyen TQ. Diverse origins of the myofibroblast-implications for kidney fibrosis. Nat Rev Nephrol. 2015;11(4):233–44. PubMed PMID: 25584804. Epub 2015/01/15. eng

11. Sargent JA, Acchiardo SR. Iron requirements in hemodialysis. Blood Purif. 2004;22(1):112–23. PubMed PMID: 14732819. Epub 2004/01/21. eng

12. Kalantar-Zadeh K, Streja E, Miller JE, Nissenson AR. Intravenous iron versus erythropoiesis-stimulating agents: friends or foes in treating chronic kidney disease anemia? Adv Chronic Kidney Dis. 2009;16(2):143–51. PubMed PMID: 19233073. Epub 2009/02/24. eng

13. Besarab A, Coyne DW. Iron supplementation to treat anemia in patients with chronic kidney disease. Nat Rev Nephrol. 2010;6(12):699–710. PubMed PMID: 20956992. Epub 2010/10/20. eng

14. Ganz T. Hepcidin, a key regulator of iron metabolism and mediator of anemia of inflammation. Blood. 2003;102(3):783–8. PubMed PMID: 12663437. Epub 2003/03/29. eng

15. Atkinson MA, Kim JY, Roy CN, Warady BA, White CT, Furth SL. Hepcidin and risk of anemia in CKD: a cross-sectional and longitudinal analysis in the CKiD cohort. Pediatr Nephrol (Berlin, Germany). 2015;30(4):635–43. PubMed PMID: 25380788. Pubmed Central PMCID: PMC4336204. Epub 2014/11/09. eng

16. Zaritsky J, Young B, Gales B, Wang HJ, Rastogi A, Westerman M, et al. Reduction of serum hepcidin by hemodialysis in pediatric and adult patients. Clin J Am Soc Nephrol CJASN. 2010;5(6):1010–4. PubMed PMID: 20299375. Pubmed Central PMCID: PMC2879302. Epub 2010/03/20. eng

17. Fried W. The liver as a source of extrarenal erythropoietin production. Blood. 1972;40(5):671–7. PubMed PMID: 4637502. Epub 1972/11/01. eng

18. Bamgbola O. Resistance to erythropoietin-stimulating agents: etiology, evaluation, and therapeutic considerations. Pediatr Nephrol (Berlin, Germany). 2012;27(2):195–205. PubMed PMID: 21424525. Epub 2011/03/23. eng

19. Borzych-Duzalka D, Bilginer Y, Ha IS, Bak M, Rees L, Cano F, et al. Management of anemia in children receiving chronic peritoneal dialysis. J Am Soc Nephrol JASN. 2013;24(4):665–76. PubMed PMID: 23471197. Pubmed Central PMCID: 3609132

20. Higuchi T, Matsukawa Y, Okada K, Oikawa O, Yamazaki T, Ohnishi Y, et al. Correction of copper deficiency improves erythropoietin unresponsiveness in hemodialysis patients with anemia. Intern Med (Tokyo, Japan). 2006;45(5):271–3. PubMed PMID: 16595992. Epub 2006/04/06. eng

21. Swaminathan S. Trace elements, toxic metals, and metalloids in kidney disease. In: J.D. Kopple, S.G. Massry, Kalantar-Zadeh K, editors. Nutritional management of renal disease. 3rd. San Diego: Elsevier Inc.; 2013. p. 339–349.

22. Duncan A, Yacoubian C, Watson N, Morrison I. The risk of copper deficiency in patients prescribed zinc supplements. J Clin Pathol. 2015;68(9):723–5. PubMed PMID: 26085547. Epub 2015/06/19. Eng

23. Richards MP, Cousins RJ. Mammalian zinc homeostasis: requirement for RNA and metallothionein synthesis. Biochem Biophys Res Commun. 1975;64(4):1215–23. PubMed PMID: 1137597. Epub 1975/06/16. eng

24. Hein MS. Copper deficiency anemia and nephrosis in zinc-toxicity: a case report. S D J Med. 2003;56(4):143–7. PubMed PMID: 12728841. Epub 2003/05/06. Eng

Chapter 24
Chronic Kidney Disease – Mineral and Bone Disorder

Rukshana Shroff

Case Presentation

A newborn male infant with an antenatal diagnosis of bilateral hydroureteronephrosis and oligohydramnios is confirmed to have posterior urethral valves. Despite valve fulguration and appropriate fluid therapy, his creatinine continues to increase with associated hyperkalaemia, metabolic acidosis, and high blood urea nitrogen and phosphate levels. He is started on peritoneal dialysis at 2 weeks of age. Following multiple episodes of peritonitis, he is transferred to haemodialysis (HD) when 8 months old. At 15 months he is noted to have a wide open anterior fontanelle, bowing of both lower limbs, inability to bear weight and no dentition. He has persistently low serum Ca levels and hyperparathyroidism. At 4 years of age, he receives a kidney transplant, but this fails after 10 years, and he returns to HD. Compliance with diet and medications is very poor, and he has high serum phosphate and PTH levels with raised serum Ca levels. A few months later, he trips and falls in the park and fractures his right tibia. At 17 years he develops ischaemic chest pain while on dialysis and is found to have extensive coronary and aortic root calcification.

Clinical Questions

1. Why do children with CKD develop bone disease?
2. What are the manifestations of bone disease in CKD, and how would you investigate it?
3. How would you manage CKD-MBD in an infant?

R. Shroff (✉)
Great Ormond Street Hospital for Children, Nephrology Unit, London, UK
e-mail: Rukshana.Shroff@gosh.nhs.uk

© Springer International Publishing AG 2017
B.A. Warady et al. (eds.), *Pediatric Dialysis Case Studies*,
DOI 10.1007/978-3-319-55147-0_24

4. How would you manage hyperphosphataemia and hyperparathyroidism in this child?
5. Why does CKD-MBD cause cardiovascular disease?

Diagnostic Discussion

1. *Mineral dysregulation in CKD*: Patients with CKD can develop bone disease due to derangements in Ca, P and vitamin D homeostasis [1, 2]. Phosphate retention begins early in CKD and results in increased PTH and fibroblast growth factor 23 (FGF23). Both will promote increased urinary P excretion, but they can also cause bone demineralisation. In parallel, there is reduced production of active 1,25-dihydroxyvitamin D [1,25(OH)2D] by the failing kidneys that causes hypocalcaemia. The body attempts to keep blood Ca levels in the normal range by mobilising Ca from bone stores into the circulation, thereby causing further bone demineralisation [1, 3]. The mineral dysregulation in CKD directly affects bone strength and architecture, and this forms the spectrum of CKD – mineral and bone disorder (CKD-MBD). Importantly, as Ca is mobilised out of the bone, and the bone loses its normal formation-resorption activity, excess Ca and P may deposit in soft tissues, causing vascular calcification [4] (Fig. 24.1).

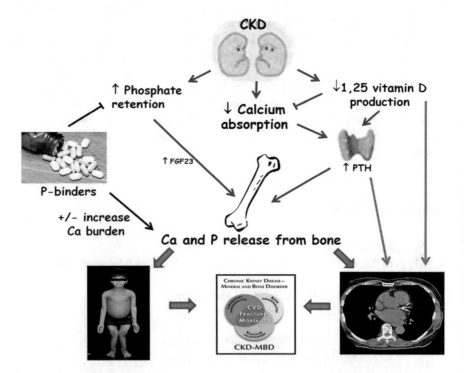

Fig. 24.1 Bone disease and arterial calcification due to dysregulated mineral homoeostasis in children with chronic kidney disease

2. *Bone disease in CKD*: Childhood CKD is associated with nearly universal distur-bances in bone and mineral metabolism that present multiple obstacles to bone accrual resulting in bone pain, deformities, growth retardation and fractures [1, 2]. On long-term follow-up of a childhood CKD cohort, 61% had severe growth retardation, 37% deforming bone abnormalities and chronic or atraumatic frac-tures and 18% were severely disabled by bone disease [5]. Approximately 35–50% of children with CKD grow up to become short adults, which reduces psychoso-cial well-being and is strongly associated with increased mortality. Abnormal bone micro-architecture and mineralisation defects are common and strongly associate with Ca status [6]. On bone biopsy, 30% of children with early CKD and >90% on dialysis have deficient mineralisation [3]. Importantly, fracture risk is associated with lower cortical volumetric bone mineral density (BMD) and low serum Ca levels: one standard deviation (SD) decrease in BMD is associated with a twofold increase in fracture risk [7]. There is a two to threefold higher fracture risk in boys and girls with CKD compared to their healthy peers [8].

   Investigations for bone disease in CKD: The diagnosis of bone disease in CKD is based on repeated biochemical analysis, along with radiographic assess-ment when required. Even though no single biochemical marker is able to pro-vide a complete assessment of renal osteodystrophy, bone biopsies are rarely performed for the clinical management of patients. In children with CKD and those undergoing chronic dialysis, high PTH and low serum calcium levels were seen in those with defective mineralisation, irrespective of their bone turnover rate. These studies suggest that a combination of serum Ca, alkaline phosphatase and PTH levels may lead to a more precise non-invasive assessment of turnover and mineralisation abnormalities. The Kidney Disease Improving Global Outcomes (KDIGO) CKD-MBD guideline places particular importance on interpreting the trend in Ca-P-PTH and vitamin D values rather than a single measure [9]. Radiological investigations are not routinely performed, although some centres prefer to do annual hand x-rays. Non-invasive assessment of BMD by peripheral quantitative CT scan [7], DEXA and bone biopsies [2, 3] are per-formed in research settings.

3. *Infant CKD*: Infancy is a period of rapid growth during which the body has a high demand for Ca and P. In healthy children, as rapid bone mass accrual occurs, the Ca content of the skeleton increases from ~25 g at birth to ~1,000 g in adults, giving rise to a greatly increased Ca and P requirement. Normal levels for serum Ca and P are highest in the first year of life and gradually decrease to the normal adult range by age 4 years. Increased Ca requirements can be met with Ca sup-plements, higher doses of vitamin D or increased dialysate calcium [10].

4. *Management of hyperphosphataemia and hyperparathyroidism in CKD*: CKD-MBD management in children must focus on maintaining normal Ca-P-vitamin D homeostasis, so as to maintain optimal bone and cardiovascular health, while correcting metabolic abnormalities such as acidosis, anaemia and malnutrition that can worsen bone disease, growth and cardiovascular disease. Prevention should be the primary objective in order to delay the development of osseous and cardiovascular sequelae.

(a) *Hyperphosphataemia* begins in early stages of CKD. Restriction of dietary P intake may be sufficient in early stages of CKD, but normophosphataemia may only be maintained at the expense of increased PTH and FGF23 levels, both of which decrease tubular phosphate reabsorption. As renal function deteriorates, dietary control of P becomes more difficult, and oral P-binders are required. P-binders are of two main types: Ca-based and Ca-free (Table 24.1). Ca-based P-binders are recommended as first-line treatment except in those with overt hypercalcaemia [10]. Ca-free P-binders have the advantage of a superior P-binding capacity (compared to Ca carbonate), and no absorption of Ca, resulting in an attenuation of coronary calcification in adult dialysis patients. Ca-free phosphate binders are especially indicated in patients with a calcium intake exceeding twice the recommended daily intake

Table 24.1 Phosphate binders

Compound	Calcium content (%)	Calcium absorbed (%)	Phosphate bound per g compound	Phosphate bound per mg Ca^{++} absorbed	Comment
Calcium carbonate	40	20–30	39	$\approx$ 1 mg / 8 mg	High Ca load; inexpensive; few GI side effects
Calcium acetate	25	22	45	$\approx$ 1 mg / 3 mg	Lower Ca load than $CaCO_3$; inexpensive; GI side effects more common, particularly in infants
Mg + Ca carbonate	variable	20–30% of Ca	NA	$\approx$ 1 mg / 2.3 mg	Lower Ca load; fewer GI side effects; unknown long-term effects
Sevelamer hydrochloride or sevelamer carbonate	0	0	NA	NA	Ca- and aluminum-free; acts as cholesterol binding resin and lowers serum cholesterol; binds fat soluble vitamins; expensive; difficult to administer to younger children; can cause metabolic acidosis (with hydrochloride preparation)
Aluminium-containing binders	0	0	Similar to calcium acetate (no studies in children)	NA	Very effective P-binding but carries risk of aluminium toxicity; can be used short-term under close monitoring of aluminium levels; recommended only for 'rescue therapy' from severe hyperphosphataemia
Lanthanum carbonate	0	0	Similar to calcium acetate (no studies in children)	NA	Hypomotility and serious cases of gastrointestinal obstruction, ileus, and faecal impaction reported in adults; Lanthanum is deposited in the growing bone and growth plate – should be used only with caution in children

NA not applicable

(which increases from 210 mg elemental calcium per day in the first 6 months of life to 1,250 mg/day in adolescents), reduced PTH levels (with likely adynamic bone disease), hypercalcaemia or even emerging soft tissue calcifications [10]. In an 8-week crossover study in children, sevelamer and calcium acetate were equally effective at reducing serum P levels, but significantly less hypercalcaemia occurred in the sevelamer group [4, 10]. However, a recent randomised clinical trial in adults with a GFR of 20–45 ml/min/1.73m^2 demonstrated an increase in arterial calcification with calcium, lanthanum and sevelamer binder therapy, but not in placebo treated patients. Similar data are not available for children. Table 24.1 describes the available P-binders, their P-binding capability and the risk of hypercalcaemia and side effects.

(b) *Vitamin D:* Children with CKD are at high risk of nutritional vitamin D deficiency. In the early stages of CKD, supplementation with ergocalciferol or cholecalciferol can delay the onset of secondary hyperparathyroidism and should be prescribed before calcitriol is considered. Although evidence is lacking, most authorities suggest that serum 25(OH)D levels should be maintained above 50–75 nMol/L. Vitamin D repletion strategies include daily, weekly, monthly and even 3-monthly dosing regimens.

(c) *Hyperparathyroidism:* If PTH levels remain elevated despite normal serum 25(OH)D and P levels, treatment with vitamin D analogues is required to compensate for reduced renal 1-α hydroxylase activity and to prevent and control secondary hyperparathyroidism. Alfacalcidol (1-α hydroxyvitamin D) or calcitriol are most commonly used. The dose of vitamin D analogue depends on initial PTH, Ca and P values. An initial dose of 5–10 ng/kg*day is effective and safe in most children with CKD, and it is suggested that the lowest dose of vitamin D analogue that maintains normal serum calcium levels is used.

Calcimimetics bind to the parathyroid Ca-sensing receptor, increase its sensitivity to Ca by allosteric modification and dose dependently decrease PTH levels by up to 80%. The effect is largely independent of baseline PTH and P levels and thus allows for control of parathyroid gland function even in patients with otherwise refractory hyperparathyroidism. Cinacalcet is the only currently approved calcimimetic agent, and paediatric trials are under way.

5. *Cardiovascular disease in CKD:* Cardiovascular mortality is dramatically increased in uremic patients. As bones decalcify, excess calcium can get deposited in soft tissues including the vessels, causing vascular calcification (Fig. 24.1). Vascular calcification is a highly regulated cell-mediated process with many promoters and inhibitors of calcification that leads to vascular stiffness and left ventricular hypertrophy [10]. More than 90% of young adults with childhood onset CKD have significant coronary artery calcifications. Alterations of the morphological and functional properties of arteries have been reported as early as in the second decade of life in children on dialysis; the presence of vascular calcification on CT scan is directly related to hyperphosphataemia, the average calcium x phosphate product over time, intake of calcium-containing phosphate binders and PTH levels [10]. This is further discussed in Chap. 27.

Clinical Pearls

1. Rickets develops from a long-standing deficiency of Ca and vitamin D. Given the high Ca requirements of growing infants, they often require high Ca intake. In an attempt to restrict dietary phosphate by limiting dairy products, Ca restriction can also occur. It is important to estimate the Recommended Nutrient Intake (or the equivalent Recommended Dietary Allowance) for Ca and ensure that these requirements are met through Ca supplementation if necessary. The routine use of dialysate Ca concentrations of 1.25 mMol/l may be inadequate in children with significant ultrafiltration-associated calcium losses. Thus, 1.5 and 1.75 mMol/L dialysate Ca concentrations are often needed, depending on the oral calcium intake from diet and P-binders, along with vitamin D treatment.

2. P-binders must always be given with meals, and the dose adjusted depending on the P content of the food. Significantly more Ca is absorbed and little P removed when Ca-containing P-binders are not given with meals. Calcium acetate and calcium carbonate contain 25% and 40% of elemental calcium, respectively. Calcium acetate binds more phosphorus per unit of calcium content and thus allows for higher doses and improved phosphate control. If given at similar doses, calcium acetate results in a reduced incidence of hypercalcaemia as compared to calcium carbonate (Table 24.1). On the other hand, less gastrointestinal side effects have been reported with calcium carbonate.

   Of note, calcium carbonate requires an acidic pH in the stomach to dissociate and bind P. Hence, calcium carbonate must not be given along with an H2-antagonist or sodium bicarbonate.

3. Active vitamin D analogues increase the intestinal absorption of Ca and P. Calcitriol increases intestinal P absorption from ~60 to 90%. Hence, it is important that serum P levels are adequately controlled with P-binder treatment when using alfacalcidol or calcitriol. Calcitriol, hypercalcaemia and hyperphosphataemia contribute to extraosseous tissue calcifications and decreased survival in children with advanced CKD and on dialysis.

4. Tertiary hyperparathyroidism (where the parathyroid glands have undergone severe hyperplasia, sometimes with adenoma formation, and escape negative feedback control via the Ca-sensing receptors) is associated with high PTH levels despite adequate or high serum Ca. This is a largely preventable condition if careful management of Ca-P-PTH and vitamin D is performed from the earliest stages of CKD. Cinacalcet reduces PTH production. Recent clinical trials in adults have shown that treatment with cinacalcet (with the addition of small doses of vitamin D analogues, if required) is effective in PTH reduction and will cause a more pronounced reduction in the progression of cardiovascular and cardiac valve calcification compared to vitamin D treatment alone [10]. Importantly, cinacalcet also reduces serum Ca levels, possibly via increased mineral deposition into bone, and a case of fatal hypocalcaemia observed in a clinical trial underlines the need for careful monitoring throughout the treatment course. With the availability of cinacalcet therapy, parathyroidectomy is now rarely required.

References

1. Bacchetta J, Harambat J, Cochat P, Salusky IB, Wesseling-Perry K. The consequences of chronic kidney disease on bone metabolism and growth in children. Nephrol Dial Transplant. 2012;27(8):3063–71.
2. Wesseling-Perry K, Salusky IB. Phosphate binders, vitamin D and calcimimetics in the management of chronic kidney disease-mineral bone disorders (CKD-MBD) in children. Pediatr Nephrol. 2013;28(4):617–25.
3. Bakkaloglu SA, Wesseling-Perry K, Pereira RC, Gales B, Wang HJ, Elashoff RM, et al. Value of the new bone classification system in pediatric renal osteodystrophy. Clin J Am Soc Nephrol. 2010;5(10):1860–6.
4. Shroff R, Long DA, Shanahan C. Mechanistic insights into vascular calcification in CKD. J Am Soc Nephrol. 2013;24(2):179–89.
5. Groothoff JW, Offringa M, Van Eck-Smit BL, Gruppen MP, Van De Kar NJ, Wolff ED, et al. Severe bone disease and low bone mineral density after juvenile renal failure. Kidney Int. 2003;63(1):266–75.
6. Borzych D, Rees L, Ha IS, Chua A, Valles PG, Lipka M, et al. The bone and mineral disorder of children undergoing chronic peritoneal dialysis. Kidney Int. 2010;78(12):1295–304.
7. Denburg MR, Tsampalieros AK, de Boer IH, Shults J, Kalkwarf HJ, Zemel BS, Foerster D, Stokes D, Leonard MB. Mineral metabolism and cortical volumetric bone mineral density in childhood chronic kidney disease. J Clin Endocrinol Metab. 2013;98:1930–8.
8. Denburg MR, Kumar J, Jemielita T, Brooks ER, Skversky A, Portale AA, Salusky IB, Warady BA, Furth SL, Leonard MB. Fracture burden and risk factors in childhood CKD: results from the CKiD Cohort Study. J Am Soc Nephrol. 2016;27:543–50.
9. Ketteler M, Elder GJ, Evenepoel P, Ix JH, Jamal SA, Lafage-Proust MH, et al. Revisiting KDIGO clinical practice guideline on chronic kidney disease-mineral and bone disorder: a commentary from a Kidney disease: improving global outcomes controversies conference. Kidney Int. 2015;87(3):502–28.
10. Rees L, Shroff R. The demise of calcium-based phosphate binders-is this appropriate for children? Pediatr Nephrol. 2015;30:2061–71.

Chapter 25
Growth Delay

Rose M. Ayoob and John D. Mahan

Case Presentation

A 23-month-old, former 37-week-old (birthweight: 3.389 kg) male with a history of chronic kidney disease (CKD) stage V secondary to bilateral renal dysplasia and right-sided grade 4 vesicoureteral reflux (VUR) presented for his monthly dialysis clinic visit. He was a new patient so previous clinic records were reviewed. His past medical history included a pneumothorax and an episode of SVT at birth. He required a left-sided nephrostomy tube for severe hydronephrosis, and he had a history of a complicated urinary tract infection for which he was placed on antibiotic prophylaxis. Feeding difficulties were noted soon after birth. Initially, he was placed on an infant renal formula (20 kcal/oz) with breast milk supplementation, but he experienced problems with poor growth. At 13 months, he was transitioned to toddler formulas with higher caloric content (24 and 27 kcal/oz), both of which were poorly tolerated, and he continued to experience poor growth.

He was evaluated and followed in feeding clinic to work with both physical and occupational therapists due to a concern regarding food aversion. Despite these interventions, he remained near the third percentile for weight and below the third percentile for height based on age. On multiple clinic visits, the parents reported problems with poor oral intake and frequent bouts of emesis. Additional medical problems included metabolic acidosis, microcytic anemia, and metabolic bone disease, all of which were managed medically. There were no problems with overall volume status or blood pressure, and he remained polyuric. Despite successful

R.M. Ayoob, MD (✉) • J.D. Mahan, MD
Nationwide Children's Hospital, Division of Nephrology, The Ohio State University,
Columbus, OH, USA
e-mail: rose.ayoob@nationwidechildrens.org

© Springer International Publishing AG 2017
B.A. Warady et al. (eds.), *Pediatric Dialysis Case Studies*,
DOI 10.1007/978-3-319-55147-0_25

medical management of electrolytes and anemia through most of his second year of life, persistent growth failure was deemed the indication to start renal replacement therapy. He initially underwent laparoscopic gastrostomy tube placement at 18 months of age with the initiation of nighttime continuous feeds, allowing him to receive PO intake during the day. At 19 months of age, he had a peritoneal dialysis catheter placed and was started on dialysis treatment 2 weeks later.

At the time of his second visit at 24 months of age, his vital signs were unremarkable, and he demonstrated good blood pressure control in addition to significant weight gain. Whereas some height gain was noted, his height remained just below the third percentile (79 cm, −2.35 SDS). He was receiving adequate dietary protein and calories based on nutritional guidelines, and his labs were all within normal ranges. The decision to initiate recombinant human growth hormone (rhGH) therapy was made after a discussion regarding growth management took place with his parents. The parents were informed that no growth hormone stimulation tests were required, despite what they had heard from family friends who had a child prescribed rhGH by endocrinology. He was started on rhGH at 0.05 mg/kg/day given subcutaneously. Over the next 21 months, he demonstrated excellent growth with a height gain of 12.65 cm per year (length 100 cm, −0.188 SDS at 45 months of age) (Figs. 25.1 and 25.2).

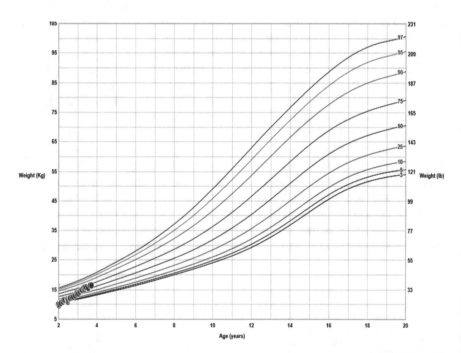

Fig. 25.1 Weight for age percentiles (boys, 2–20 years). Weight for age for this patient demonstrating improved outcome after 24 months of age, coincident with the initiation of recombinant human growth hormone (rhGH) therapy

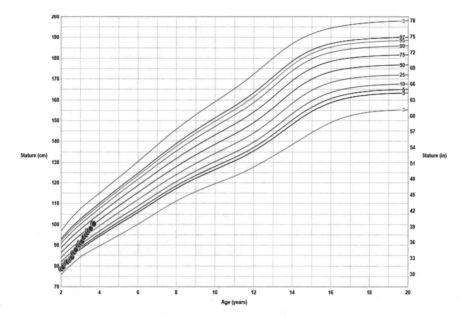

Fig. 25.2 Height for age percentiles (boys, 2–20 years). Height for age for this patient demonstrating improved outcome after 24 months of age, coincident with initiation of recombinant human growth hormone (rhGH) therapy

Clinical Questions

1. What are the short- and long-term consequences of growth delay in children who receive chronic dialysis?
2. What are the possible causes of growth delay in a child on dialysis?
3. Is there a need for growth hormone (GH) stimulation tests when evaluating a pediatric dialysis patient for recombinant human growth hormone (rhGH) therapy?
4. What are the factors that cause a state of GH resistance in children with chronic kidney disease/end-stage renal disease and what are the mechanisms that explain how rhGH therapy improves growth in these children?
5. What is the best way to administer and monitor rhGH therapy in a child on dialysis?

Diagnostic Discussion

1. Growth failure is a common and significant clinical problem in patients with chronic kidney disease (CKD) [1]. Patients with CKD-associated growth failure can exhibit a range of potentially serious medical and psychological complications.

Table 25.1 Etiology of growth failure in CKD

Age of onset of CKD[a]
Primary renal disease[a]
Severity of renal insufficiency[a]
Water and electrolyte problems
Calorie deficiency and abnormal protein metabolism
Metabolic acidosis
Metabolic bone disease
Abnormal GH/IGF1 axis
Treatment modalities and treatment effects
Genetic factors[a]

[a]Non-modifiable factors

Poor growth during CKD that leads to short stature at dialysis initiation is a marker for a more complicated clinical course and worse long-term outcomes. Growth failure in children with CKD and in children on dialysis is associated with an increased number of hospitalizations and even increased mortality, double that of children with CKD and no growth failure [2]. Early intervention for growth failure is critical since measures, such as the correction of malnutrition and CKD-mineral bone disease (CKD-MBD) abnormalities, and treatment with recombinant human growth hormone (rhGH) are considerably more effective in promoting growth and good health when started before the initiation of dialysis [1].

Long-term outcomes have been studied in adults who had CKD in childhood. Studies have shown that a greater final adult height in these individuals correlates with higher educational attainment, better employment rates, more successful marriages, and greater rates of independent living [3]. Better quality of life has also been strongly correlated with overall height satisfaction in adults who experienced CKD as children [4].

2. The etiology of growth failure in children with CKD is usually multifactorial and includes both modifiable and non-modifiable risk factors (Table 25.1). Complicating the approach to evaluation and treatment of growth failure in these patients is, in turn, its multifactorial pathogenesis in most affected children [1]. Congenital and acquired renal abnormalities can exert their effects on the child's growth and development either early or late in the course of the kidney disease, primarily dependent on the severity of the CKD. Additional clinical problems that affect growth include fluid and electrolyte abnormalities, metabolic acidosis, abnormal bone metabolism, and malnutrition. Moreover, the severity of the growth hormone (GH)-insulin-like growth factor-1 (IGF-1) axis abnormalities (cellular resistance, IGF-1 binding protein accumulation) vary greatly in these children and can significantly affect growth, independent of nutrition and medical therapies [5].

Children also undergo a variety of medical interventions at different times during the course of their disease management that can impact growth and development positively (e.g., correction of acidosis) or negatively (e.g., corticosteroid therapy, poor control of hyperphosphatemia, etc.). The choice and effectiveness of renal replacement therapy may also influence growth in children with advanced

CKD since effective dialysis can reduce uremia and both promote and permit better nutrition [6].

Thus, growth in children with CKD or end-stage renal disease (ESRD) may be influenced by (1) patient genetic factors and nonrenal comorbidities; (2) specific aspects of the timing, type, and severity of the underlying renal disorder; (3) specific types and severity of CKD complications; and (4) the different types and timing of renal therapies [6–8]. In children with CKD (on dialysis or not) who have growth failure, careful assessment and evaluation for modifiable factors should be pursued. Once the modifiable causes have been successfully addressed for a sufficient period of time (usually 3–4 months), continued growth failure as reflected by little or no improvement in growth velocity or height SDS should prompt consideration for addressing the GH-IGF-1 axis abnormalities of CKD with exogenous rhGH therapy [1].

3. There is no need for growth hormone stimulation testing when caring for a patient with CKD who is a potential candidate for rhGH therapy. Children with CKD typically demonstrate normal to high normal levels of GH, normal IGF-1 levels, and normal responses to GH stimulation. Children with CKD and poor growth respond well to exogenous GH therapy despite normal GH and IGF-1 serum levels. However, before initiating rhGH treatment, assessment of serum electrolytes, renal function, glucose, calcium, phosphorus, alkaline phosphatase, parathyroid hormone (PTH), thyroid status, bone disease (hip and knee radiographs), bone age, and funduscopic examination should be performed [1]. If the intact PTH is >900 pg/ml in CKD 5 or >400 pg/ml in CKD 2–4, enhanced treatment of CKD-MBD to lower intact PTH below these values should occur before initiating rhGH therapy [9].

4. In children with CKD there are multiple functional abnormalities in the GH-IGF-1 axis, even though circulating levels of GH and IGF-1 are not reduced, that contribute to a state of GH resistance [8] (Fig. 25.3):

   (a) There is less free circulating IGF-1 because of increased binding to IGF-1 binding proteins (IGF-1 BPs) due to both increased production and decreased renal clearance of IGF-1 BPs. While IGF-1 BP 3 is the most prominent IGF-1 BP, in uremia, IGFPB-1, 2, 4, and 6 accumulate and thus there is less free IGF-1 available to stimulate cartilage and bone cells to promote growth. In fact, in uremia free IGF-1 levels are decreased by as much as 50%.

   (b) Increased proteolysis of IGFBP-3 leads to a reduction in the level of IGF-1 circulating in the IGF-1/acid labile subunit (ALS)/IGFBP-3 complex which results in reduced IGF-1 receptor activation and reduced feedback to the hypothalamus and pituitary.

   (c) Cellular resistance to the effects of GH and IGF-1 occurs, and this is at least partially due to alterations in the post-receptor GH-activated Janus kinase/signal transducer and activator of the transcription (JAK/STAT) signaling pathway. An intact JAK2-STAT signaling pathway is needed for GH stimulation of IGF-1 gene expression. In renal failure, impairment of phosphorylation of JAK2 and STAT proteins leads to diminished IGF-1 gene expression.

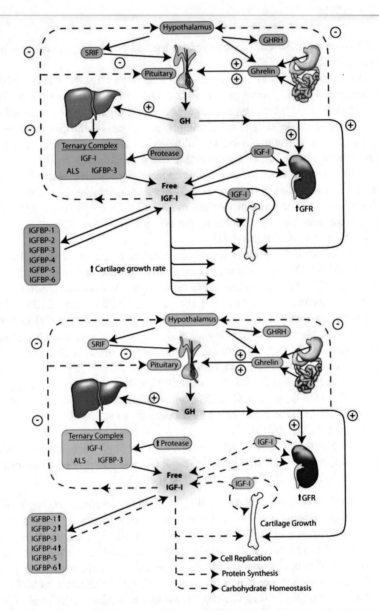

Fig. 25.3 The growth hormone-insulin-like growth factor-1 (GH-IGF-1) axis in CKD. In CKD, the GH-IGF-1 axis is markedly deranged. Circulating GH level is high normal due to increased pituitary pulsatile release and reduced renal GH clearance. Total IGF-1 levels are normal, not elevated as expected in relation to circulating GH levels. Free, bioactive IGF-1 is reduced due to increased levels of most circulating IGF binding proteins (IGFBPs), especially high-affinity forms IGFBP-1, 2, 4, and 6, related to decreased renal clearance. Increased proteolysis of IGFBP-3 leads to less IGF-1 in association with the IGFBP-3 and ALS ternary complex resulting in less cellular IGF-1 receptor activation. There is also marked GH and IGF-1 resistance; the mechanisms responsible for IGF-1 resistance in CKD are not completely understood, but appear to involve a defect in the post-receptor GH-activated Janus kinase 2 (JAK2) signal transducer and activator of the transcription (STAT) pathway. This signaling pathway is critical to the process of stimulated IGF-1 gene expression which is the key cellular response to GH receptor activation. A decrease in cellular GH receptors also appears to exist and may also contribute to the blunted IGF-1 response to GH seen in CKD. (Reprinted from Janjua and Mahan [8], with permission from Elsevier)

Clinical and experimental studies have demonstrated that the state of GH resistance in uremia can be overcome by supraphysiologic levels of GH produced by exogenous rhGH therapy. In addition, the alterations in GH secretion that occur during glucocorticoid treatment can also be overcome by rhGH therapy. These observations provide the rationale for treating children with CKD and growth failure unresponsive to nutritional/medical measures with rhGH. Administration of rhGH to children with CKD increases the production of IGF-1 to a greater extent than that of IGF-1 binding proteins (IGF-1 BPs), thereby raising the availability of free IGF-1 at the tissue level to a degree that overcomes intracellular resistance and promotes the anabolic growth processes.

5. In children with CKD, rhGH should be provided as subcutaneous injections of 0.05 mg/kg/day. Less frequent dosing is associated with a suboptimal response. The timing of rhGH injections is also important; in most cases, the injection is recommended to be given in the evening. For children on dialysis, the following considerations regarding the timing of injections apply:

   (a) Hemodialysis patients should receive their injections at bedtime or at least 3–4 h after dialysis treatment to avoid the possibility of hematoma formation from prior heparin use.
   (b) Continuous cycling peritoneal dialysis (CCPD) patients should receive injections in the morning after dialysis to minimize the removal of rhGH by dialysis.
   (c) Continuous ambulatory peritoneal dialysis (CAPD) patients should receive their injections in the evening, at the time of the overnight exchange since this is the longest dwell and is associated with less clearance of rhGH over a 24 h period.

The typical growth velocity associated with rhGH therapy in children with CKD stages 2–4 ranges from 7 to 10 cm/year; responses are less vigorous in children on dialysis. Serum IGF-1 levels can be monitored to assess compliance and response to rhGH administration [10]. In children with less than the desired growth response (which is more than 2 cm/year greater than the rate of the previous year [8], or below values depicted in growth response charts [11]), evaluation for other modifiable factors that may be impairing the growth response should be performed. Monitoring the growth response every 3–4 months is recommended in order to permit adjustment of the dose of rhGH for weight and to check for side effects. Most notable side effects include the possibility of mild hyperglycemia, intracranial hypertension, and slipped capital femoral epiphysis.

Clinical Pearls

1. Poor growth is a sign of problems in a child with CKD on or not on dialysis. Addressing growth failure in a systematic manner can be associated with better outcomes during childhood (fewer hospitalizations, better survival and better quality of life) and into adulthood (greater life satisfaction and quality of life).

2. Growth failure in childhood in patients with CKD is usually multifactorial in origin, and modifiable factors that appear to be involved must be remedied to enhance growth; if growth continues to be suboptimal over a 3–4 month time span, evaluation for rhGH therapy should be pursued.
3. There are multiple abnormalities of the GH-IGF-1 axis in uremia, including increased levels of IGF-1 BPs and increased proteolysis of IGFBP-3 in the IGF-1/ALS/IGFBP-3 complex, which contribute to the development of resistance at the cellular level to GH and IGF-1. Administration of rhGH increases the level of free IGF-1 in the serum.
4. GH stimulation testing is not required for children with CKD who are being considered for rhGH therapy. However, a number of baseline studies should be obtained before embarking on rhGH therapy.
5. The standard dose of rhGH for children with CKD and poor growth is 0.05 mg/kg/day. The best time for administration in children on dialysis is affected by the type of dialysis modality. Regular monitoring through follow up visits every 3–4 months should be conducted to assess the growth response, to adjust the dose for weight gains, and to survey for side effects of therapy.

References

1. Mahan JD, Warady BA. Assessment and treatment of short stature in pediatric patients with chronic kidney disease: a consensus statement. Pediatr Nephrol. 2006;21:917–30.
2. Furth SL, Hwang W, Yang C, Neu AM, Fivush BA, Powe NR. Growth failure, risk of hospitalization and death for children with end-stage renal disease. Pediatr Nephrol. 2002;17:450–5.
3. Broyer M, Le BC, Charbit M, Guest G, Tete MJ, Gangnadoux MF, Niaudet P. Long-term social outcome of children after kidney transplantation. Transplantation. 2004;77:1033–7.
4. Rosenkranz J, Reichwald-Klugger E, Oh J, Turzer M, Mehls O, Schaefer F. Psychosocial rehabilitation and satisfaction with life in adults with childhood-onset of end-stage renal disease. Pediatr Nephrol. 2005;20:1288–94.
5. Mahesh S, Kaskel F. Growth hormone axis in chronic kidney disease. Pediatr Nephrol. 2007;23:41–8.
6. Ingulli EG, Mak RH. Growth in children with chronic kidney disease: role of nutrition, growth hormone, dialysis, and steroids. Curr Opin Pediatr. 2014;26:187–92.
7. Stefanidis CJ, Klaus G. Growth in prepubertal children on dialysis. Pediatr Nephrol. 2007;22:1251–9.
8. Janjua HS, Mahan JD. Growth in chronic kidney disease. Adv Chronic Kidney Dis. 2011;18(5):324–31. http://dx.doi.org/10.1053/j.ackd.2011.02.005
9. Langman C, Work Group. K/DOQI clinical practice guidelines for bone metabolism and disease in children with chronic kidney disease. Am J Kidney Dis. 2005;46(Supplement 1):1–122.
10. Bacchetta J, Harambat J, Cochat P, Salusky IB, Wesseling-Perry K. The consequences of chronic kidney disease on bone metabolism and growth in children. Nephrol Dial Transplant. 2012;27:3063–71.
11. Mahan JD, Warady BA, Frane J, Rosenfeld RG, Swinford RD, Lippe B, Davis DA. First-year response to rhGH therapy in children with CKD: a national cooperative growth study report. Pediatr Nephrol. 2010;25:1125–30.

Chapter 26
Hypertension

Joseph T. Flynn

Case Presentation

The patient is a 12-year-old girl with end-stage renal disease (ESRD) from obstructive uropathy related to neurogenic bladder. Hemodialysis (HD) had been started 6 months prior to presentation due to persistent metabolic acidosis and weight loss. At the time of HD initiation, a feeding gastrostomy was inserted for provision of overnight enteral nutritional supplementation. Dialysis access was a right internal jugular hemocatheter; transplant evaluation had been initiated and a potential living donor was currently being worked up at the adult hospital.

On the day of presentation, the patient had reported feeling short of breath and had coughed up blood-tinged sputum. She was evaluated in the emergency department where she was found to have a blood pressure (BP) of 162/100 mm Hg, pulmonary edema on chest X-ray, and a dilated left ventricle on bedside echocardiography. She was admitted to the pediatric intensive care unit (PICU) where initial management included a nicardipine infusion and continuous renal replacement therapy (CRRT). After 48 h of CRRT, nicardipine was able to be weaned off, and she was transitioned to intermittent HD, which she received daily for the next 5 days.

While in the PICU, her HD records from the past month were reviewed. She frequently had requested that HD be stopped early, and her estimated dry weight (EDW) had been reached only six times over the past month. Pre-dialysis BPs were usually 130–140/85–95, but post-dialysis BPs were in the 120s/70s. The patient also admitted that she had stopped giving herself her overnight feedings because she did not like waking up early to disconnect herself from the feeding pump. At the time of discharge from the hospital, her BP was 110/72 and her weight was 3.5 kg below her prior EDW.

J.T. Flynn, MD, MS (✉)
University of Washington School of Medicine, Division of Nephrology, Seattle Children's
Hospital, Seattle, WA, USA
e-mail: joseph.flynn@seattlechildrens.org

© Springer International Publishing AG 2017   203
B.A. Warady et al. (eds.), *Pediatric Dialysis Case Studies*,
DOI 10.1007/978-3-319-55147-0_26

Clinical Questions

1. What is the likely cause or causes of hypertension in a dialysis patient?
2. How common is hypertension in pediatric dialysis patients?
3. In addition to the short-term effects of hypertension as illustrated in the case, are there any long-term consequences to be concerned about?
4. How should hypertension in dialysis patients be evaluated and treated?
5. What is the best way of making sure that a dialysis patient has controlled hypertension?
6. In a pediatric dialysis patient similar to the one presented, what factors can complicate assessment of blood pressure control?

Diagnostic Discussion

1. Hypertension (HTN) in dialysis patients can be multifactorial, but volume overload, usually related to inadequate dietary sodium restriction or insufficient fluid removal on dialysis, is the most important etiology, and one of the most difficult to manage. Other contributing factors may include inappropriate activation of the renin-aldosterone-angiotensin system (RAAS), overactivity of the sympathetic nervous system (SNS), and iatrogenic causes such as medication use (including over-the-counter and illicit substances). In patients with ESRD from glomerular disease, there may also be a significant contribution from the native kidneys, although this can also be the case in patients with ESRD from congenital diseases such as obstructive uropathy and renal dysplasia. In long-term dialysis patients, chronic vascular changes, including stiffening of the aorta and other central vessels, may further contribute to HTN; this is especially true in patients with predominantly systolic HTN and a wide pulse pressure [1, 2].
2. Registry data from both the United States and Europe have demonstrated that a significant proportion (67–69%) of pediatric dialysis patients have uncontrolled BP, defined as BP above the 90th percentile for age, gender, and height [3]. Patients were hypertensive despite widespread use of antihypertensive medications (e.g., ~58% in American children). Similar rates of HTN were seen in HD and peritoneal dialysis (PD) patients. Interestingly, rates of uncontrolled BP appear to be highest in the youngest children (<6 years of age), perhaps reflecting a reluctance among providers to aggressively treat HTN in this age group, or an unfamiliarity with normal BP values in younger children [4, 5].
3. Large cohort studies in the United States and the Netherlands have established that cardiovascular (CV) disease is the leading cause of death in young adults with childhood-onset ESRD. Rates of death from CV events such as myocardial infarction and stroke are between 30 and 100 times greater in these patients than in the general population. It is thought that the combination of traditional (BP, lipids, smoking) and nontraditional (hyperparathyroidism, anemia, proteinuria) CV risk factors, especially over many years of chronic kidney disease and renal

replacement therapy, leads to an acceleration in various pathophysiologic processes, chief among them atherosclerosis and myocardial hypertrophy [6]. The task for the clinician is to identify which CV risk factors are present in an individual patient and institute appropriate changes in management to reduce the patient's overall CV risk. HTN is felt to be a potentially modifiable CV risk factor; thus, aggressive control of BP should be a priority in all dialysis patients.

4. Control of volume status is the first step in the treatment of hypertensive children undergoing chronic dialysis. If fluid overload has not been addressed, the use of multiple antihypertensive drugs is inappropriate and frequently ineffective. Therefore, in every hypertensive patient newly started on dialysis therapy, one should try to gradually withdraw any antihypertensive medication and institute a reasonable sodium and fluid restriction until the patient's true EDW has been established. In our experience, long-acting vasodilators such as amlodipine make achievement of EDW particularly difficult, and they are the first class of antihypertensive medication that we discontinue. Noninvasive blood volume monitoring (BVM), if available, may enable accurate establishment of EDW in HD patients and has been shown to facilitate discontinuation of antihypertensive medications [7].

Once fluid overload has been addressed and EDW attained, if the patient is still hypertensive, addition of antihypertensive medications should be considered. We tend to use angiotensin-converting enzyme inhibitors or cardioselective beta-adrenergic blockers, as they may address some of the other causes of HTN such as RAAS or SNS activation. Drug-resistant HTN is rare and usually the result of inadequate ultrafiltration, but may also be due to a paradoxical (heightened) response of the RAAS to fluid removal. Noncompliance with the recommended fluid and sodium restriction can be other reasons for poor BP control in dialyzed children. In compliant patients who are oligo-anuric and remain hypertensive despite achievement of EDW, bilateral native kidney nephrectomy should be considered. A suggested treatment algorithm for HTN in pediatric dialysis patients is presented in Fig. 26.1 [2].

5. As illustrated in the case presentation, reliance on post-dialysis BP readings can mislead the clinician into thinking that BP is being adequately controlled on dialysis. Following dialysis, fluid will re-equilibrate from the extravascular to the intravascular compartment, and BP may rise significantly after the patient leaves the HD unit (or completes overnight PD). Ambulatory BP monitoring (ABPM) has been shown to better correlate with CV outcomes in patients with or without ESRD and, in the case of dialysis patients, allows assessment of BP in the interdialytic period, revealing whether a patient has masked HTN (normal casual BP but abnormal ambulatory BP). In HD patients, ABPM is recommended to be done over the entire 44-h interdialytic period. Studies of 44-h ABPM in both adult and pediatric HD patients have shown a better correlation than post-dialysis casual BP measurements with intermediate CV outcomes such as left ventricular hypertrophy, with nighttime BP parameters being especially predictive of increased left ventricular mass [1, 8].

6. The major unique aspect of children undergoing chronic dialysis that may complicate efforts at treating HTN is that somatic growth is expected (at least in

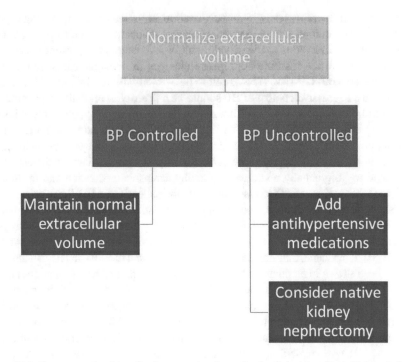

Fig. 26.1 Treatment algorithm for hypertension in pediatric dialysis patients (Adapted from Seeman 2013)

school-aged children and younger adolescents), which can confuse assessment of EDW. Additionally, ESRD in children is almost always complicated by anorexia, so that even if a patient's weight appears to be stable (and EDW achieved following each dialysis session), the patient's lean body mass may be decreasing due to inadequate caloric intake. This phenomenon is extremely common in pediatric dialysis patients and is not limited to HD (although perhaps more common in HD than PD). The use of BVM may help to avoid this problem in HD patients; in PD patients, the use of more sophisticated techniques of body composition analysis such as bioimpedance may be needed to determine lean body mass and establish EDW [1, 7]. In the presented case, HTN was likely the result of these factors and was further complicated by nonadherence to the prescribed HD session length.

Clinical Pearls

1. Hypertension in a dialysis patient can have a variety of etiologies, with volume overload the most likely and the first potential cause that should be addressed.
2. Treatment with long-acting vasodilating medications may impede the ability to achieve EDW; these agents should be discontinued first during efforts to achieve EDW.

3. Once EDW has been achieved, if the patient is still hypertensive, other potential etiologies should be sought out and treated as appropriate.
4. Cardiovascular disease is the leading cause of mortality in adults with childhood-onset ESRD, making control of hypertension during childhood a priority.
5. Periodic 44-h ambulatory blood pressure monitoring in HD patients allows for the optimal assessment of BP control; shorter monitoring periods may be sufficient in PD patients.
6. In children on dialysis, assessment of EDW can be complicated by the assumption that weight gain increases represent somatic growth, not fluid retention, increasing the risk of inadequate fluid removal on dialysis and contributing to chronic hypertension.

References

1. Agarwal R, Flynn J, Pogue V, Rahman M, Reisin E, Weir MW. Assessment and management of hypertension in patients on dialysis. J Am Soc Nephrol. 2014;25:1630–46.
2. Seeman T. Hypertension in end-stage renal disease. In: Flynn JT, Ingelfinger J, Portman RM, editors. Pediatric hypertension. 3rd ed. New York: Springer Science + Business Media; 2013. p. 343–66.
3. National High Blood Pressure Education Program Working Group on High Blood Pressure in Children and Adolescents. The fourth report on the diagnosis, evaluation, and treatment of high blood pressure in children and adolescents. Pediatrics. 2004;114:555–76.
4. Halbach SM, Martz K, Matoo T, Flynn J. Control of hypertension in pediatric dialysis patients. J Pediatr. 2012;160:621–625.e1.
5. Kramer AM, van Stralen KJ, Jager KJ, et al. Demographics of blood pressure and hypertension in children on renal replacement therapy in Europe. Kidney Int. 2011;80:1092–8.
6. Flynn JT. Hypertension and future cardiovascular health in pediatric ESRD patients. Blood Purif. 2012;33:138–43.
7. Patel HP, Goldstein SL, Mahan JD, Smith B, Fried CB, Currier H, Flynn JT. A Standard non-invasive monitoring of hematocrit algorithm improves blood pressure control in pediatric hemodialysis patients. Clin J Am Soc Nephrol. 2007;2:252–7.
8. Katsoufis CP, Seeherunvong W, Sasaki N, Abitbol CL, Chandar J, Freundlich M, Zilleruelo GE. Forty-four-hour interdialytic ambulatory blood pressure monitoring and cardiovascular risk in pediatric hemodialysis patients. Clin Kidney J. 2014;7:33–9.

Chapter 27
Cardiovascular Disease

Mark M. Mitsnefes

Case Presentation

A 16-year-old male has been on maintenance hemodialysis (three times per week, 4 h treatment) for the last 6 months as he progressed to end-stage renal disease (ESRD) secondary to focal segmental glomerulosclerosis (FSGS). His dialysis course has been complicated by nonadherence: he admits frequently forgetting to take his medications; occasionally, he does not show up for his hemodialysis session.

He presented in the emergency department (ED) complaining of severe headache and vomiting that had developed over the last 24 h. The initial evaluation in ED showed a BP of 180/100 mm Hg, heart rate of 112/min, respiratory rate 32/min, and oxygen saturation 92%. His weight was 6 kg above his estimated dry weight. Physical examination demonstrated bibasilar rales and an S3 gallop, no peripheral edema except eye puffiness. The laboratory results were: Hg 7.9 g/dL, BUN 123 mg/dL, serum creatinine 10.2 mg/dL, K 5.9 mEq/L, HCO3 16 mEq/L, Ca 7.8 mg/dL, P 7.3 mg/dL, and albumin 2.6 mg/dL. Echocardiography showed diffuse chamber enlargement and depressed biventricular function with shortening fraction of 18%. The patient was treated for hypertension in the ED and then admitted to the hospital for acute hemodialysis treatment. His last hemodialysis treatment prior to the ED visit had been 5 days ago.

His routine monthly evaluation 2 weeks before had shown Hg 9.2 g/dL, BUN 93 mg/dL, serum creatinine 12.4 mg/dL, K 5.1 mEq/L, HCO3 18 mEq/L, Ca 8.2 mg/dL, P 8.3 mg/dL, iPTH 560 pg/ml, and albumin 3.1 mg/dL. Lipid profile demonstrated LDL cholesterol 152 mg/dL and triglycerides 274 mg/dL. Over the last few months, BP has been elevated despite two prescribed antihypertensive medications.

M.M. Mitsnefes, MD, MS (✉)
Cincinnati Children's Hospital Medical Center, Division of Nephrology and Hypertension, Cincinnati, OH, USA
e-mail: mark.mitsnefes@cchmc.org

© Springer International Publishing AG 2017
B.A. Warady et al. (eds.), *Pediatric Dialysis Case Studies*,
DOI 10.1007/978-3-319-55147-0_27

Echocardiography demonstrated concentric left ventricular hypertrophy (LVH). He has no available kidney transplant living donor. Active listing for deceased donor kidney transplantation is currently on hold due to nonadherence.

Clinical Questions

1. Why is monitoring of cardiovascular risk essential in children on maintenance dialysis?
2. How should a child on maintenance dialysis be evaluated for cardiovascular risk? What are the most common cardiovascular abnormalities in children on maintenance dialysis?
3. What are appropriate targets and treatment options to control cardiovascular risk?
4. What is the best strategy to prevent progression of cardiovascular disease (CVD) in pediatric patients on maintenance dialysis?

Diagnostic Discussion

1. Young adults who develop ESRD during childhood have a significantly diminished life expectancy. Upon reaching adulthood, dialysis patients live 40–50 years less compared to the age- and race-matched general population [1]. Cardiovascular disease (CVD) is the leading cause of death in children and young adults on maintenance dialysis, accounting for one third of all causes [2]. However, the causes of death in children are different from those in adults. In young adults with childhood-onset ESRD, coronary artery disease and congestive heart failure due to cardiomyopathy are two leading causes of mortality from CVD [3]. The mortality from these causes is extremely low in pediatric patients. Of the specific causes of cardiovascular deaths in children, cardiac arrest is the most common, followed by arrhythmia and cardiomyopathy.
2. The prevalence of traditional cardiovascular risk factors in children on maintenance dialysis is similar to that in adults on dialysis. Thus, cardiovascular diagnostic evaluation is focused on identifying children with hypertension, dyslipidemia, and obesity. In contrast to adults, diabetes as a cause of ESRD is very rare in children. However, hyperglycemia and insulin resistance could be seen in dialyzed children, especially in the obese and those on steroid therapy.

   Hypertension is the most frequent risk but is also the likely modifiable factor. Poor BP control in children on maintenance dialysis is multifactorial, but the major cause is fluid overload. Thus, the first step in the diagnosis and management of hypertension should be evaluation of volume status. Unfortunately, many children on dialysis do not achieve their dry weight. Volume status assessment in very young patients is frequently inaccurate. This is one of the reasons why the frequency of hypertension is higher in young children. In addition, correct assessment of BP is difficult in small children, and consequently it is frequently underdiagnosed and therefore not adequately treated. Another group of children who present with significant fluid overload and hypertension is adolescents, who are almost always non-compliant with fluid and salt restriction. Significant fluid overload, likely due to nonadherence, can lead to acute hypertension and congestive heart failure, as was seen in the case presentation above.

Chronic fluid overload with secondary hypertension (volume and pressure overload) is also a major cause of left ventricular hypertrophy (LVH), the most common intermediate cardiovascular abnormality seen in children on maintenance dialysis. As a result of pressure overload that occurs with hypertension, concentric LV remodeling and hypertrophy develop, whereas volume overload and severe anemia result in eccentric LVH (Fig. 27.1). Abnormal mineral metabolism, specifically increased fibroblast growth factor 23 (FGF23), also plays an important role in inducing concentric LVH. Initially, LVH is compensatory and adaptive. However, if untreated, LVH might become maladaptive with development of myocardial fibrosis. All this leads to myocyte death and, finally, to diastolic and systolic dysfunction. If LVH is diagnosed at the time of dialysis initiation, routine echocardiographic monitoring every 6 months is advisable. If the initial echocardiogram is normal, yearly echocardiographic follow-up to reassess cardiac structure and function is suggested.

In addition to cardiac changes, children on dialysis might develop intermediate vascular abnormalities such as increased carotid artery intima-media thickness, increased arterial stiffness, and even coronary artery calcification – all markers of

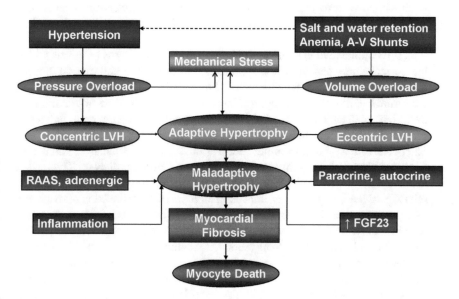

Fig. 27.1 LVH in dialysis: pathogenesis

early atherosclerosis and arteriosclerosis [3]. In addition to hypertension and dyslipidemia, abnormally high serum phosphorus and increased calcium-phosphorus product are important causes of these vascular abnormalities.

3. The target blood pressure in children with CKD should be less than the 90th percentile adjusted for age, gender, and height, or less than 120/80 mm Hg, whichever is lower [4]. Aggressive management of fluid overload and achievement of dry weight is the most effective treatment of hypertension and LVH in children on chronic dialysis. If BP remains elevated despite adequate volume control, antihypertensive medications should be optimized. Angiotensin-converting enzyme inhibitors or angiotensin II receptor blockers should be considered as a first line of therapy in children on dialysis because of their reno- and cardioprotective effects. Addition of calcium channel blockers or beta-blockers should be tried next. It is important to remember that if effective dry weight is not achieved, antihypertensive meds, especially vasodilators and beta-blockers, will likely not work and may further impair the ability to remove fluid.

The assessment of dyslipidemias should include a complete fasting lipid profile with total cholesterol, LDL, HDL, and triglycerides. The definition of dyslipidemia differs in children and adults. Hyperlipidemia in children is defined as lipid levels greater than the 95th percentile for age and gender. For adolescents with Stage 5 CKD and a level of LDL cholesterol $\geq$130 mg/dl, KDOQI recommends treatment to reduce LDL to <130 mg/dl. If LDL is <130 mg/dl, fasting triglycerides $\geq$200 mg/dl, and non-HDL cholesterol (total cholesterol minus HDL) $\geq$160 mg/dl, treatment should be considered to reduce non-HDL cholesterol to <160 mg/dl [5]. All children with dyslipidemias should follow the recommendations for therapeutic lifestyle changes (TLC), which include diet modification with reduction in saturated fat intake and increase in fiber intake, and moderate physical activity. Adolescents should be counseled about avoiding smoking.

It is recommended to maintain calcium (Ca) and phosphorus (P) levels within the normal range and the Ca $\times$ P product <55 mg^2/dl^2 in children on chronic dialysis. The use of non-calcium-based phosphate binders, careful monitoring of the serum calcium level, and appropriate adjustment of the dose of vitamin D to avoid hypercalcemia are essential in the management of children on dialysis to prevent development and progression of cardiovascular abnormalities [6].

4. The overall strategy in preventing cardiovascular complications in children with advanced chronic kidney disease is avoidance of long-term dialysis. The goal is to prevent development and delay the progression of cardiomyopathy and atherosclerosis. Even though kidney transplantation poses a continued cardiovascular risk (hypertension, hyperlipidemia, allograft dysfunction), it eliminates many uremia-related risks, reduces the risk of cardiac death by approximately 80%, and prolongs life span by 20–30 years. Graft failure after the first kidney transplantation is associated with an almost five times higher mortality rate as compared to children with a functioning graft. Having maintenance dialysis even for a few months before transplant is also associated with worse survival. Thus, preemptive kidney transplantation should be the ultimate goal to minimize cardiovascular morbidity and mortality.

For those patients who must have long-term dialysis, the strategy is directly linked to the achievement of adequate dialysis outcomes which includes aggressive monitoring and management of hypertension, dyslipidemia, calcium-phosphorus metabolism, anemia, nutrition, systemic inflammation, and other dialysis complications. Unfortunately, achieving recommended Kt/V urea as measurement of adequacy does not necessarily lead to control of the above problems. Longer and more frequent dialysis sessions are typically needed to avoid or reduce cardiovascular complications.

Clinical Pearls

1. Children with ESRD are among the populations with the highest cardiovascular risk due to an extremely high prevalence of traditional and uremia-associated risk factors.
2. LVH is the most common cardiac abnormality found in children on maintenance dialysis. Other early cardiac (LV dysfunction) and vascular abnormalities (increased carotid artery IMT, arterial stiffness, coronary artery calcification) may also be detected, especially in patients with uncontrolled hypertension and abnormal calcium-phosphorus metabolism.
3. Young adults with childhood onset of ESRD and poorly controlled cardiovascular risk frequently develop accelerated cardiovascular disease, the major cause of premature death in this population.
4. Longer and more frequent dialysis sessions are a proven strategy to minimize cardiovascular risk.
5. Kidney transplantation, preferably performed preemptively, is the best treatment option to prevent development and progression of cardiovascular disease in children with ESRD.

References

1. Renal Data System US. USRDS 2014 annual data report: atlas of chronic kidney disease and end-stage renal disease in the United States. National Institutes of Health, National Institute of Diabetes and Digestive and Kidney Diseases: Bethesda; 2014.
2. Mitsnefes MM, et al. Mortality risk among children initially treated with dialysis for end-stage kidney disease, 1990-2010. JAMA. 2013;309(18):1921–9.
3. Mitsnefes MM. Cardiovascular disease in children with chronic kidney disease. J Am Soc Nephrol. 2012;23(4):578–85.
4. Agarwal R, et al. Assessment and management of hypertension in patients on dialysis. J Am Soc Nephrol. 2014;25(8):1630–46.
5. KDIGO. Clinical practice guideline for lipid management in chronic kidney disease. Kidney Int Suppl. 2013;3(3):259–305.
6. Kidney Disease: Improving Global Outcomes (KDIGO) CKD-MBD Work Group. KDIGO clinical practice guideline for the diagnosis, evaluation, prevention, and treatment of chronic kidney disease-mineral and bone disorder (CKD-MBD). Kidney Int Suppl. 2009;76:S1–130.

Chapter 28
Sleep Disorders

Annabelle N. Chua

Case Presentation

A 12-year-old female has a past medical history significant for end-stage renal disease secondary to bilateral renal dysplasia. Her mother presented to the dialysis unit with complaints of her child's poor school performance. The patient had been on chronic hemodialysis (HD) for 3 years, and her mother reported that the patient had increasing problems with her behavior at school. The teachers relate that over the past year, she has been falling asleep during class, does not pay attention, and repeatedly has failed her tests. She demonstrates apathy when questioned about her school performance and states that she feels tired all of the time. Upon further questioning, she admits that she has trouble sleeping at night and that her legs feel "funny" at night which leads her to constantly have to move her legs for relief, symptoms consistent with restless legs syndrome (RLS). Her mother wants to know if her daughter would have less trouble sleeping at night if she were switched to peritoneal dialysis. Monthly labs were notable for hemoglobin 9 g/dL, total iron 27 mcg/dL, transferrin saturation 14%, and serum ferritin 18 ng/mL. Consultation with the sleep clinic was carried out, and polysomnography was performed and revealed less slow-wave sleep and a higher arousal index. After treating with IV iron and carrying out a recommended reduction in caffeine intake, the patient has started to feel more rested throughout the day with less symptoms of restless legs syndrome. The patient also anxiously awaits deceased donor kidney transplantation and the hope that the RLS symptoms will further subside.

A.N. Chua (✉)
Duke University, Department of Pediatrics/Division of Pediatric Nephrology,
Durham, NC, USA
e-mail: annabelle.chua@duke.edu

© Springer International Publishing AG 2017
B.A. Warady et al. (eds.), *Pediatric Dialysis Case Studies*,
DOI 10.1007/978-3-319-55147-0_28

Clinical Questions

1. How likely is it that a sleep disorder is contributing to the patient's apathy and poor behavior at school?
2. How common is restless legs syndrome? What are some therapeutic interventions for restless legs syndrome?
3. What are other types of sleep-related disorders that can be seen in patients with ESRD? How common are these conditions in children with CKD and ESRD?
4. Is there any relationship between the dialysis modality and the risk for sleep disorders?

Diagnostic Discussion

1. In this scenario, the patient's apathy and problems at school are likely related to poor sleep. Sleep disturbances in children have been associated with daytime behavioral problems, inattention, poor school performance, and reduced health-related quality of life [1]. Insufficient sleep time (<9 h of sleep nightly in school-age child) has been associated with a range of behaviors such as hyperactivity, irritability, aggression, and other conduct problems [2]. Sleep deprivation studies in adults suggest that sleep loss impairs the functional connectivity between the prefrontal cortex (area involved in voluntary control) and the amygdala (area involved in emotional reactions) [3]. In contrast, increased sleep time has been associated with decreased aggressive ideation and actions during conflicts. Sleep disorders in pediatric hemodialysis patients have been characterized by polysomnography, which demonstrates lower slow-wave sleep values and higher values of arousal index, respiratory disturbance index, and periodic limb movement disorder (PLMD) as compared to the control group. These findings correlate with subjective symptoms in the pediatric hemodialysis patients which include excessive daytime sleepiness, limb pains, difficult morning arousals, more night-time awakening, and the need for sleep medications [4].
2. Restless legs syndrome (RLS) is a neurological disorder characterized by an irresistible urge to move the legs. Onset is typically at night and at rest. Movement of an individual's legs results in improvement in symptoms. The restlessness can result in difficulty initiating and maintaining sleep. While the prevalence of RLS in children aged 12–17 years in the general population is estimated to be 2%, the prevalence in children with CKD and ESRD is reported to be 10–35% [1, 5–8]. CKD patients with restless legs syndrome have poorer sleep quality, lower emotional health-related quality of life, and are more likely to be using sleep medications [7]. Restless legs syndrome is possibly secondary to uremia, anemia, iron deficiency in the brain (iron is a cofactor for dopamine production in the brain), and/or the peripheral neuropathy associated with uremia [1, 9, 10]. Management of restless legs syndrome includes changes in lifestyle (reduction in caffeine

intake, exercise), correction of anemia, and treatment with iron to correct iron deficiency, particularly if the serum ferritin is <30 ng/mL [5, 11, 12]. Medications such as dopamine agonists and antidepressants have been shown to be effective in adults, but are not approved for use in children with this disorder [5, 13].

3. Sleep-related disorders in patients with CKD and ESRD include sleep-disordered breathing (SDB) and obstructive sleep apnea, excessive daytime sleepiness (EDS), poor sleep quality, insomnia, and insufficient sleep time, in addition to restless legs syndrome and/or PLMD. Only a limited number of studies have evaluated the prevalence of sleep disturbances in pediatric patients with CKD and ESRD. Davis and colleagues noted a sleep disturbance prevalence rate of 85% in a group of 21 children and adolescents on chronic dialysis, with 46% having SDB, 60% with EDS, 25% with insufficient sleep time, and 30% with RLS [6].

4. Hemodialysis-associated elevations in body temperature may activate cooling mechanisms, which in turn may result in increased daytime sleep propensity during the post-hemodialysis period. Increased daytime sleep propensity may then lead to delayed sleep onset and decreased nighttime sleep [14]. However, data are limited in pediatrics to suggest that switching dialysis modality from HD to peritoneal dialysis would prove beneficial to a HD patient's sleep disorder. On the contrary, a study in adult patients with ESRD reported that RLS was more prevalent among patients receiving automated peritoneal dialysis, with a prevalence of 50% as compared to 23% in HD patients and 33% in patients receiving continuous ambulatory peritoneal dialysis (CAPD) [15]. Finally, in two studies, pediatric renal transplant recipients had lower rates of restless legs syndrome than dialysis patients, but the difference was not statistically significant [1, 7]. In adults, however, renal transplantation has been associated with an improvement in restless legs syndrome [16, 17].

Clinical Pearls

1. Sleep disorders are commonly reported in adult dialysis patients, with a prevalence of 60–80%. These disorders include sleep-related breathing disorders and obstructive sleep apnea, restless legs syndrome (RLS) and periodic limb movements during sleep (PLMD), poor sleep quality, excessive daytime sleepiness, insomnia, and insufficient sleep time. As many as 86% of children on dialysis may exhibit a sleep disturbance.

2. Polysomnography may be a useful tool in helping characterize sleep disorders in pediatric CKD and ESRD patients.

3. The etiology of sleep disorders in pediatric CKD and ESRD patients is not known. Possible contributing factors leading to excessive daytime sleepiness include uremia, sleep disruption from RLS/PLMD, arousals associated with obstructive sleep apnea, neurochemical imbalances, and altered sleep-wakefulness rhythms [10, 18].

4. Sleep disorders in children with CKD can be associated with a decrease in health-related quality of life scores. Early identification of sleep disturbances with appropriate intervention might, in turn, lead to an improvement in quality of life, in addition to improved behavior and school performance.

References

1. Davis ID, Greenbaum LA, Gipson D, et al. Prevalence of sleep disturbances in children and adolescents with chronic kidney disease. Pediatric nephrology (Berlin/Germany). 2012;27(3):451–9.
2. Aronen ET, Paavonen EJ, Fjallberg M, Soininen M, Torronen J. Sleep and psychiatric symptoms in school-age children. J Am Acad Child Adolesc Psychiatry. 2000;39(4):502–8.
3. Schmidt RE, Van der Linden M. The relations between sleep, personality, behavioral problems, and school performance in adolescents. Sleep Med Clin. 2015;10(2):117–23.
4. El-Refaey AM, Elsayed RM, Sarhan A, et al. Sleep quality assessment using polysomnography in children on regular hemodialysis. Saudi J Kidney Dis Transpl: Off Publ Saudi Cent Org Transpl, Saudi Arabia. 2013;24(4):714–8.
5. Applebee GA, Guillot AP, Schuman CC, Teddy S, Attarian HP. Restless legs syndrome in pediatric patients with chronic kidney disease. Pediatr Nephrol (Berlin/Germany). 2009;24(3):545–8.
6. Davis ID, Baron J, O'Riordan MA, Rosen CL. Sleep disturbances in pediatric dialysis patients. Pediatr Nephrol (Berlin/Germany). 2005;20(1):69–75.
7. Riar SK, Leu RM, Turner-Green TC, et al. Restless legs syndrome in children with chronic kidney disease. Pediatr Nephrol (Berlin/Germany). 2013;28(5):773–95.
8. Sinha R, Davis ID, Matsuda-Abedini M. Sleep disturbances in children and adolescents with non-dialysis-dependent chronic kidney disease. Arch Pediatr Adolesc Med. 2009;163(9):850–5.
9. Trenkwalder C, Paulus W. Restless legs syndrome: pathophysiology, clinical presentation and management. Nat Rev Neurol. 2010;6(6):337–46.
10. Perl J, Unruh ML, Chan CT. Sleep disorders in end-stage renal disease: 'Markers of inadequate dialysis'? Kidney Int. 2006;70(10):1687–93.
11. Dye TJ, et al. Outcomes of long-term iron supplementation in pediatric restless legs syndrome/periodic limb movement disorder (RLS/PLMD). Sleep Med. 2017. http://dx.doi.org/10.1016/j.sleep.2016.01.008.
12. Amos LB, Grekowicz ML, Kuhn EM, et al. Treatment of pediatric restless legs syndrome. Clin Pediatr. 2014;53(4):331–6.
13. Hanly P. Sleep disorders and end-stage renal disease. Curr Opin Pulm Med. 2008;14(6):543–50.
14. Koch BC, Nagtegaal JE, Kerkhof GA, ter Wee PM. Circadian sleep-wake rhythm disturbances in end-stage renal disease. Nat Rev Nephrol. 2009;5(7):407–16.
15. Losso RL, Minhoto GR, Riella MC. Sleep disorders in patients with end-stage renal disease undergoing dialysis: comparison between hemodialysis, continuous ambulatory peritoneal dialysis and automated peritoneal dialysis. Int Urol Nephrol. 2015;47(2):369–75.
16. Molnar MZ, Novak M, Ambrus C, et al. Restless Legs Syndrome in patients after renal transplantation. Am J Kidney Dis: Off J Natl Kidney Found. 2005;45(2):388–96.
17. Beecroft JM, Zaltzman J, Prasad GV, Meliton G, Hanly PJ. Improvement of periodic limb movements following kidney transplantation. Nephron Clin Pract. 2008;109(3):c133–9.
18. Parker KP. Sleep disturbances in dialysis patients. Sleep Med Rev. 2003;7(2):131–43.

Chapter 29
The Highly Sensitized Dialysis Patient

Paul C. Grimm

Case Presentation

A 15-year-old male has been on maintenance hemodialysis and waiting for his second renal allograft for more than 2 years. The disease that caused his original ESRD was renal dysplasia. He received his first kidney as a preemptive deceased donor transplant with a 0 HLA antigen match at age 7 years. Over the next 4 years, social problems in the family led him to be poorly supervised, frequently running out of medications and culminating in cellular rejection and graft loss at the age of 11 years. He was placed in foster care and returned to dialysis where his baseline immunosuppression medications were weaned over the following 2 months. Shortly after that, he developed pain and tenderness in the rejected kidney and required an urgent allograft nephrectomy with a blood transfusion.

Over the subsequent 2 years, his foster parents adopted him, and he thrived under their supervision. He was considered to be a good candidate for a second kidney transplant but was found to be highly HLA sensitized with 80% cPRA (calculated panel reactive antigen) with antibodies to HLA A2, B7, and DQ 7. Neither the adoptive parents nor his biological relatives were able to be kidney donors due to medical issues, so he was placed on the deceased donor list. Two years passed without a successful transplant offer. It was decided he would undergo desensitization to improve his chance of receiving a donor renal allograft. He was treated with a protocol of monthly IVIG (2 g/kg/dose) and one dose of rituximab [1]. Three months after the IVIG was initiated, HLA testing was repeated. The MFI (mean fluorescence intensity, a measure of HLA antibody strength measured using bead technology) of the anti-A2 antibody surprisingly

P.C. Grimm (✉)
Division of Pediatric Nephrology, Department of Pediatrics, Stanford University School of Medicine, Lucile Packard Childrens Hospital Stanford, Stanford, CA, USA
e-mail: pgrimm@stanford.edu

© Springer International Publishing AG 2017
B.A. Warady et al. (eds.), *Pediatric Dialysis Case Studies*,
DOI 10.1007/978-3-319-55147-0_29

increased from 10,000 prior to initiating desensitization to 25,000 after the third dose of IVIG. The MFI of the other two antibodies had fallen. At this time, the team transiently considered abandoning desensitization or switching to a protocol of plasmapheresis with bortezomib; however, they elected to carry on with three more doses of monthly IVIG. The anti-A2 antibody MFI fell after the sixth dose of IVIG to 2,000.

A few weeks later, a deceased donor kidney became available, but a cause for concern was the fact that this donor kidney was positive for HLA A2.

Clinical Questions

1. What is the effect of the HLA match of the first renal allograft with the recipient on the risk of sensitization and success of a subsequent kidney transplant?
2. Did the graft nephrectomy and blood transfusion that followed the failure of the first transplant affect the sensitization status?
3. Why did the patient have to wait more than 2 years for a kidney transplant to become available?
4. Why did the titer of one of the antibodies go up after three doses of IVIG?
5. Was the patient able to receive a kidney which carried HLA A2, when he had detectable levels of anti-A2?

Diagnostic Discussion

1. Over the last 30 years, successful short-term renal transplant outcomes have surpassed 95%. It is now common for patients who are waiting on dialysis to receive kidneys with no HLA match. We rely on the effectiveness of immuno-suppression to prevent rejection. However, the trade-offs we as clinicians make do have long-term effects. In an attempt to shorten or avoid dialysis (with its associated higher mortality than living with a transplant), the choice of a poorly matched kidney can have long-term consequences. Registry studies now show that children and adults who received a poorly matched kidney for the first transplant have higher levels of sensitization when they return to the waiting list for a second kidney transplant [2]. In the situation where the family is trying to decide between an available living donor and taking their chances with deceased donation, in most situations it is preferable to take the living donor first. Studies show the outcomes from a poorly matched living donor are better than the outcomes from a well-matched deceased donor [3].
2. Data show that having an allograft nephrectomy is a risk factor for subsequent sensitization; however, it is a relatively minor risk unless combined with blood transfusion. If a blood transfusion occurs in the context of an allograft nephrec-

tomy, especially if there is little or no immunosuppression, then there is a high risk for the development of new HLA sensitization [4]. Although there is limited data on this topic, at least one study suggests a minimum of 3 months of immunosuppression following return to dialysis due to allograft rejection is necessary to reduce the risk of excessive HLA sensitization. If a patient is likely to receive a second kidney transplant very quickly (e.g., if they have a willing living donor and they are medically qualified), it may be prudent to maintain the patient on immunosuppression during their dialysis interval to minimize the risk of developing de novo sensitization to the next donor [5].

3. Prior to desensitization, this patient had a cPRA of 80%. This means that 80% of the typical transplant donors would be incompatible based on his HLA sensitization. He would be further limited by his blood group, as blood group match is a requirement for the allocation system. If he was 99% or 100% sensitized, i.e., less than 1% of random donors would be an acceptable match, he would qualify for regional or national sharing in the United States. This means that a potentially crossmatch negative kidney is mandated to be allocated to your patient even if it has to travel from one coast to another. Patients who are 99% sensitized have mandated regional but not national sharing. This also gives them availability of substantially more kidneys. At 80% sensitization, he is caught in a "doughnut hole" where there are few donors in the local area who would be compatible, but he is not able to compete at a regional nor national level. This is the usual explanation for a patient such as this who has to wait many years on dialysis.

4. When an antibody against HLA antigens is at a very high titer, it may inhibit the reaction that measures the MFI of the antibody with the bead – the "prozone effect." In this situation, the test may read out that there is no antibody or that the antibody has a low MFI using undiluted "neat" serum. When the patient's serum is diluted, you would expect the MFI to fall, but, counter-intuitively, it goes up, revealing the strength of this antibody [6]. In the case of this patient, the A2 was a very high-level antibody with a prozone effect. When the IVIG was starting to reduce the strength of that antibody, the prozone effect diminished, allowing the beads to more accurately reflect the strength of the antibody, so the reported MFI went up. This is not a sign of desensitization failure, as one can go back to earlier samples and perform serial dilutions to prove the antibody titer was at much higher levels in earlier serum samples. By continuing to infuse IVIG as part of the desensitization protocol, the antibody titer continued to fall in this patient.

Some HLA labs test whether or not a specific HLA antibody activates C1q in a bead-based assay. In some labs, C1q positivity is more specific than the standard IgG bead testing to predict how dangerous a specific anti-HLA antibody is. A recent publication suggested that C1q antibody testing is not susceptible to the prozone effect, so it may reflect more accurately the degree of sensitization [7]. Some have suggested that regularly doing serial dilutions can give the same information that C1q antibody testing can give. This is an area of substantial controversy, but hopefully further study will provide clarity to this area.

5. High levels of HLA-specific antibody will bind to the target cell surface and activate the complement cascade leading to cell death. This is the basis for the cytotoxicity crossmatch which is the in vitro surrogate for the in vivo catastrophe of hyperacute rejection. This is now avoided at all costs in the modern era. Lower levels of antibody may be detectable using a flow crossmatch, and even lower levels may be detectable using solid phase bead technology. But alone, these lower levels of antibody detected using more sensitive techniques are likely not enough to trigger the complement cascade and cause cell death. In patients with relatively little sensitization, the presence of low levels of antibody may be enough to identify these antigens as "avoids," which means a donor kidney carrying this antigen will not be offered to your patient. In patients who have substantial sensitization, the clinician should work with the HLA lab to identify antibodies which have a low enough MFI to likely not cause a positive crossmatch and make these acceptable, leaving as "avoids" only the higher MFI antibodies that are more likely to cause a positive crossmatch. The HLA lab specialists have the unique experience to determine what is a safe cutoff threshold which may be different from other labs based on their technology and even individual antibodies. During the process of desensitization, in a collaborative and often iterative process, the HLA lab staff and clinicians identify antigens that can be removed from the patient's list of "avoids" as the sensitization levels hopefully respond to therapy. As the avoided antigens are removed, a larger fraction of the potential donor pool is theoretically acceptable, and hopefully one will lead to a negative crossmatch that can allow a transplant to proceed.

This patient received a "past-positive current-negative" crossmatch transplant. The previous high levels of donor-specific antibody warn the clinician of the presence of long-term immunological memory. Donor-specific B cells may be powerful antigen-presenting cells, so cellular rejection or recurrent antibody is likely, especially with any lapse in immunosuppressive coverage. Patients who have received a kidney transplant after desensitization are at long-term increased risk of graft loss compared to those who have not undergone desensitization [8]. They therefore often require a more intensive immunosuppression protocol and long-term posttransplant monitoring.

Epilogue

In spite of the presence of an anti-A2 antibody with an MFI of 2,000 (and a history of this same antibody having an MFI of 25,000 in the not too distant past), the prospective flow crossmatch with fresh patient serum was negative, and the transplant was successfully carried out with thymoglobulin induction and with maintenance immunosuppression including tacrolimus, mycophenolate, and steroids. Three months after the transplant, there was no evidence of anti-A2 antibody, and graft function remains excellent.

Clinical Pearls

1. A blood transfusion at the time of allograft nephrectomy is strongly associated with new onset of sensitization. This should be avoided if possible and if unavoidable, should be performed under the cover of immunosuppression.
2. In a patient who has sensitization against alloantigens, finding a suitable donor kidney can be a challenge. The best outcomes are with a crossmatch negative kidney, so exploring living donation, paired exchange, and waiting for a crossmatch negative kidney are the first choices. If these strategies are unsuccessful, desensitization should be considered to facilitate transplantation.
3. HLA labs vary in their technique and protocols used to provide the clinician with actionable HLA data. Thresholds for "calling" an antigen in determining whether the level of antibody sensitization would lead to a positive crossmatch are laboratory specific. It is important for clinicians to have a close working relationship with their HLA lab. The use of some assays such as the C1Q antibody assay is controversial with the role of this assay yet to be determined.
4. An antibody subject to the prozone effect will be reported to have a lower titer or MFI than it really has. This can be recognized by testing serial dilutions of patient sera or when the MFI substantially increases during the process of desensitization.
5. It is possible to perform a kidney transplant where the kidney contains an antigen to which the patient has previously formed an antibody or currently is expressing an antibody, as long as the MFI is low enough so the crossmatch is not positive. This is a high-risk situation which warrants substantial immunosuppression and close long-term surveillance.

References

1. Vo AA, Lukovsky M, Toyoda M, et al. Rituximab and intravenous immune globulin for desensitization during renal transplantation. N Engl J Med. 2008;359(3):242–51.
2. Gralla J, Tong S, Wiseman AC. The impact of human leukocyte antigen mismatching on sensitization rates and subsequent retransplantation after first graft failure in pediatric renal transplant recipients. Transplantation. 2013;95(10):1218–24.
3. Marlais M, Hudson A, Pankhurst L, Fuggle SV, Marks SD. Living donation has a greater impact on renal allograft survival than HLA matching in pediatric renal transplant recipients. Transplantation. 2016;100(12):2717–2722.
4. Scornik JC, Kriesche HU. Human leukocyte antigen sensitization after transplant loss: timing of antibody detection and implications for prevention. Hum Immunol. 2011;72(5):398–401.
5. Casey MJ, Wen X, Kayler LK, Aiyer R, Scornik JC, Meier-Kriesche HU. Prolonged immunosuppression preserves nonsensitization status after kidney transplant failure. Transplantation. 2014;98(3):306–11.
6. Weinstock C, Schnaidt M. The complement-mediated prozone effect in the Luminex single-antigen bead assay and its impact on HLA antibody determination in patient sera. Int J Immunogenet. 2013;40(3):171–7.
7. Tambur AR, Herrera ND, Haarberg KM, et al. Assessing antibody strength: comparison of MFI, C1q, and titer information. Am J Transplant. 2015;15(9):2421–30.
8. Orandi BJ, Garonzik-Wang JM, Massie AB, et al. Quantifying the risk of incompatible kidney transplantation: a multicenter study. Am J Transplant. 2014;14(7):1573–80.

Chapter 30
Health-Related Quality of Life in Youth on Dialysis

Shari K. Neul

Case Presentation

The patient is an 18-year-old Hispanic bilingual female with ESRD secondary to renal dysplasia. She currently undergoes thrice-weekly hemodialysis treatments after transitioning from peritoneal dialysis due to multiple exit site infections and poor adherence. Communication between the patient and her dialysis treatment team has been deteriorating, reflecting conflicts arising from her ongoing nonadherence, the minimal involvement of her parent, and growing staff perception of the patient as generally uninterested in her medical care. In addition, she recently dropped out of high school due to failing grades and a lack of peer relationships.

Dialysis plan of care meetings have recently focused on transferring the patient's care to an adult program where the medical team hopes she can have a new start and may be more motivated to participate in her treatment. During these discussions, some members of the interdisciplinary team raise concerns that transfer of care may place the patient at increased risk of medical complications due to adult care requiring substantially more patient autonomy. Further, it is noted that when the topic of transferring to an adult program has been broached with the patient, she becomes upset and refuses to talk about it.

As a result of the above history and concerns, a referral was made to the renal psychologist. Findings from the psychosocial assessment revealed concerns for overall poor psychosocial adjustment to living with ESRD. Relative strengths were noted in a desire for autonomy and for pursuing goals appropriate to navigating the path to becoming a young adult. An age- and gender-normed assessment of behavior, emotional, and adaptive functioning (BASC-2: Behavior Assessment System for Children – 2nd edition, Adolescent Self-Report Form) revealed at-risk levels of concern for depression, anxiety, social interaction skills, independence in daily activities, communication, and

S.K. Neul (✉)
Department of Neurosciences, University of California San Diego, La Jolla, CA, USA
e-mail: sharineulphd@gmail.com

© Springer International Publishing AG 2017   225
B.A. Warady et al. (eds.), *Pediatric Dialysis Case Studies*,
DOI 10.1007/978-3-319-55147-0_30

withdrawal from others [1]. Additional information was obtained from a review of results from the most recent semiannually administered 36-item Kidney Disease Quality of Life (KDQOL-36) assessment [2]. While average scores were noted on the Physical Component Summary (PCS) and Symptoms and Problems subscale, the KDQOL-36 showed below average scores on the Mental Component Summary (MCS) and Burden of Kidney Disease and Effects of Kidney Disease on Daily Life subscales.

More encouraging findings from the clinical interview conducted by the renal psychologist included a warm relationship with her mother, along with several age-appropriate goals: attaining a GED, obtaining a driver's license, and securing employment to contribute to household finances. Interests included dating, making more friends, cooking gourmet meals, and spending time with pets.

The renal psychologist summarized these findings for the treatment team as showing emotional, social, and adaptive functioning concerns that are likely the result of dealing with the HRQOL-related challenges of the emotional, social, and physical burden of chronic kidney disease and its impact on daily functioning. Despite these concerns, the renal psychologist noted the resiliency and potential for growth in the patient as evidenced by having good parental support, future- and goal-directed plans, and developmentally appropriate interests she pursues and enjoys. As a result, a comprehensive treatment plan involving the patient, her mother, and her interdisciplinary treatment team was developed that included continued close monitoring by the renal psychologist. Transfer to an adult program was delayed indefinitely in order to give this plan an opportunity to yield results.

Clinical Questions

1. How does the status of this young adult's health-related quality of life (HRQOL) functioning compare to that of other young adults with ESRD who are on dialysis?
2. What should one consider in the assessment of HRQOL functioning in older youth on dialysis?
3. How can intervention planning be helpful in improving HRQOL functioning in older youth on dialysis?
4. How can the dialysis team be involved in better supporting HRQOL functioning in older youth on dialysis?

Diagnostic Discussion

1. HRQOL is generally defined as a multidimensional construct tapping domains related to physical, mental, emotional, and social functioning and focuses on the subjective and objective impact that health status has on a person's quality of life [3]. This patient's overall HRQOL functioning is indeed poor; her emotional, social, and academic life reflects the negative impact of her disease and its demanding medical care on her ability to function. Further impacting this

patient's HRQOL is poor patient-dialysis team communication, lack of caregiver support and involvement, and history of poor adherence to self-care.

Depending upon the patient's length of time on dialysis, treatment course, and psychosocial history, HRQOL functioning in the older adolescent and young adult patient can be significantly compromised, particularly in the realms of experiencing intimate relationships, completing academic or other vocational training programs, and being gainfully employed to be able to live independently. Likewise, medical management of ESRD in the older pediatric patient can be fraught with challenges as the patients go through what has been termed a medical adolescence [4]. During this time, the dialysis team, patient, and caregivers must continually negotiate shared tasks in ways that encourage patient autonomy and responsibility for ESRD self-care, yet monitor patient care closely to avoid medical endangerment. Further, barriers to care often exist (e.g., complex healthcare systems, cultural factors impacting patient-healthcare provider communication, health beliefs, skills and knowledge, financial resources) increasing the risk of marginalization of socioeconomically disadvantaged groups [5]. Indeed, these barriers tend to be disproportionately represented in the pediatric ESRD population and can impact HRQOL functioning and hinder collaboration between youth with ESRD, caregivers, and the medical team in providing optimal care.

2. Annual assessment of HRQOL in pediatric dialysis patients is now mandated in the United States by the Centers for Medicare and Medicaid Services (CMS); however, little guidance is offered regarding what measure(s) to use, how to interpret assessment results, and how to develop interventions to improve HRQOL outcomes. Preliminary norms now exist for relative comparisons of pediatric patients in global and disease-specific aspects of HRQOL functioning (e.g., PedsQL™4.0 Generic Core Scales and PedsQL™3.0 ESRD Module, respectively) [6, 7]. The KDQOL-36 offers gender- and age-based norms for comparisons of young adult patient functioning. With few to no measures spanning the pediatric through the young adult years, psychometric continuity is compromised, which makes it difficult to meaningfully track HRQOL over time. However, proper planning and awareness of various practical and methodological considerations can help to augment the reliability and validity of the information obtained from assessing the young adult patient. Practical considerations can include patient characteristics (e.g., level of insight, cognitive functioning), proximal (e.g., dialysis side effects, time of day) and distal factors (e.g., disease-related factors impacting overall mood and cognitive functioning), and program-based factors (e.g., having trained staff, cost of measures, and acceptance by dialysis team). Methodological considerations can include assessing either or both global and disease-specific HRQOL and continuing with parent-proxy assessments (if young adults continue to live at home and give informed consent to have parent involved). Attention must be given to the frequency of assessments and its impact on respondent fatigue in obtaining valid and reliable responses. When collecting and analyzing longitudinal data, it can be difficult to tease apart response shift phenomena (i.e., shifts in internal standards in terms of how one thinks about adjustment to chronic disease) from normative developmental changes in the young adult patient (e.g., more future-oriented thinking and

increased awareness of the disease severity) [8]. Interpreting statistical versus clinically meaningful change in scores across time can also be difficult [9, 10].

3. Intervention planning is key to improving HRQOL functioning; however, the literature is generally focused on assessment findings rather than examining how to utilize assessment information and translate it into intervention efforts for youth with ESRD. In the adult world, HRQOL functioning is considered a patient-reported outcome (PRO) with benchmarks to help translate assessment findings into opportunities for patient-centered care practices. In the pediatric world, PROs for HRQOL assessment are in a relatively nascent stage, as are the use of patient-centered care practices. Patient-centered care practices can be devised to actively involve patients and caregivers in better understanding HRQOL assessment results: easy-to-understand language and graphical displays, jointly discussing what is of most importance to the patient and/or caregivers regarding HRQOL, collaboratively identifying ways to address their needs, and then seeking feedback on whether the needs are indeed being addressed, problem-solving barriers, and whether the efforts positively influence their HRQOL functioning [11]. Ideally, as pediatric units amass more HRQOL data and incorporate more patient-centered care approaches, young adult patients will benefit in that they will have been involved more actively in their care over time. In turn, they will be more prepared as they enter young adulthood to transition to actively collaborating with the dialysis team regardless of whether they remain in the pediatric setting or transition to an adult program.

4. Ideally, the patient-healthcare provider relationship grows and adapts with the patient's developmental needs to support and encourage autonomy in self-care, including sensitively addressing burgeoning areas of need (e.g., sexual health, risk-taking behavior, transitioning to adult care). This can be best facilitated via the interdisciplinary team comprised of attending physicians, fellows, nurses, social workers, child life specialists, psychologists, and other professionals who may be involved (e.g., quality of life coordinators, arts in healthcare professionals, academic tutors). Patient-centered care practices (e.g., exchanging versus imparting information, encouraging discussion, problem-solving, and creating a reasonable plan with patient input) particularly lend themselves to forging an effective patient and dialysis team relationship [12]. Finally, it will be important to ensure that HRQOL assessment data, pertinent details of conversations regarding HRQOL functioning, and forms documenting assessment feedback and intervention planning can all be made available via the electronic medical record. Having such information readily available to the interdisciplinary team can increase awareness of patient strengths and concerns, as well as facilitate engagement in meaningful discussions across multiple patient contacts. When more intensive intervention may be needed, mental health professionals (e.g., social workers, psychologists) can serve to improve communication between patients and the dialysis team, promote patient advocacy during patient care planning meetings, and foster learning and implementing important life skills to better navigate the demands of young adulthood while dealing with a serious, life-limiting chronic medical condition. Such efforts serve to promote HRQOL functioning and can help improve medical outcomes.

Clinical Pearls

1. Pediatric-onset chronic health conditions can pose significant challenges to the overall development of the functioning of the affected child and family. Poor rates of adherence, financial strain, and a myriad of psychosocial stressors are often present and thus pose challenges to attempt to improve HRQOL functioning. For the emerging young adult, opportunities for developing resiliency and improving HRQOL functioning can present themselves in the form of increased capability for insight and more future-oriented thinking. The latter is more likely if a good relationship already exists between the patient and the dialysis team or intervention is sought as early as possible to address concerns more preemptively rather than allowing frustrations to fester.
2. Efforts to ensure patient understanding of the purpose of HRQOL assessment, how to complete the measure(s), and more importantly, how the patient may benefit from thoughtfully participating in the assessment are vital to obtaining reliable and valid information, as well as devising a programmatic approach to HRQOL assessment and intervention. After providing feedback on HRQOL scores to patients and/or caregivers, it is important to seek feedback regarding what is of highest priority to them, as these concerns do not always reveal themselves in the pattern of scores.
3. Gathering information from patients about their HRQOL priorities creates "buy in" for the patient in discussing and identifying interventions to improve HRQOL functioning. Further, identifying concrete steps and delineating patient and dialysis team responsibilities to implement the intervention, along with building in repeated, brief check-ins with patients, fosters accountability and allows for problem-solving to overcome barriers to implementing interventions. Implementing

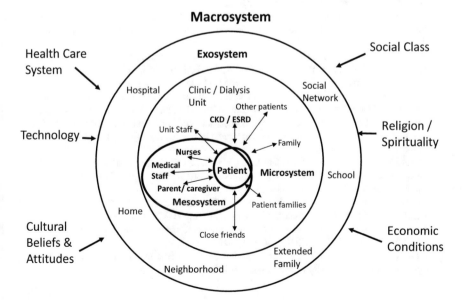

Fig. 30.1 Schematic representation of "there is life outside the dialysis unit"

such intervention planning strategies will help maintain patient engagement and ensure better success in improving the young adult's HRQOL functioning.

4. "There is life outside of the dialysis unit." This speaks volumes regarding the importance of keeping in mind all that impacts patients and their families, how they may interact with various members of the dialysis team on any given day, and if and when they are more or less capable of following through on various aspects of disease self-care (Fig. 30.1). In general, it is best to assume there is a skill deficit (i.e., a "can't") instead of a performance deficit (i.e., a "won't") at play when a problem arises. Assuming it is a lack of skill or knowledge allows for an open-mind in problem-solving and fostering collaboration and providing support to patients. Assuming it is a lack of willingness or motivation serves to label the patient and/or family as "difficult" and essentially shuts down the opportunity to effectively ameliorate the concern. Taking the right approach, pooling the talents and efforts of the interdisciplinary team and proactively facilitating referrals for psychosocial intervention will help to optimize HRQOL functioning in older youth with ESRD.

References

1. Reynolds CR, Kamphaus R. Behavior assessment system for children. 2nd ed. Circle Pines, MN: AGS; 2004.
2. Schatell DW. B. Measuring dialysis patients' health-related quality of life with the KDQOL-36. Med Educ Inst, Inc. 2008;3:1759–68.
3. Offie of Disease Prevention and Health Promotion. Health-related quality of life and well-being. www.healthypeople.gov/2020/topics-objectives/topic/health-related-quality-of-life-well-being.
4. Goldstein SL, Gerson AC, Goldman CW, Furth S. Quality of life for children with chronic kidney disease. Semin Nephrol. 2006;26(2):114–7.
5. Seid M, Sobo EJ, Gelhard LR, Varni JW. Parents' reports of barriers to care for children with special health care needs: development and validation of the barriers to care questionnaire. Ambul Pediatr. 2004;4(4):323–31.
6. Varni JW, Burwinkle TM, Seid M, Skarr D. The PedsQL 4.0 as a pediatric population health measure: feasibility, reliability, and validity. Ambul Pediatr. 2003;3(6):329–41.
7. Goldstein SL, Graham N, Warady BA, Seikaly M, McDonald R, Burwinkle TM, et al. Measuring health-related quality of life in children with ESRD: performance of the generic and ESRD-specific instrument of the pediatric quality of life inventory (PedsQL). Am J Kidney Dis. 2008;51(2):285–97.
8. Brossart DF, Clay DL, Willson VL. Methodological and statistical considerations for threats to internal validity in pediatric outcome data: response shift in self-report outcomes. J Pediatr Psychol. 2002;27(1):97–107.
9. de Vet H, Terwee C, Ostelo R, Beckerman H, Knol D, Bouter L. Minimal changes in health status questionnaires: distinction between minimally detectable change and minimally important change. Health Qual Life Outcomes. 2006;4(1):54.
10. Guyatt GH, Osoba D, Wu AW, Wyrwich KW, Norman GR. Methods to explain the clinical significance of health status measures. Mayo Clin Proc. 2002;77(4):371–83.
11. Neul SK. Quality of life intervention planning: pilot study in youth with kidney failure who are on dialysis. Nephrol Nurs J. 2015;42(5):487–96. quiz 97.
12. Lohr KN, Zebrack BJ. Using patient-reported outcomes in clinical practice: challenges and opportunities. Qual Life Res. 2009;18(1):99–107.

Chapter 31
Nonadherence

Rebecca J. Johnson

Case Presentation

A 14-year-old male with ESRD secondary to atypical hemolytic uremic syndrome, receiving home peritoneal dialysis, had a history of good adherence to his prescribed treatment regimen. He lived at home with his mother and younger sister. His father was not involved in his care. Two months after transition from primary to secondary school, it was discovered he was taking few (if any) of his prescribed oral medications. The nephrology team reviewed pertinent education and basic reminder strategies with the patient and his mother and encouraged better adherence. Subsequent follow-up indicated that he continued to be nonadherent to his medications and also revealed increased parent-child conflict surrounding medication administration and adherence. The family was referred to psychology. Interview with the patient and his mother revealed that the onset of nonadherence had coincided with the patient returning to school and changes to the mother's work schedule, resulting in cessation of parental monitoring and an abrupt transition of responsibility for medication adherence from the parent to the patient. During the interview, the parent expressed her belief that "He is old enough to remember his own medications." Patient and parent reported that since the onset of nonadherence, parent reminders and queries had increased ("Did you take your medications?") as had lecturing and scolding. The patient felt increasingly defensive and stressed by these interactions and became more argumentative with his mother. To avoid negative interactions, he acknowledged sometimes lying to his mother about his adherence.

When asked about barriers to adherence, the patient reported that he missed doses of his medications for a variety of reasons: sometimes he simply forgot, other times he felt too tired or rushed during his morning routine, and sometimes he felt "fed up"

R.J. Johnson, PhD, ABPP (✉)
Division of Developmental and Behavioral Sciences, Children's Mercy Hospital,
Kansas City, MO, USA
e-mail: rejohnson@cmh.edu

© Springer International Publishing AG 2017   231
B.A. Warady et al. (eds.), *Pediatric Dialysis Case Studies*,
DOI 10.1007/978-3-319-55147-0_31

with taking medications and coping with his chronic health condition. He stated that it "wasn't fair" that he had to deal with the additional responsibilities associated with his ESRD, and at times he "just didn't care" about taking his medications.

Clinical Questions

1. How are baseline adherence and barriers to adherence determined?
2. How are parent-child interactions determined?
3. What assessments should be considered for evaluation of patient functioning?
4. How are targeted interventions to nonadherence designed?

Diagnostic Discussion

1. When first-line interventions such as education and encouraging the patient to use basic reminder strategies have not resulted in improved adherence, a thorough assessment of baseline adherence and barriers to improved adherence is needed. Information can be obtained from a variety of sources, including self-report, pharmacy refill records, lab results, and, rarely, electronic monitoring. The most frequent source of adherence information is obtained during patient and parent interview. While research shows that patients often overestimate adherence, an interview that is matter of fact, free of reprimands and judgment, focuses on a specific time frame and asks specific questions is most likely to yield information that is clinically useful [1]. In the research setting, diary measures (such as 24-h recall or daily phone diaries) have been used and appear to yield more accurate information than traditional self-report [2]. However, these methods can be challenging to implement in the clinical setting. When deciding which adherence behaviors should be selected for assessment, a number of different approaches can be used, including obtaining baseline data on all relevant behaviors, selecting the behaviors that are perceived as most problematic by parents or providers, selecting the most "critical" adherence behaviors, or selecting the behaviors that are the easiest to change, to build behavioral momentum [1].

   The clinician may also utilize questionnaires and structured interviews to assist with the assessment of barriers to adherence [3–5]. The Parent Medication Barriers Scale (PMBS) and Adolescent Medication Barriers Scale (AMBS) are short paper-and-pencil measures that assess barriers to adherence from both the parent and patient perspective, and responses at baseline have been shown to predict adherence at 18-month follow-up [6]. In one study using the AMBS, pediatric dialysis patients reported a high number of prescribed pills, aversive taste of medications, difficulty remembering the medication schedule, and psychological fatigue related to taking medications and having a chronic health condition as barriers to adherence [7]. Recommendations exist for selecting and using self-report measures of adherence [8].

Providers assessing nonadherence to oral medications should also ask the parent and the patient to talk about the pill-swallowing routine in detail. How many pills can the child take at one time? How long does it take the child to swallow all of his or her medications? Does the child have problems swallowing medications of certain tastes, textures, shapes, or sizes? Indications of concern may include the child taking more than a few seconds to swallow pills, only being able to swallow one pill at a time or requiring multiple attempts to successfully swallow pills.

2. The best way to gather information about parent-child interactions surrounding medication administration or other aspects of care is to perform a thorough diagnostic interview. Such an interview will elicit specific information about patient behaviors that are undesired (e.g., talking back, fussing), antecedents of those behaviors (e.g., parent request or instruction), information regarding aspects of the setting that might influence behavior (e.g., television on during parental instructions), and the consequences that follow the behavior (e.g., parent reprimands, lecturing). The psychologist can then identify targets for intervention. Other assessment methods include behavioral observation of parent-child interactions, either in person or through a one-way mirror, standardized behavior questionnaires or checklists, and gathering information about the child's behavior from other informants such as teachers.

3. Assessing a patient's general psychological functioning can also inform adherence interventions. Cognitive executive functioning has been shown to predict adherence [9], and symptoms of depression can include difficulty concentrating, lack of motivation, apathy, and hypersomnia, all symptoms that may interfere with adherence. Assessment includes evaluating for symptoms of depression, anxiety, and other psychopathology via interview or interview combined with parent- and self-report measures, and a brief assessment of cognitive executive functioning, including learning, memory, and attention. If indicated, a more thorough neurocognitive evaluation can be performed.

4. Once baseline adherence has been estimated and barriers to adherence have been identified, interventions can be designed to target specific concerns. Assessment of targeted adherence behaviors should be ongoing, in order to evaluate treatment effects.

   (a) *Unintentional nonadherence*: Unintentional nonadherence includes accidental forgetting and patient or parent misunderstanding of the treatment regimen. It is commonly reported as a reason for nonadherence. Reminder strategies are often used to address barriers related to forgetting to take medications. These include alarms or apps on electronic devices such as smartphones, increasing parental monitoring and prompting, visual cues, pairing medication administration with another aspect of the patient's routine, or self-monitoring (e.g., use of tracking sheet or calendar). To prevent unintentional nonadherence due to misunderstanding of the treatment regimen, written information might be provided to the family, or health literacy interventions, such as teach-back, may be used [10]. It is also important to consider the complexity of the treatment regimen. There is evidence that increased complexity is related to decreased adherence. For example, medications that are prescribed greater than two times per day are associated with higher rates of nonadherence [11]. Whenever possible, simplify the medication schedule or other aspects of the treatment regimen to improve adherence.

(b) *Volitional nonadherence*: In contrast to unintentional nonadherence, such as forgetting, up to one-third or more of patients engage in volitional nonadherence [12], which has also been referred to as intentional or adaptive nonadherence [13]. Research has identified a number of reasons that patients intentionally make changes to their treatment regimens. These include trying to reduce aversive side effects; the drug or treatment is not producing the desired result; the patient's or parent's treatment goals are not aligned with those of the provider; the prescribed regimen does not fit the patient or family's lifestyle or routine; or the family wishes to reduce the treatment burden [1, 13, 14]. Volitional nonadherence may be associated with greater disease activity and poorer patient quality of life [12]. Interventions that target volitional nonadherence include changes to the treatment regimen to reduce medication side effects; adapting the treatment to better fit the family's lifestyle or reduce the treatment burden; patient education about why a medication or treatment is prescribed; and review of treatment goals from both the provider's and the family's perspective, to identify discrepancies and work toward improved understanding and collaboration.

(c) *Problems with parent-child interactions*: It is important to examine parent-child interactions surrounding delivery of the prescribed treatment regimen. Negative parent-child interactions can be a precursor to, or a result of, nonadherence. When parents adopt an authoritative parenting style [15], versus one that is permissive or authoritarian, they are more likely to gain consistent behavioral compliance from their children and parent-child relationships tend to be more positive. Adaptive maternal parenting behaviors are associated with better adherence [9]. Particularly within the context of a chronic disease with a high treatment burden, such as ESRD, the use of effective parenting strategies and development of functional parent-child relationships is key. Interventions to improve parent-child interactions may include teaching parents and patients more effective communication behaviors, setting clear guidelines for parental reminders or prompts that are agreed upon by both parent and patient, eliminating undesirable parent behavior such as lecturing or repeated reminders (typically perceived as "nagging" by the patient), and inclusion of positive reinforcement, such as verbal praise or token reinforcement, of the patient's behavioral compliance. There may be a need to more broadly address the parent-child relationship, utilizing behavioral parent-training to promote effective parenting or referral to a family therapist.

(d) *Problems with transition of responsibility from parent(s) to patient*: Unfortunately, decisions to decrease parental monitoring of adherence are often be related to chronological age or family circumstances versus the patient's actual performance. Sometimes, an abrupt transition occurs secondary to repeated, frustrating interactions between caregivers and adolescents, with caregivers ultimately "giving up" and adopting a hands off approach. However, parental involvement and monitoring is related to adherence during adolescence [16, 17]. Although not yet sufficiently tested empirically, "best practice" clinical guidelines strongly suggest that gradual, versus abrupt, transition of responsibility for adherence from parent(s) to the patient is a desirable goal (see American Academy of Pediatrics [18]). Rather than being withdrawn abruptly, transition of responsibility should evolve over the course of the child's development. Parent involvement should be faded gradually and be contingent on the child's performance. Interventions to promote successful transition of responsibility from parent to patient, within the context of nonadherence, include increasing parental involvement initially, such as increased monitoring or the parent directly observing medication administration; contingency management, including positive reinforcement of the patient's desired adherence behaviors; gradual fading of parental involvement based on child performance; and providing support to the parent, who may be experiencing disease-related psychological "fatigue." Psychoeducation may be necessary, as some parents have expectations of their children that are not consistent with what is known about child development.

(e) *Problems coping with a chronic health condition*: Clinical interview and the PMBS/AMBS or other questionnaires can shed light on the patient's perceptions of medical care, including their thoughts and feelings regarding taking medications and other treatments. A not infrequent barrier to adherence is negative self-talk surrounding medical care. Adolescents may report having frequent thoughts such as "I hate taking meds," "I am sick of taking meds," "I avoid meds because I don't like to be reminded that I have kidney disease," and "I just want to be like everyone else." Treatment can help adolescents identify negative thoughts or self-talk regarding their disease and its treatment; provide psychoeducation regarding the link between thoughts, feelings, and behavior; and utilize cognitive-behavioral strategies to promote more neutral or helpful self-talk regarding kidney disease and adhering to the prescribed treatment regimen. In addition, other therapeutic strategies can be employed to promote more adaptive, positive coping, including scheduling of pleasant activities, stress management, increasing social support, and positive reinforcement of coping behaviors. In addition to cognitive-behavioral approaches, other treatment approaches to reduce distress and increase adaptive coping and adherence behaviors include motivational interviewing techniques [19] and acceptance and commitment therapy [20].

(f) *Difficulty swallowing medications*: Pill-swallowing difficulties were not a concern in the case discussed in this chapter, but it is worth noting that problems with pill swallowing can occur at any point in treatment and can be successfully treated, following functional assessment, using a behavioral approach [21, 22, 23]. Key components of behavioral treatment typically include modeling, stimulus fading, contingency management, and generalization. For patients who exhibit anxiety or conditioned aversive responses to taking medication, additional behavioral intervention may be necessary [23, 24].

(g) *Problems with patient functioning*: If assessment reveals clinically significant symptoms of psychopathology for the patient, such as depression or anxiety, the patient should be referred for evidence-based psychotherapy. For problems related to cognitive executive functioning or learning, psychotherapy can target interventions such as teaching organizational strategies, memory aids, and implementation of other home- and school-based accommodations to promote success with healthcare tasks.

Epilogue

This case illustrates the importance of a thorough assessment of baseline adherence and barriers to improved adherence. Assessment in this case included consultation with the medical team, a detailed interview with the patient and parent regarding current circumstances surrounding medication administration, and completion of the AMBS/PMBS. The evaluation revealed a number of factors contributing to this patient's nonadherence, including situational factors (changes to his routine, abrupt transition of responsibility for medication adherence from the parent to the patient), parent-child interaction problems (increased conflict surrounding medication administration), and barriers related to the patient's difficulty coping with his chronic health condition. A treatment plan was developed that included parent education targeting successful transition of responsibility and, subsequently, increased parental monitoring; recommendations to improve communication between the parent and patient with regard to medication adherence; and examination of the patient's routine and modifications to promote adherence. Treatment also included cognitive-behavioral therapy aimed at improving his coping skills and targeting maladaptive cognitions and motivational interviewing techniques to enhance his motivation to change.

Clinical Pearls

1. Nonadherence has a number of negative consequences for children and adolescents receiving dialysis, including compromising their health and growth [25], and it is a barrier to kidney transplant. It is also common in pediatric populations. It is estimated that children who have chronic illnesses take, on average, 50% of their medications [26, 27]. However, there are a number of evidence-based interventions and treatment approaches that have been shown to improve adherence [28].

2. Assessment of adherence behaviors includes selection of behaviors on which to obtain baseline data and selection of an assessment method. This is most commonly patient or parent self-report, which can result in overestimates of adherence. However, there are ways to optimize the quality of the information obtained via self-report. Information should be elicited in a manner that is matter of fact, free of reprimands and judgment, focuses on a specific time frame, and asks specific questions. Providers may also employ structured interviews or paper-and-pencil assessment measures.

3. Barriers to adherence take many forms, from simple forgetting to intentional changes to the prescribed treatment regimen, as well as patient characteristics such as difficulties with pill swallowing, psychopathology, neurocognitive deficits, and poor adjustment and coping. When appropriate, broad screening leading to targeted assessment will assist in identifying important opportunities for intervention.

4. In pediatrics, parents and caregivers play a key role in the care delivered to children. Assessment and intervention must include parents, and parent behavior itself is often a target of intervention. Parent-child interactions surrounding healthcare tasks may need to be modified by improving communication and teaching parents how to use effective behavior management strategies.

5. It is important that transition of responsibility for healthcare from parents to patient occurs gradually and that transition is based on the patient's level of development and performance with regard to healthcare tasks. Too often, transition of responsibility occurs abruptly or is precipitated by factors other than the patient's ability to perform tasks independently. Parental monitoring predicts adherence during adolescence, often needs to be increased in cases of nonadherence, and should be phased out gradually.

6. Even when intervention results in improved adherence, too often treatment gains do not persist [29]. Close follow-up and continued attention to adherence behaviors may help maintain treatment gains. Integrating behavioral healthcare with medical care is one way to improve access to behavioral health consultation. Training multiple members of the healthcare team to deliver adherence interventions is another promising strategy [30].

References

1. Rapoff MA. Adherence to pediatric medical regimens. 2nd ed. New York: Springer; 2011.
2. Quittner AL, Modi AC, Lemanek KL, Ievers-Landis CE, Rapoff MA. Evidence-based assessment of adherence to medical treatments in pediatric psychology. J Pediatr Psychol. 2008;33:916–36.
3. Modi AC, Quittner AL. Barriers to treatment adherence for children with cystic fibrosis and asthma: what gets in the way? J Pediatr Psychol. 2006;31:846–58.
4. Simons LE, Blount RL. Identifying barriers to medication adherence in adolescent transplant recipients. J Pediatr Psychol. 2007;32:831–44.
5. Zelikovsky N, Schast AP, Palmer JA, Meyers KAC. Perceived barriers to adherence among adolescent renal transplant candidates. Pediatr Transplant. 2008;12:300–8.
6. Simons LE, McCormick ML, Devine K, Blount RL. Medication barriers predict adolescent transplant recipients' adherence and clinical outcomes at 18-month follow-up. J Pediatr Psychol. 2010;35:1038–48.
7. Silverstein DM, Fletcher A, Moylan K. Barriers to medication adherence and its relationship with outcomes in pediatric dialysis patients. Pediatr Nephrol. 2014;29:1425–30.
8. Stirratt MJ, Dunbar-Jacob J, Crane HM, et al. Self-report measures of medication adherence behavior: recommendations on optimal use. TBM Pract Publ Health Policies. 2015;5:470–82.
9. O'Hara LK, Holmbeck GN. Executive functions and parenting behaviors in association with medical adherence and autonomy among youth with spina bifida. J Pediatr Psychol. 2013;38:675–87.

10. American Medical Association Foundation and American Medical Association. Health literacy and patient safety: help patients understand. Chicago, IL: AMA Foundation; 2007.
11. Blydt-Hansen TD, Pierce CB, Cai Y, Samsonov D, Massengill S, Moxey-Mims M, Warady BA, Furth SL. Medication treatment complexity and adherence in children with CKD. Clin J Am Soc Nephrol. 2014;9:247–54.
12. Schurman JV, Cushing CC, Carpenter E, Christenson K. Volitional and accidental nonadherence to pediatric inflammatory bowel disease treatment plans: initial investigation of associations between quality of life and disease activity. J Pediatr Psychol. 2011;36:116–25.
13. Adams CD, Dreyer ML, Dinakar C, Portnoy JM. Pediatric asthma: a look at adherence from the patient and family perspective. Curr Allergy Asthma Rep. 2004;4:425–32.
14. Graves MM, Adams CD, Bender JA, Simon S, Portnoy AJ. Volitional nonadherence in pediatric asthma: parental report of motivating factors. Curr Allergy Asthma Rep. 2007;7:427–32.
15. Baumrind D. The influence of parenting style on adolescent competence and substance use. J Early Adolesc. 1991;11:56–95.
16. Ellis DA, Podolski CL, Frey M, Naar-King S, Wang B, Moltz K. The role of parental monitoring in adolescent health outcomes: impact on regimen adherence in youth with type 1 diabetes. J Pediatr Psychol. 2007;32:907–17.
17. Ellis DA, Templin TN, Naar-King S, Frey MA. Toward conceptual clarity in a critical parenting construct: parental monitoring in youth with chronic illness. J Pediatr Psychol. 2008;33:799–808.
18. American Academy of Pediatrics. American Academy of Family Physicians, and American College of Physicians, Transitions Clinical Report Authoring Group. Clinical report – supporting the health care transition from adolescence to adulthood in the medical home. Pediatrics. 2011;128:182–202.
19. Miller WR, Rollnick S. Motivational interviewing: preparing people for change. 2nd ed. New York: Guilford; 2002.
20. Hayes SC, Strosahl KD, Wilson KG. Acceptance and commitment therapy: the process and practice of mindful change. 2nd ed. New York: Guilford; 2011.
21. Anderson CM, Ruggiero KJ, Adams CD. The use of functional assessment to facilitate treatment adherence: a case of a child with HIV and pill refusal. Cogn Behav Pract. 2000;7:282–7.
22. Walco GA. A behavioral treatment for difficulty in swallowing pills. J Behav Ther Exp Psychiatry. 1986;17:127–8.
23. Blount RL, Dahlquist LM, Baer RA, Wuori D. A brief, effective method for teaching children to swallow pills. Behav Ther. 1984;15:381–7.
24. Johnson RJ. Organ transplantation. In: Wu Y, Aylward B, Roberts MC, editors. Clinical practice of pediatric psychology: cases and service delivery. New York: Guilford; 2014.
25. Akchurin OM, Schneider MF, Mulqueen L, Brooks ER, Langman CB, Greenbaum LA, Furth SL, Moxey-Mims M, Warady BA, Kaskel FJ, Skversky AL. Medication adherence and growth in children with CKD. Clin J Am Soc Nephrol. 2014;9:1519–25.
26. Drotar D. Promoting adherence to medical treatment in chronic childhood illness: concepts, methods, and interventions. Mahwah NJ: Lawrence Erlbaum Associates; 2000.
27. Rapoff MA, Barnard MU. Compliance with pediatric medical regimens. In: Cramer JA, Spilker B, editors. Patient compliance in medical practice and clinical trials. New York: Raven Press; 1991. p. 73–98.
28. Graves MM, Roberts MC, Rapoff M, Boyer A. The efficacy of adherence interventions for chronically ill children: a meta-analytic review. J Pediatr Psychol. 2010;35:368–82.
29. Rapoff MA. Commentary: adherence matters. J Pediatr Psychol. 2013;38:688–91.
30. Wu YP, Pai ALH. Health care provider-delivered adherence promotion interventions: a meta-analysis. Pediatrics. 2014;133:1698–707.

Chapter 32
Transition to Adult Care

Lorraine E. Bell

Case Presentation

An 18-year-old girl receiving hemodialysis will soon need to transfer to adult care.

She began renal replacement therapy when she was 17 years old, after years of slowly progressive chronic kidney disease due to severe Shiga toxin-associated hemolytic uremic syndrome during infancy. Her past medical history is also significant for tetralogy of Fallot, successfully repaired in the neonatal period.

Prior to starting dialysis, she excelled in team sports but always found school-work challenging. She is 1 year behind her peers in school and may not pass this academic year. She lives with her parents, but their involvement in her care is limited and they rarely accompany her to the hospital.

In the dialysis unit, she is unfailingly polite and pleasant, charming almost everyone she meets. Unfortunately, there are ongoing challenges with her treatment. She has difficulty arriving on time for dialysis, limiting her fluid intake and controlling her phosphorus levels. Occasionally she is very late and the dialysis nurses need to call and remind her of her treatment. She always promises to try harder. Her listing for transplant has been delayed because of concerns regarding her adherence.

She is seen annually by the pediatric cardiology team because of her tetralogy of Fallot repair and will require long-term follow-up in a specialized center for adult congenital heart disease. Most likely this will be in a different location from her future adult dialysis unit.

Her oral medications are $CaCO_3$ with lunch and supper, sevelamer with all three meals, and a renal multivitamin; in addition she receives IV darbepoetin, IV iron, and IV calcitriol. She was previously on several antihypertensive agents, but they were no longer needed once her dry weight was achieved. Her pre-dialysis blood

L.E. Bell (✉)
Division of Nephrology, Department of Pediatrics, McGill University Health Centre,
Montreal Children's Hospital, Montreal, QC, Canada
e-mail: lorraine.bell@mcgill.ca

© Springer International Publishing AG 2017
B.A. Warady et al. (eds.), *Pediatric Dialysis Case Studies*,
DOI 10.1007/978-3-319-55147-0_32

pressure is usually in the target range of 110–120/70–80 mmHg, but when she is very fluid overloaded, it can be as high as 150/100 mmHg. With rapid ultrafiltration she experiences headache, nausea, abdominal pain, leg cramps, and hypotension. Therefore, when a large volume of fluid must be removed, her treatment time needs to be extended; on occasion it requires an extra dialysis session.

Her laboratory results are generally as follows:

Hgb 110–115 g/L
Phosphorus 1.8–2.6 mmol/L (5.6–8.0 mg/dL)
Ionized calcium 1.2–1.3 mmol/L
Potassium 4.5–5.5 mmol/L, occasionally 6 mmol/L on Mondays
PTH 10–30 pmol/L (normal values: 1.6–9.3 pmol/L)

The pediatric dialysis nurses are worried about what will happen when she transfers to adult care and have asked you about transition preparation.

Clinical Questions

1. What is the difference between transfer and transition to an adult unit?
2. When should transition planning begin?
3. What potential treatment–related problems and complications do you foresee when she transfers to the adult unit?
4. What measures can you take now to try to mitigate these risks?
5. What other aspects of her medical care need coordination?

Diagnostic Discussion

1. Transition is a process spanning several years, whereas transfer is the actual move from one unit to another. Ideally the transition process begins well in advance of the date of transfer and continues after, until the young person is fully integrated into adult care (Fig. 32.1).
2. Some would say *transition planning* begins shortly after diagnosis. Parents often need coaching on ways to empower their child and still provide structured support [1, 2]. This is embodied in a parenting model of leadership transition, beginning with parents as "CEOs" of care, then "managers," "supervisors," and finally "consultants," [3] as their children mature and become progressively more autonomous (Fig. 32.2, Table 32.1). The actual *transition preparation process* should begin between 10 and 14 years of age and involve the patient, parent/guardian, and healthcare team. It is multifaceted and includes attention to social determinants of health, such as education and vocational planning, peer and social support networks, and psychological well-being [4]. When there is more

The Transition Process

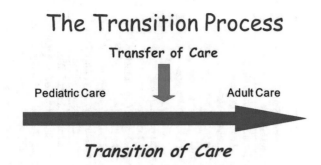

Fig. 32.1 Transfer is just one stage in the process of transition to adult care (Adapted from: Rosen DS. Grand Rounds: all grown up and nowhere to go: transition from pediatric to adult healthcare for adolescents with chronic conditions. Presented at: Children's Hospital of Philadelphia; 2003; Philadelphia, PA)

Fig. 32.2 A model of leadership transition for health management responsibility between parents and their children with special healthcare needs. Adapted from Kieckhefer and Trahms [3]

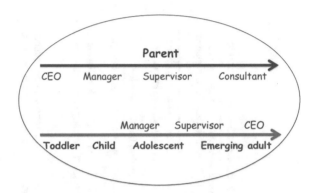

than one medical problem, integration of healthcare is key. A dedicated family doctor can be an important facilitator of the process.

3. Major concerns relate to our patient's ability and/or desire to take charge of her medical management and to adhere to her current treatment. With a very supportive dialysis team, she is doing well, particularly for treatments supervised by her nurses such as blood pressure control (ultrafiltration, extended dialysis sessions), anemia management, and PTH levels (intravenous medications). In contrast, her phosphorus management, which requires her active participation, is suboptimal. When she transfers to an adult unit, and loses the personalized support of her pediatric team, her condition may suffer. In adult dialysis units, patient volumes are higher, nurse-to-patient ratios lower, and schedules less flexible than those of pediatric centers. If our patient arrives late, her treatment will probably be shortened. Missed treatments may be difficult to make up, with progressive fluid overload and hypertension likely and increased risk for left ventricular hypertrophy. Poor phosphorus control will add to her cardiovascular risk factors.

Table 32.1 Approach to the development of child and adolescent leadership/self-management skills

Child Age/Developmental Stage	Parent Role	Child/Adolescent Role	Child Capabilities/Actions forming basis for leadership skills (with kidney disease-related examples)	Parents' Leadership Actions Supporting Child/Youth's increasing capabilities
Toddler (1–3 years)	*Parent* as "CEO"	Child receives parent's care	• Cooperates in routine treatment with limited acting out (e.g., help hold treatment supplies) • Understands firm limits of parents	• Develop rituals for treatment so child knows what to expect and can learn by repetition • Identify treatment roles to share with child • Emphasize hygiene for infection prevention
Preschool (4–5 years)		Child learns some basic self-care	• Assists further in self-care (e.g., helps gather treatment supplies) • Participates in medical play (e.g., nurse, doctor kits, doll or teddy bear that undergoes treatments) • Learns name of health condition • Learns simple terms for condition-related problems (e.g., for feeling unwell, nausea, painful urination)	• Acknowledge child's need for control over body (e.g., explain what will happen at hospital visit) • Set fair and appropriate limits (e.g., taking medication, dietary/fluid requirements) • Allow appropriate choices (e.g., which medicine to swallow first) • Reassure that child is not being punished if treatment causes discomfort (e.g., injections, blood drawing, enteral feeding tube)
Early school age (6–9 years)	*Parent* becomes "Manager" of care	Child provides some self-care	• Recognizes 1–2 major internal body cues of a problem (e.g., fever, pain, dysuria) • Participates actively in care and monitoring of condition (e.g., fluid intake, recording medications on personal record) • Increases simple understanding of health condition and treatment	• Label body cues and reward recognition • Negotiate child's tasks and "rules" to get all treatment done (e.g., taking medication on time in parent's presence) • Encourage healthy active living • Support activities (sports, other organized activities) to encourage fitness, teamwork, and sense of achievement • Model telling others about medical condition

Developmental stage	Role	Adolescent tasks	Interventions
Early adolescence (10–13 years)	*Adolescent performs greater self-care and some self-management*	• Increases understanding of health condition and its effect on daily life • Begins to discuss issues with healthcare providers in parents' presence • Independently completes specific self-management tasks (e.g., alarm watch for medication, agenda with appointments, learns medication names, times, and allergies) • Prepares medication dose boxes with parental supervision • Actively participates, with parental supervision, in more complex tasks (e.g., dialysis machine setup, growth hormone injections) • Learns how to respond to peer pressure and still take care of self	• Provide tools to aid self-management (e.g., alarm watch, notebook to record medication taken) • Delegate components of more complex tasks to adolescent • Shadow or observe performance closely; offer immediate corrective feedback • Remain involved in care and decision-making • Be there for new symptoms, changes in treatment, and emergencies • Ensure adolescent has told important others (e.g., friends, teachers, coaches) of health condition and assistance they could provide if needed • Further encouragement of healthy living and normative activities
Mid adolescence (14–16 years)	*Adolescent becomes "Manager" of care* *Parent becomes "Supervisor" of care*	• Achieves more abstract knowledge of health condition and complication prevention • Develops strategies to complete routine tasks, e.g., taking medication on time (alarm watch, cues linked to daily routine) • Learns roles of each medication and major side effects • Participates in appointment making • Assumes active role in complex treatments (e.g., self-injections of ESA, setting up home-dialysis machine) • Able to effectively ask for assistance in complex situations	• Negotiate and renegotiate who does what • Continue to be present for/supervise treatments • Discuss new issues (e.g., sex, drugs, and alcohol) particularly as they relate to peer group activities/pressures and health condition • Begin to discuss vocational and educational aspirations and insurance issues • Encourage community involvement (club, volunteer work, extracurricular activity groups) • Consider adolescent's participation in limited part-time or summer employment

(continued)

Table 32.1 (continued)

Child Age/ Developmental Stage	Parent Role	Child/ Adolescent Role	Child Capabilities/Actions forming basis for leadership skills (with kidney disease-related examples)	Parents' Leadership Actions Supporting Child/ Youth's increasing capabilities
Late adolescence (17–19 years)	*Parent* becomes "Consultant" to adolescent	*Adolescent* becomes "Supervisor" of care	• Achieves sense of self as capable manager of the health condition • Takes responsibility for routine and complex health self-management tasks • Integrates realities of health condition care with the "invincible" nature of peers • Continues to develop more independent clinical and community support network with transition to adult-based services	• Remain informed but not interfering • Be present for support and problem solving • Provide encouragement and guidance as the youth transitions from pediatric to adult care services • Encourage vocational, college, or university training and/or integration into the workforce

Adapted from Bell et al. [2], Kieckhefer and Trahms [3]

A framework for the progressive development of self-management skills in children and adolescents with chronic kidney disease

4. A multifaceted approach is needed; key components are outlined below.

   (a) *Transition preparation*

   Intensive transition preparation is needed for both our patient and her parents. Ideally, this would have begun much earlier [2, 5]. Now it is essential to help her parents understand that, although their daughter is almost 18, she still requires support, structure, and encouragement.

   The pediatric healthcare team needs to give our patient increasing responsibility and progressively help her adapt to the expectations of an adult unit. This may involve more limit setting in terms of late arrivals and helping her achieve greater motivation and responsibility for her health.

   An assessment of our patient's understanding of her underlying disease, her current health issues, and her treatment plan is also key. A transition checklist can facilitate this and identify areas in need of focused interventions to help her attain autonomy [6, 7]. From this an action plan can be developed. Areas where ongoing support may be required after transfer to adult care should be clearly specified. Examples of transition checklists and other tools are available on the Got Transition™ website, a program of the National Alliance to Advance Adolescent Health (www.gottransition.org) [6].

   (b) *Cognitive assessment*

   Good social skills can sometimes mask cognitive deficits, leading to an overestimate of a patient's ability to understand. Our patient is charming and adept at casual communication, but may lack a depth of understanding of her condition. Patients with renal failure from an early age are at increased risk of subtle cognitive problems [8], as are patients who have undergone cardiac surgery in infancy [9]. A neurocognitive assessment can help better understand our patient's abilities and guide ways to coach and teach. Ideally this is done early in care, allowing timely educational supports and interventions, but it will still be useful at this point in time.

   (c) *Adherence*

   The basis for our patient's poor adherence needs to be explored (see Chap. 31). Causes of nonadherence are multifaceted and include (1) the patient (e.g., development, knowledge, self-efficacy, comorbidities, psychological/psychiatric conditions, attitudes, quality of care, trust in the treating team), (2) social and economic factors (e.g., family functioning, social supports, medication costs), (3) therapy-related issues (e.g., symptoms, treatment complexity, and side effects), and (4) health system-related determinants [10]. A careful analysis of major factors involved in this patient's nonadherence could help direct and target interventions.

   (d) *Health summary*

   A *succinct* health summary needs to be prepared and shared with our patient. This can help her achieve a sense of ownership for her health. Many youth with a childhood onset of chronic health conditions haven't learned the details of their health history, since it was their parents who received the initial teaching, often many years earlier. This is especially important when the disease began in infancy, as with our patient.

Preparation of a *comprehensive* transfer summary for the adult treating team is also essential.

(e) *Vocational planning*

Employment is an important socioeconomic determinant of health. Our patient already has challenges at school, which may be exacerbated by time missed for dialysis treatments. Her strengths include her excellent communication and interpersonal skills. The nephrology social worker and hospital educators could help her develop a strategy to complete high school and assist her in choosing further training in a field that might foster her talents [2, 7, 11].

(f) *Communication and collaboration with the adult team*

This is a central element. If possible, the pediatric healthcare team should identify adult nephrology units with an interest in transitioning youth. Ideally our patient would visit one or more of these units prior to transfer and choose the one she prefers. Participation in the decision-making process is empowering [7]. Once she has selected her adult unit, her pediatric physicians and nurses need to communicate with the new treating team. In addition to a comprehensive health summary, a phone call or meeting is very helpful. A copy of the most recent transition checklist should be part of the transfer documents, communicating areas where ongoing assistance and support will be required. It is important for the receiving adult unit to understand that transfer is but one step in the transition process and that transition activities should continue until the young person is fully integrated into adult care [2, 12]. The adult physicians and nurses may also benefit from information on adolescent/emerging adult brain development, and how full adult functions are not usually attained until the mid- to late twenties [12, 13].

5. What other aspects of her medical care need coordination?

(a) *Cardiology*

Her continuing cardiology follow-up and her future listing for kidney transplant need to be integrated with her transfer. Many young adults with congenital heart disease have been lost to follow-up, often with serious consequences. Ideally, she will be followed in an adult cardiology unit with expertise in congenital heart disease [9]. Transfer arrangements need to be made in collaboration with the pediatric cardiology team, and a summary of her cardiac condition should accompany her dialysis transfer package. Her new dialysis unit may be in a different location from the adult congenital heart disease clinic, making coordination more challenging.

(b) *Transplant planning*

Communication with the adult transplant unit where she will eventually be listed for kidney transplant should take place prior to transfer and an introductory appointment arranged. As with the dialysis unit, it will be useful to identify transplant programs that are interested in receiving transitioning youth [14]. The transplant unit will also need a copy of her comprehensive medical summary, including both the renal and cardiac history.

(c) *Tracking mechanism and/or registry*

  A system is needed to track her progress, both during the transition preparation phase and after her transfer to adult care [6]. It should include documentation of attendance at her first adult site appointments. Optimally it would incorporate a mechanism for longer-term outcome assessment. A registry for all the pediatric nephrology division's patients with chronic kidney disease, in need of transition planning, would be helpful for evaluation of patient progress, transfer plans, and future outcomes.

Epilogue

An accelerated transition preparation process was implemented for our patient. The nephrology interdisciplinary team worked intensively with her on issues related to understanding of her health condition, her adherence, her motivation, and her further educational plans. After 8 months there was a tangible improvement in her treatment adherence, and it was decided to list her for transplant. For this she was referred to an adult transplant center with a dedicated program for young adult transplant recipients; it provided youth-friendly services with extra attention, more frequent appointments, and a peer support network [14]. Shortly after transferring to her adult dialysis unit, she received a deceased donor kidney. One-year posttransplant she has excellent graft function. Her continuing care at a specialized adult congenital heart disease unit is also on track. She completed high school through an adult education program and has applied to college to become a teacher.

Clinical Pearls

1. Transition to adult care for youth with special healthcare needs is a process spanning several years, whereas transfer is a single point in time. The transition process begins in early adolescence and continues beyond transfer, until the young person is fully integrated into the adult milieu.
2. Children with special healthcare needs benefit from developmentally appropriate progressive responsibility for management of their healthcare condition, beginning early in the course of their illness.
3. Education is an important social determinant of health. Youth with chronic health conditions are at risk for lower educational achievement, due to a multiplicity of factors. Early evaluation and intervention are key in helping them achieve their potential.
4. Communication, collaboration, and teamwork, involving the pediatric and adult healthcare teams, the patient, and the patient's family, are essential elements of successful pediatric transition to adult healthcare.
5. A system to track transition preparation and its process, both before and after transfer to adult care, is central to patient safety and quality assurance.

References

1. Beacham BL, Deatrick JA. Health care autonomy in children with chronic conditions: implications for self-care and family management. Nurs Clin N Am. 2013;48:305–17.
2. Bell LE, Bartosh SM, Davis CL, et al. Adolescent transition to adult care in solid organ transplantation: a consensus conference report. Am J Transplant. 2008;8:2230–42.
3. Kieckhefer GM, Trahms CM. Supporting development of children with chronic conditions: from compliance toward shared management. Pediatr Nurs. 2000;26:354–63.
4. Foster BJ, Bell L. Improving the transition to adult care for young people with chronic kidney disease. Curr Pediatr Rep. 2015;3:62–70.
5. Bell LE, Ferris ME, Fenton N, Hooper SR. Health care transition for adolescents with CKD-the journey from pediatric to adult care. Adv Chronic Kidney Dis. 2011;18:384–90.
6. Six core elements of health care transition (2.0). 2014. Accessed 10 Dec 2016, at http://www.gottransition.org/resources/index.cfm.
7. Gleeson H, Turner G. Transition to adult services. Arch Dis Child Educ Pract Ed. 2012;97:86–92.
8. Warady BA, Neu AM, Schaefer F. Optimal care of the infant, child, and adolescent on dialysis: 2014 update. Am J Kidney Dis. 2014;64:128–42.
9. Williams RG. Transitioning youth with congenital heart disease from pediatric to adult health care. J Pediatr. 2015;166:15–9.
10. Foster BJ. Heightened graft failure risk during emerging adulthood and transition to adult care. Pediatr Nephrol. 2015;30:567–76.
11. Lewis H, Marks S. Differences between paediatric and adult presentation of ESKD in attainment of adult social goals. Pediatr Nephrol. 2014;29:2379–85.
12. Gleeson H, McCartney S, Lidstone V. 'Everybody's business': transition and the role of adult physicians. Clin Med. 2012;12:561–6.
13. Colver A, Longwell S. New understanding of adolescent brain development: relevance to transitional healthcare for young people with long term conditions. Arch Dis Child. 2013;98:902–7.
14. Harden PN, Walsh G, Bandler N, et al. Bridging the gap: an integrated paediatric to adult clinical service for young adults with kidney failure. BMJ (Clin Res ed). 2012;344:e3718.

Chapter 33
Pregnancy in a Woman Approaching End-Stage Kidney Disease

Talal Alfaadhel and Michelle A. Hladunewich

Case Presentation

A 20-year-old female was referred to our clinic at 12 weeks' gestation with stage 5 chronic kidney disease (CKD; eGFR 10 ml/min/1.73 m^2). She was born with a solitary kidney. She had multiple episodes of urinary tract infections in her childhood. At 8 years of age, she had severe pyelonephritis. This was complicated by acute kidney injury and subsequently chronic renal impairment. Her additional medical history included childhood asthma, hypothyroidism, and a history of smoking. She had been on salbutamol puffer, thyroxin, ferrous fumarate, prenatal vitamins, and low-dose aspirin (started a week before her nephrology assessment). During her first visit in our clinic, she complained of anorexia, nausea, and vomiting. She also complained of fatigue with a decrease in her functional capacity.

On physical examination, her blood pressure was 110/79 mmHg, and her heart rate was 84 beats per minute. Her jugular venous pulsation was 2 cm above the sternal angle. Auscultation of her heart and lungs were normal. Routine laboratory investigations are summarized in Table 33.1. Other pertinent investigations showed a PTH of 46.9 pg/ml and a hemoglobin A1C 5.4%. Her previous workup included a negative ANA and negative HIV, HBV, and HCV screening. On abdominal ultrasound, her right (solitary) kidney measured 8 cm in length with a thin cortex and increased echogenicity of the corticomedullary junction.

T. Alfaadhel
Division of Nephrology, Sunnybrook Health Sciences Centre, University of Toronto, Toronto, ON, Canada

M.A. Hladunewich (✉)
Divisions of Nephrology and Obstetric Medicine, Department of Medicine, Sunnybrook Health Sciences Centre, University of Toronto, Toronto, ON, Canada
e-mail: michelle.hladunewich@sunnybrook.ca

© Springer International Publishing AG 2017
B.A. Warady et al. (eds.), *Pediatric Dialysis Case Studies*,
DOI 10.1007/978-3-319-55147-0_33

Table 33.1 Relevant clinical parameters monitored during pregnancy

Clinical parameter	Prepregnancy	First trimester	Second trimester	Third trimester	Postpartum
Blood pressure (mmHg)	120/60	110/79	150/90	130/80	120/70
Urea (mmol/L)	18	*20*	14	16	13
Creatinine (umol/L)	380	413	NA	NA	NA
Hemoglobin (g/L)	119	112	104	110	105
Ferritin (ug/L)	50	48	30	40	30
Iron saturation (%)	32	30	20	31	29
Albumin (g/L)	41	42	36	35	32
HCO3$^-$ (mmol/L)	21	20	22	22	23
K$^+$ (mmol/L)	4.6	4.8	4.3	4.2	4.5
Phosphate (mmol/L)	1.54	1.68	1.2	0.9	1.1
Intervention	NA	Hemodialysis initiated	Labetalol initiated; iron sucrose loading and erythropoietin started	Dialysis frequency increased to 5 days per week	

After counseling her on the maternal and fetal risks related to her advanced kidney disease, and discussion of her management, she decided to carry on with her pregnancy. She also agreed to initiate renal replacement therapy, the decision being made based on her increased serum urea and aforementioned symptoms. A tunneled hemodialysis (HD) catheter was inserted within a week of her assessment, and in-center HD was initiated with a schedule of three sessions per week (4 h per session).

For the remainder of her first trimester, her nausea and vomiting started to improve after initiating HD and adding pyridoxine/doxylamine therapy. In the second trimester, epoetin alfa and IV iron sucrose were initiated for a decreasing hemoglobin. At the same time, her blood pressure gradually increased, reaching 150/90 mmHg at 22 weeks gestation, but subsequently improved after instituting antihypertensive management with labetalol. At 30 weeks gestation, her obstetrical ultrasound revealed an amniotic fluid index greater than the 95th percentile; this was in keeping with polyhydramnios. Given this finding and her high urea nitrogen level, her frequency of HD was increased to five times per week. She was also seen weekly at the high-risk pregnancy clinic to monitor fetal well-being and to guide her dialysis requirements. Finally, she was induced and delivered vaginally at 38 weeks' gestation; her baby boy weighed 5 lbs. and 13 oz. at birth. Post delivery she continued HD. She had poor milk production and her son had to be supplemented with formula. Her transplant workup was started soon thereafter.

Clinical Questions

1. What was the likelihood of this woman becoming pregnant given her GFR?
2. What are the maternal risks associated with pregnancy and CKD?
3. What are the fetal risks associated with pregnancy and CKD?
4. How does the delivery of HD differ in a woman who is pregnant?

Diagnostic Discussion

1. Fertility often decreases in women with advanced kidney disease [1]. This is due to the disturbance of the sexual hormonal milieu as GFR declines. Many women with advanced kidney disease also report sexual inactivity; uremia is often associated with a decreased sexual drive, lack of sexual pleasure, and dyspareunia [2]. The absence of the pulsatile release of GnRH, increased prolactin activity, and dampening of the mid-cycle LH and FSH peaks result in disrupted menstrual cycles and anovulation [3]. Just as recognizing pregnancy can be challenging in the uremic state, early pregnancy loss can go unrecognized, and early miscarriages may not be reported [4]. Based on limited registry data among women of childbearing age who are on maintenance conventional HD, only 1–7% ever become pregnant [5]. Despite these low rates, it appears that the rate of pregnancy in women on maintenance HD has increased in the past decade [6]. This may be related to improved dialysis delivery, especially in women receiving a higher dialysis dose, such as on nocturnal HD.
2. Pregnancy can be associated with a considerable risk of morbidity and even mortality in women with CKD (Table 33.2). Women with kidney disease can have difficulty adapting to the necessary physiological changes of pregnancy, such as hyperfiltration and reduced vascular resistance [7]. In women who fail to adapt to these changes, systemic hypertension and renal impairment may ensue. Additionally, placental implantation and vascularization can be poor in the setting of underlying CKD. Practitioners should, therefore, review the risk of CKD progression during pregnancy and after delivery, in addition to highlighting the risk of preeclampsia and its complications. These risks are shown to be incrementally

Table 33.2 Maternal and fetal risks associated with pregnancy in CKD

Maternal risks	Fetal risks
Deterioration of renal function	Intrauterine growth restriction
Hypertension	Small for gestational age
Worsening of proteinuria	Polyhydramnios
Preeclampsia	Premature birth
Flare of underlying kidney/systemic disease	Low birth weight
Peripartum acute kidney injury	Neonatal mortality

related to the degree of renal impairment [8]. It is also likely that the cause of kidney disease plays a significant role in the development of adverse maternal outcomes. Specifically, women who become pregnant with uncontrolled diabetic nephropathy (with reduced GFR and increased albuminuria) appear to have a high risk of developing complications [4]. Other kidney diseases that can be associated with considerable risk include non-remitting IgA nephropathy and active lupus nephritis [4, 9]. In the latter, a systemic flare can be devastating and may require aggressive immunosuppression, which can add further risk to the mother and fetus. In women with mild renal impairment (eGFR more than 60 ml/min/1.73 m²) and low-grade proteinuria (less than 0.5 g per day), the risk is slightly increased compared to the general population [8, 10]. However, women with moderate to severe kidney disease (serum creatinine 168 umol/L or more) have a significant risk of worsening of their underlying kidney disease during pregnancy (20%) and after delivery (23%) [11]. As such, some women with severe renal impairment will subsequently require renal replacement therapy during pregnancy or after delivery.

Preeclampsia can be severe and may occur earlier in women with advanced kidney disease [12]. Due to the overlapping signs of kidney disease and pre-eclampsia, the latter can be difficult to diagnose in its early stage, especially when proteinuria and hypertension are present preconception. Severe preeclampsia can be associated with multi-organ involvement manifesting as worsening hypertension and proteinuria, pulmonary edema, neurologic impairment, HELLP, or eclampsia [13]. Low-dose aspirin has been shown to reduce the risk of adverse maternal and fetal outcomes related to preeclampsia and has been recommended for women who are at risk [14].

3. Historically, advanced maternal kidney disease was associated with poor fetal outcomes (Table 33.2). This likely reflects the poor adaptation to pregnancy in the setting of kidney disease. Several studies have reported intrauterine growth restriction in women with renal impairment [15]. There is also an increased risk of intrauterine fetal death. The risk of preterm birth increases as GFR declines [8]. This is likely to be multifactorial in origin, with a higher rate of uncontrolled maternal hypertension, worsening kidney function, and higher rates of pre-eclampsia often resulting in the need for early delivery. As a result, pregnant women with kidney disease require close monitoring of fetal development, ideally in a high-risk pregnancy clinic. Routine ultrasounds are employed to assess placental health, fetal growth, and amniotic fluid indices. Uremia, in the setting of end-stage kidney disease (ESKD), is a rare cause of polyhydramnios. This is potentially related to urea solute diuresis by the fetus [16]. In such pregnancies, intensified dialysis may limit the progression of polyhydramnios and potentially avert its complications [16].

4. Dialysis requirements are increased in pregnant women. In the past, the dialysis prescription had been tailored to reduce the serum urea nitrogen to less than 17 mmol/L, with most women receiving 3–4 dialysis sessions per week [17, 18]. Recent studies have shown improved maternal and fetal outcomes with intensi-

fied dialysis (often reaching 6–7 sessions per week) [19]. The live birth rate has been as high as 85% among those who have been dialyzed more than 36 h per week. In comparison, women dialyzed less than 20 h per week have a live birth rate of only 48%. The median duration of pregnancy is longer in women receiving intensified dialysis, often reaching 36 weeks of gestation [19]. Although these results are encouraging, it can be difficult to achieve such high doses of HD either at an in-center dialysis facility or with home dialysis.

A particular challenge related to dialysis during pregnancy is fluid management. Although blood pressure control is advised, it is important to avoid maternal hypotension during dialysis. Assessment of the fluid status prior to each dialysis session is recommended, and fluid removal during dialysis should be tempered. Dialysis hypotension can compromise the fetoplacental circulation, and in women receiving many hours of dialysis per week, the development of hypotension can be associated with a resultant significant time of impaired blood supply to the fetus.

There is also a marked increase in the requirement for iron during pregnancy that must be addressed as part of dialysis management. The increased requirement may result from the increase in maternal blood volume. Fetal growth and development also leads to an increased consumption of iron. Many women with end-stage kidney disease will, thus, require iron supplementation, more often in the form of intravenous iron. There is also a higher erythropoietic-stimulating agent (ESA) requirement, and monitoring of hemoglobin is necessary to tailor erythropoietin dosing. Supplementation of water-soluble vitamins is needed as these can be consumed by increased maternal metabolism and fetal growth, as well as from loss due to frequent dialysis. Finally, diet can often be liberalized and a higher potassium bath is often required along with phosphate supplementation (oral or added to the dialysate). Given the rare incidence of pregnancy in dialysis, referral to a nephrologist with experience in managing such high-risk women is recommended.

Clinical Pearls

1. Pregnancy is rare in ESKD, as the fertility of women with advanced kidney disease is impaired. However, pregnancy can occur, and discussions regarding family planning in young women with ESKD are required.
2. In women with CKD/ESKD, there is an increased risk of maternal and fetal complications. Planned pregnancies and close follow-up in a high-risk clinic may help reduce these complications.
3. There is no consensus on the optimal management of pregnant women on dialysis. There is more experience in pregnancy outcomes in women on hemodialysis compared to peritoneal dialysis. It is likely that intensive HD improves fetal outcomes. See Table 33.3.

Table 33.3 Recommendations for management of ESKD in pregnancy

Issue	Intervention
Dialysis adequacy	Target frequent hemodialysis (>36 h per week) especially in later pregnancy. Ensure appropriate functioning access. Anticoagulation with heparin
OB monitoring	Follow-up in a high-risk maternal-fetal clinic. Frequent ultrasounds for monitoring of placental heath, amniotic fluid levels, as well as fetal growth and well-being
Hypertension	Consider therapy with pregnancy safe antihypertensive agents. Avoid aggressive fluid removal during dialysis
Anemia	Treat iron deficiency adequately. Consider IV iron treatment if unable to tolerate oral iron or in cases of severe deficiency. Erythropoietin requirements may increase. Adjust dose accordingly
Nutrition	Ensure adequate intake of water-soluble vitamins. Dietary consultation can be helpful
Fluid and electrolyte management	Clinical assessments of volume status to determine ultrafiltration needs. Frequent monitoring of electrolytes, calcium and phosphate with supplementation as required

References

1. Holley JL, Schmidt RJ. Changes in fertility and hormone replacement therapy in kidney disease. Adv Chronic Kidney Dis. 2013;20:240–5.
2. Palmer BF. Sexual dysfunction in men and women with chronic kidney disease and end-stage kidney disease. Adv Ren Replace Ther. 2003;10:48–60.
3. Rathi M, Ramachandran R. Sexual and gonadal dysfunction in chronic kidney disease: pathophysiology. Indian J Endocrinol Metab. 2012;16:214–9.
4. Jungers P, Chauveau D. Pregnancy in renal disease. Kidney Int. 1997;52:871–85.
5. Schmidt RJ, Holley JL. Fertility and contraception in end-stage renal disease. Adv Ren Replace Ther. 1998;5:38–44.
6. Jesudason S, Grace BS, McDonald SP. Pregnancy outcomes according to dialysis commencing before or after conception in women with ESRD. Clin J Am Soc Nephrol. 2014;9:143–9.
7. Williams D, Davison J. Chronic kidney disease in pregnancy. BMJ. 2008;336:211–5.
8. Piccoli GB, et al. Risk of adverse pregnancy outcomes in women with CKD. J Am Soc Nephrol. 2015;26:2011–22.
9. Huong DLT. Pregnancy in past or present lupus nephritis: a study of 32 pregnancies from a single Centre. Ann Rheum Dis. 2001;60:599–604.
10. Zhang J-J, et al. A systematic review and meta-analysis of outcomes of pregnancy in CKD and CKD outcomes in pregnancy. Clin J Am Soc Nephrol. 2015;10:1964–78.
11. Jones DC, Hayslett JP. Outcome of pregnancy in women with moderate or severe renal insufficiency. N Engl J Med. 1996;335:226–32.
12. Maruotti GM, et al. Preeclampsia in women with chronic kidney disease. J Matern Fetal Neonatal Med. 2012;25:1367–9.
13. ACOG. Executive summary: hypertension in pregnancy. Obstet Gynecol. 2013;122:1122–31.
14. Henderson JT, et al. Low-dose aspirin for the prevention of morbidity and mortality from preeclampsia. At <http://www.ncbi.nlm.nih.gov/books/NBK196392/>.
15. Nevis IF, et al. Pregnancy outcomes in women with chronic kidney disease: a systematic review. Clin J Am Soc Nephrol. 2011;6:2587–98.

16. Reddy SS, Holley JL. The importance of increased dialysis and anemia management for infant survival in pregnant women on hemodialysis. Kidney Int. 2009;75:1133–4.
17. Holley JL, Reddy SS. Pregnancy in dialysis patients: a review of outcomes, complications, and management. Semin Dial. 2003;16:384–8.
18. Asamiya Y, et al. The importance of low blood urea nitrogen levels in pregnant patients undergoing hemodialysis to optimize birth weight and gestational age. Kidney Int. 2009;75:1217–22.
19. Hladunewich MA, et al. Intensive hemodialysis associates with improved pregnancy outcomes: a Canadian and United States cohort comparison. J Am Soc Nephrol. 2014;25:1103–9.

Chapter 34
Withholding and Withdrawal of Dialysis

Aaron Wightman

Case Presentation

A 2-week-old boy born with severe kidney disease due to renal dysplasia is referred from an outside neonatal intensive care unit for possible dialysis. The birth weight was 2 kg. The neonate has had no urine output, but an improving pulmonary status on mechanical ventilation. The pulmonologist has evaluated the child's pulmonary hypoplasia and believes that the child will likely require prolonged mechanical ventilation, but may eventually be able to be extubated. The cranial ultrasound shows a unilateral grade 1 intraventricular hemorrhage.

The neonatologist has recommended withholding dialysis because of concerns over the lifelong burdens of dialysis and the high mortality rate. The nephrology team disagrees, citing recent improvements in survival and quality of life among neonatal recipients of dialysis. The family is uncertain how to proceed, but "want everything done" for their child.

After a series of conversations involving the parents, neonatologists, nephrologists, surgeons, chaplain, and bioethics specialists, the parents were able to identify goals of care for their baby focused on maximizing quality of life while limiting burdens. A consensus was reached among the medical team to pursue dialysis with regular assessment about whether the benefits of continued dialysis still exceeded the burdens for the child.

Peritoneal dialysis was initated; however, after two weeks, the newborn developed fever and abdominal distention. Further evaluation was concerning for the development of necrotizing enterocolitis. Surgical exploration revealed evidence of massive bowel necrosis necessitating significant bowel resection. Peritoneal dialysis was halted. In the postoperative setting, the newborn continued to have worsening pain and hypotension and required increased respiratory support. After a series

A. Wightman, MD, MA (✉)
University of Washington School of Medicine, Seattle, WA, USA
e-mail: aaron.wightman@seattlechildrens.org

© Springer International Publishing AG 2017
B.A. Warady et al. (eds.), *Pediatric Dialysis Case Studies*,
DOI 10.1007/978-3-319-55147-0_34

of discussions involving the parents, nephrologist, neonatologist, and surgeons, consensus was reached that any benefit of further life-sustaining therapies such as dialysis no longer outweighed their associated burdens and were no longer in the child's interests. The decision was made to forego further dialysis and transition to comfort measures only.

Clinical Questions

1. Is it ever permissible to withdraw or withhold dialysis?
2. Are withholding and withdrawing dialysis the same?
3. What factors may be considered in decisions to withhold or withdraw dialysis?
4. What approaches should be taken when there is disagreement between the medical team and the family or among the medical team?

Diagnostic Discussion

1. Withholding dialysis is defined as foregoing dialysis in a patient for whom dialysis has yet to be initiated. Withdrawal of dialysis means the discontinuation of ongoing dialysis therapy. Both are examples of foregoing life-sustaining treatments. The 2010 Renal Physicians Association (RPA) Guidelines on Shared Decision-Making in the Appropriate Initiation of and Withdrawal from Dialysis recommend, 1) foregoing dialysis if the initiation or continuation of dialysis is deemed to be harmful or of no benefit and, 2) to strongly consider foregoing dialysis in a patient with a terminal illness whose long-term prognosis is poor [1]. It is important to recognize that a decision to forgo life-sustaining treatments is not the same as foregoing care. An intensification of palliative treatments should occur in conjunction with any decision to forgo dialysis.

   Withdrawal of dialysis is common. In the United States, approximately one quarter of all deaths among individuals who receive chronic dialysis occur after a decision has been made to withdraw dialysis. In fact, withdrawal of dialysis is the second leading cause of death among all adult chronic dialysis patients in the United States [2]. Less is known about the withdrawal from pediatric dialysis; however, withdrawal of life-sustaining treatments is a leading cause of death in neonatal and pediatric intensive care units [3, 4]. An analysis of French-speaking pediatric nephrology centers from 1995 to 2001 found 50 cases where dialysis was withheld or withdrawn among 440 children with end-stage kidney disease (11.5%) [5]. The most common reasons for withdrawal included concerns of subsequent quality of life, severe neurological handicap, and consequences of the disease on the family [5].

   In adult nephrology the patient's wishes may dictate withholding or withdrawing from dialysis. This is supported by the principle of respect for autonomy which holds that competent patients should be well informed and then be allowed to decide for themselves within the range of choices in accordance with their own values and beliefs [6]. This allows a competent adult to refuse all medical therapies. Indeed, the unwanted provision of dialysis would be considered battery.

When the patient is unable to express his or her wishes, a surrogate may make that decision, appealing to an advanced directive or substituted judgment. Substituted judgment requires the surrogate to choose as the patient would if he/she were competent. Children are generally considered to lack the competence required to clearly state preferences regarding life-sustaining interventions. As a result, the Best Interests Standard is used when questions regarding withholding or withdrawing therapy arise, rather than a standard of substituted judgment [7, 8]. The Best Interests Standard considers the interests to the child *alone* and requires weighing the current and future interests of the child and selecting the option that maximizes the child's overall benefit and minimizes the child's overall risks of harm [9]. The importance of evaluating the potential harms and benefits of dialysis is further supported by the physician's primary obligation to first do no harm [10]. Reflecting this, the RPA guidelines state that dialysis should be withheld or withdrawn if it is deemed to be overwhelmingly harmful or of no benefit to the child [1].

2. It is generally accepted that there is no ethical distinction between withholding and withdrawing care, even if there may be an emotional distinction for the patient, family, and medical team [1, 6]. A 2005 survey of pediatric intensivists and subspecialists showed that many providers do not feel that withholding and withdrawing life-sustaining treatments are the same [11]. Providers may sense that withdrawing dialysis or other life-sustaining treatments feels more distressing than simply withholding the treatment. This may reflect a perception of greater moral agency, responsibility, and culpability on the part of the healthcare provider for a patient's death associated with withdrawal of treatment (commission) vs. never initiating life-sustaining treatment (omission). There is a tendency to describe a situation in which treatment has begun as "the train has left the station" and cannot be stopped. Once treatment has begun, it cannot be stopped. Implicit belief in this distinction can result in the creation of an "up-front barrier" to appropriate treatment which may lead to both inappropriate overtreatment (continuation of treatment that is no longer beneficial or desirable for the patient) and undertreatment (hesitancy to initiate treatment because of concerns about being trapped by biomedical technology that once begun cannot be stopped) [12]. Others may claim that to withhold therapy is more problematic than to withdraw therapy. For example, if a patient appears to be dying and has a low likelihood of benefiting from dialysis treatment, withholding the dialysis precludes the possibility of an unexpected recovery. If dialysis is provided and later withdrawn, the treatment is forgone only after its lack of utility has been confirmed [13].

The distinction between withdrawing and withholding dialysis is, in fact, morally and legally irrelevant. Both not initiating and stopping life-sustaining therapy can be justified, depending upon the circumstances. Both can be instances of allowing to die, and both can be instances of killing [14]. Courts recognize that individuals can commit a crime by omission if they have an obligation to act, just as a physician can commit a wrong by omission in medical practice. In situations where the physician has a clear duty to treat, omission of treatment by withholding or withdrawing violates that duty. Conversely, if there is no clear duty to treat, then both withholding and withdrawing could be considered to be permissible.

3. There is no universally accepted criterion for withholding or withdrawing life-sustaining treatments such as dialysis. Decisions made to withhold or withdraw dialysis in pediatrics should be individualized and consistent with the interests of the child and with consideration of the benefits and burdens resulting from continued renal replacement therapy. Choices should reflect the patient's and family's goals of care that are achievable and should be centered upon the patient's quality of life [1, 8, 15].

The RPA guideline, along with the American Academy of Pediatrics, recommends that physicians develop a patient-physician relationship that promotes family-centered shared decision-making [1, 15]. Shared decision-making involves clinician-family collaboration and culminates in a decision arrived at through consensus of the involved groups [16]. Family-centered shared decision-making respects parental authority in medical decision-making for children and is supported by the ethical principles of beneficence, nonmaleficence, and respect for autonomy. If parents request involvement of other family members, these requests should be respected. Although children generally do not have legal authority to make independent healthcare decisions, it is important to involve children in the decision-making process to the extent it is developmentally appropriate. In addition, other members of the medical team, potentially including the patient's pediatrician, intensivist, and any other relevant subspecialist, should be encouraged to participate in coordinating care related to treatment decisions made by the family. In the setting of a child with multiple medical comorbidities, decisions about dialysis should be made in the context of other life-sustaining treatments, including ventilators, parenteral nutrition, and the provision of intensive care.

Parents should be provided with information regarding the risks, discomforts, side effects, and benefits of treatment alternatives including dialysis and comfort care only. As part of these discussions, the nephrologist should provide recommendations of the best options for the child, citing medical, experiential, and moral factors [7]. Importantly, changes in a patient's prognosis may change the nephrologist's recommendations. The family should be informed of this change without delay [8].

The ethical concept of futility is rarely, if ever, a sufficient basis to withhold dialysis. A claim of futility is supported by the principle that a doctor is under no moral obligation to do to a patient that which is of no benefit to the patient. Unfortunately, there is no single agreed upon definition of futility, and the concept has different meanings to physicians, parents, and the press [6, 17]. *Physiologic futility* claims that an intervention cannot achieve the desired outcome [17]. An example of this would be dialysis in a child for whom it is impossible to obtain vascular or peritoneal access. *Quantitative futility* claims that while it is possible for an intervention to achieve the desired goal, it is so unlikely that it should not be pursued [18]. An example may be providing dialysis to an exceptionally small newborn (i.e., <1 kg) who is too small for traditional forms of vascular or peritoneal access. While it may be possible to obtain dialysis access in the case of a 1 kg neonate, it is very unlikely but not impossible to be successful. So long as access may be obtained, dialysis will almost always provide improved metabolic clearance and volume control and thus will not meet a standard of physiologic or quantitative futility. This is not to claim that in every instance dialysis should be pursued; rather that futility is an inappropriate reason not to do so. The assessment of benefit in such cases goes beyond whether dialysis will provide renal clearance and ultrafiltration to more global questions focused on quality of life for the patient. These considerations are inherently value based and should be determined by the child's parents [8, 17, 19].

4. In the setting of disagreement between medical team and family, instead of pursuing unilateral decisions, it is the duty of the medical team to continue to engage in respectful dialogue with the child's family [10]. These discussions should include revisiting the family's goals of care for the child and education about the child's expected prognosis and treatment options. Discussions should also acknowledge the degree of uncertainty related to prognosis [1]. It is highly recommended to involve additional medical teams, including palliative medicine and pastoral care, early in this process [1, 8]. The RPA guideline recommends that medical teams explicitly describe comfort measures and other components of palliative care that are available [1]. The purpose of these discussions is to develop consensus (not unanimity) among the medical team and the family.

   The RPA also recommends the establishment of a systematic due process approach for conflict resolution if there is disagreement between parents and the medical team or within the medical team itself about what decision should be made with regard to dialysis. Potential interventions could include consultation with colleagues not involved in the child's direct medical care or convening of multidisciplinary conferences to discuss different perspectives related to treatment. In some instances it may be appropriate to consider a time-limited trial of dialysis for patients requiring dialysis, but who have an uncertain prognosis or for whom consensus cannot be reached about providing dialysis. A trial of dialysis therapy may allow for further information to be gathered to make more informed decisions; however, these trials must have clearly defined end points. Otherwise, they risk simply adding further burden to a child who will not benefit from the intervention. Finally, if consensus still cannot be reached or if the treating nephrologist believes that the parents are making decisions inconsistent with the best interests of the child, consultation with a hospital ethics committee is highly recommended [1]. Court involvement to order dialysis treatment over parental objections represents a serious challenge to parental authority and autonomy and may permanently alter a family's future interactions with medical providers. Pursuit of state intervention should be considered only as a last resort.

Some parents may request that withdrawal of dialysis occur in the hospital setting. In most circumstances this request should be respected. The goal of medical care is not limited to treatment and cure; medical teams also carry an obligation to ease their patient's pain and suffering associated with dying. In some circumstances those obligations may best be met in the hospital setting.

Some providers may be concerned over the allocation of resources to children with poor prognoses; or conversely, they may be concerned about the "waste" of withholding or withdrawing dialysis therapy in a child in whom enormous resources have been invested. It is important to acknowledge that there are limited resources available for healthcare and that society should utilize these resources in the most efficient manner possible for the benefit and greater good of the population. However, in a society with resources available to fund medical care, rationing decisions should not be left to doctors at the bedside; rather they should be considered at a societal level. In addition, studies of the neonatal and pediatric intensive care units suggest that few resources are "wasted" on those children with even the most futile diagnoses [20, 21]. Similarly, the degree of previous resource utilization or medical effort is irrelevant to a discussion of the justification of ongoing treatments.

Clinical Pearls

1. Withdrawal of dialysis is common in adult nephrology, but little information pertaining to pediatric nephrology is available. Withdrawal of life-sustaining treatments is the most common reason for death in the neonatal and pediatric intensive care unit.
2. A decision to forgo life-sustaining treatments is not the same as forgoing care. There is a continued duty to provide effective palliative care. Death following withdrawal of dialysis is rarely immediate. Withdrawal of life-sustaining treatment is not a withdrawal of care. A decision to withdraw dialysis should include provision of palliative care for the patient and continued support for the patient, family, and medical team.
3. Withholding and withdrawing therapies are generally considered to be ethically equivalent. Both may be acceptable in the setting of proposed dialysis for end-stage kidney disease depending on an individualized assessment of the benefits and burdens of dialysis therapy for the child.
4. Decision-making regarding forgoing initiation or continuation of dialysis should be made using a model of shared decision-making. Parents should be fully informed of the risks, discomforts, side effects, and benefits of treatment alternatives and the physician's recommendation of the best option based upon medical, experiential, and moral factors. It is highly recommended to involve palliative medicine early in the decision-making process. In settings of disagreement, continued discussions are warranted, and other interventions such as a trial of therapy or ethics committee involvement should be considered. Court intervention should be sought only as a last resort.

References

1. RPA. Shared decision making in the appropriate initiation of and withdrawal from dialysis. 2nd ed. Rockville: RPA; 2010.
2. System USRD. 2015 USRDS annual data report: epidemiology of kidney disease in the United States. Bethesda: National Institutes of Health, National Institute of Diabetes and Digestive and Kidney Diseases; 2015.
3. Vernon DD, Dean JM, Timmons OD, Banner Jr W, Allen-Webb EM. Modes of death in the pediatric intensive care unit: withdrawal and limitation of supportive care. Crit Care Med. 1993;21(11):1798–1802. PubMed
4. Carter BS, Howenstein M, Gilmer MJ, Throop P, France D, Whitlock JA. Circumstances surrounding the deaths of hospitalized children: opportunities for pediatric palliative care. Pediatrics. 2004;114(3):e361–6. PubMed PMID: 15342898.
5. Fauriel I, Moutel G, Moutard ML, Montuclard L, Duchange N, Callies I, et al. Decisions concerning potentially life-sustaining treatments in paediatric nephrology: a multicentre study in French-speaking countries. Nephrol Dial Transplantat Off Publ Eur Dial Transplant Assoc Eur Renal Assoc. 2004;19(5):1252–7. PubMed Pubmed Central PMCID: 1890006. Epub 2004/03/03.
6. Beauchamp TL, Childress JF. Principles of biomedical ethics. 8th ed. New York City: Oxford University Press; 2012. 480 p.
7. Association AM. AMA code of medical ethics opinion 2.20 – withholding or withdrawing life-sustaining medical treatment. 1996 [cited 2016 4/17/16]. Available from: http://www.ama-assn.org/ama/pub/physician-resources/medical-ethics/code-medical-ethics/opinion220.page?
8. American Academy of Pediatrics Committee on Bioethics. Guidelines on foregoing life-sustaining medical treatment. Pediatrics. 1994;93(3):532–6. PubMed PMID: 8115226.
9. Kopelman LM. Using the best interests standard to generate actual duties. AJOB Prim Res. 2013;4(2):11.
10. Dionne JM, d'Agincourt-Canning L. Sustaining life or prolonging dying? Appropriate choice of conservative care for children in end-stage renal disease: an ethical framework. Pediatr Nephrol. 2015;30(10):1761–9. PubMed PMID: 25330877.
11. Solomon MZ, Sellers DE, Heller KS, Dokken DL, Levetown M, Rushton C, et al. New and lingering controversies in pediatric end-of-life care. Pediatrics. 2005;116(4):872–83. PubMed PMID: 16199696. Epub 2005/10/04.
12. Derse AR. Limitation of treatment at the end-of-life: withholding and withdrawal. Clin Geriatr Med. 2005;21(1):223–38, xi. PubMed PMID: 15639048.
13. Orentlicher D. Matters of life and death: making moral theory work in medical ethics and the law. Princeton: Princeton University Press; 2001. p. 8, 234.
14. Levine DZ, Truog RD. Discontinuing immunosuppression in a child with a renal transplant: are there limits to withdrawing life support? Am J Kidney Dis Off J Nat Kidney Found. 2001;38(4):901–15. PubMed PMID: 11576900.
15. Committee On Hospital C, Institute For P, Family-Centered C. Patient- and family-centered care and the pediatrician's role. Pediatrics. 2012;129(2):394–404. PubMed PMID: 22291118.
16. Charles C, Gafni A, Whelan T. Decision-making in the physician-patient encounter: revisiting the shared treatment decision-making model. Soc Sci Med. 1999;49(5):651–61. PubMed PMID: 10452420.
17. Helft PR, Siegler M, Lantos J. The rise and fall of the futility movement. N Engl J Med. 2000;343(4):293–6. PubMed PMID: 10911014.
18. Schneiderman LJ, Jecker NS, Jonsen AR. Medical futility: its meaning and ethical implications. Ann Intern Med. 1990;112(12):949–54. PubMed PMID: 2187394.
19. Fetus CO, Newborn T. The initiation or withdrawal of treatment for high-risk newborns. Pediatrics. 1995;96(2):362–3.

20. Sachdeva RC, Jefferson LS, Coss-Bu J, Brody BA. Resource consumption and the extent of futile care among patients in a pediatric intensive care unit setting. J Pediatr. 1996;128(6):742–7. PubMed PMID: 8648530.
21. Lantos JD, Mokalla M, Meadow W. Resource allocation in neonatal and medical ICUs. Epidemiology and rationing at the extremes of life. Am J Respir Crit Care Med. 1997;156(1):185–9. PubMed PMID: 9230745.

Chapter 35
Peritoneal Dialysis as Treatment for Acute Kidney Injury (AKI)

Mignon I. McCulloch

Case Presentation

A 2-year-old African boy presented to his local clinic with a 5-day history of fever, diarrhoea and vomiting. He had not been able to keep any solids or liquids down for the prior 2 days, and he was drowsy. His mother was uncertain whether he had passed any urine in view of the diarrhoea potentially being mixed with urine. He lives in a very rural part of Africa and had never been ill previously, apart from occasional upper respiratory tract infections. His immunization status was up to date.

The boy's initial evaluation revealed the following: weight 10 kg (in contrast to usual weight of 12 kg), pulse rate 140 beats/min, respiratory rate 30 breaths/min, blood pressure 80/40 mmHg and temperature 39 °C. Clinically, he appeared profoundly unwell and was very dehydrated with cool peripheries, a capillary refill time of 4 s and reduced skin turgor.

An intravenous cannula was placed, and blood was taken for complete blood count, malaria screen, electrolytes and kidney function. No blood culture bottles were available, and the blood gas analyser had run out of cartridges and had been non-functional for 2 months.

A urine bag was placed but remained empty. Broad spectrum antibiotics (e.g., ampicillin and gentamicin) were given as per routine practice. The patient's rapid malaria screen was positive, and antimalarial therapy was initiated.

He was resuscitated with bolus intravenous fluids followed by maintenance intravenous fluid and kept under observation in the casualty area of the clinic overnight. Venous blood gas showed pH 7.0 PCO_2 5.5 kPa PO_2 12 kPa Bicarb 8 BE −25.

M.I. McCulloch (✉)
Red Cross Children's Hospital, Department of Paediatric Nephrology and Paediatric ICU, Cape Town, South Africa
e-mail: mignon.mcculloch@uct.ac.za

© Springer International Publishing AG 2017
B.A. Warady et al. (eds.), *Pediatric Dialysis Case Studies*,
DOI 10.1007/978-3-319-55147-0_35

Over the next 24 h, the child was rehydrated but continued to be anuric. The results of his blood tests, which only became available 24 h later, were as follows:

Sodium 165 mmol/l, potassium 7.5 mmol/l, chloride 140 mmol/l, urea 25 mmol/l and creatinine 450 umol/l (5.1 mg/dl)

The haemoglobin was 4 g/dl, white blood cell count 22 × 109/l and platelets 600 × 109/l

He was given a blood transfusion and subsequently began to look fluid overloaded with evidence of peripheral oedema.

A trial of furosemide, 1 mg/kg, was given followed by a second dose, 2 mg/kg. Aminophylline 1 mg/kg was given as an additional diuretic with no resultant urine output. His intravenous fluid infusion was reduced to insensible losses only.

At the same time, a cardiac monitor revealed evidence of peaked T waves; he was promptly given Kayexalate (potassium binding/ion-exchange resin) per rectum, calcium gluconate and intravenous sodium bicarbonate.

Over the next 6 h, the patient had no urine output, and his T waves were looking taller. Whereas blood was obtained during the evening for repeat evaluation, results were not available until the next morning, and so a decision was made to initiate acute peritoneal dialysis (PD). This choice was made despite the fact that there was no dialysis facility at this clinic and no transport to the regional hospital (8 h away) was available at night. Although no surgeon was available, the paediatrician had received training in bedside peritoneal dialysis catheter insertion. She used a chest drain set as a 'makeshift' PD catheter and a Y connector with a three-way tap and prepared dialysis fluid with 1 l of Ringer's lactate and added dextrose. She initially used a fill volume of 10 ml/kg per cycle and later increased the volume to 20 ml/kg using 2 h cycles (e.g. fill 30 min, dwell 1 h, drain 30 min), as she conducted the dialysis and cared for others in the clinic simultaneously as a result of staff shortages.

Acute PD was performed for 36 h prior to the time the patient started passing urine spontaneously. He eventually became polyuric, but required 3 days of dialysis. The patient made a full recovery and was discharged home with the diagnosis of septicaemic shock, malaria and acute kidney injury (AKI).

Clinical Questions

1. What are the key aspects of treatment for hypovolaemic shock?
2. What diuretic medications should be considered in the setting of acute kidney injury and oliguria?
3. In a healthcare facility with limited resources, what materials can be used to serve as a PD access for a patient requiring acute PD?
4. In the same locale with limited resources, what steps would be required to constitute a "PD set"?
5. What fluids can be used to prepare a 'home-made solution' for PD? What precautions need to be considered when doing so?
6. What are the basic principles to be addressed when conducting acute PD?

Diagnostic Discussion

1. Fluid replacement is the key management step for treatment of hypovolaemic shock, with identification of the cause for the presentation a key factor (crystalloid for diarrhoea or blood products in the case of bleeding) in determining the preferred approach to therapy associated with the greatest likelihood of preventing the development of AKI.

    This is not to be confused with fluid replacement for septic shock where more recently caution has been advocated with respect to recommendations in the sepsis guidelines [1] following the FEAST trial [2] in East Africa. In this trial, intravenous fluid boluses were found to be deleterious in low-resource settings where no cardiac or respiratory support was available. Thus, new guidelines are being published by WHO [3], as well as by European and American organizations.

2. Diuretics such as furosemide have not been shown to improve long-term outcome, but do make the management of AKI easier if the use of the agents results in converting a patient from an anuric to polyuric state, especially if renal replacement is not readily available. Aminophylline is an old-fashioned diuretic which works well in combination with furosemide [4]. Furosemide provided as a slow bolus of 1–2 mg/kg/dose is the recommended starting dose, but can also be given as an infusion of 0.1–1 mg/kg/h in cases of treatment-resistant severe oliguria/anuria. Aminophylline at a dose of 1 mg/kg/dose every 6 h can be used provided there is no contraindication in terms of cardiac arrhythmias.

3. The gold standard for a PD catheter to be used for treatment of AKI is a surgically inserted Tenckhoff catheter with cuffs. Ideally, the catheter is also tunnelled and inserted by an experienced surgeon. In the absence of such resources, bedside PD catheters can be placed using a sterile technique at the bedside in a paediatric intensive care or paediatric ward setting. These can be placed by any provider who has received the proper training to be able to place a well-functioning catheter using a technique that is designed to limit the risk of placement and infectious-related complications [5].

    In the absence of PD catheters which are designed for this purpose, alternative materials have been used and include central lines or multipurpose drainage catheters inserted by Seldinger technique, chest drains and even nasogastric catheters in extreme situations [6, 7].

4. Ideally, a closed system which is designed for acute peritoneal dialysis (such as systems manufactured by Fresenius or Baxter with measuring devices as part of the system) should be used as the PD set.

    In the absence of this resource, a 'self-made' device using a fill system and a drain system via a three-way tap can be constructed. Development of the set is initiated using a fluid bag with a measuring buretrol connected to a drainage system which, in turn, attaches to a three-way tap connected to the PD catheter; this permits passage of the dialysis fluid into the abdomen.

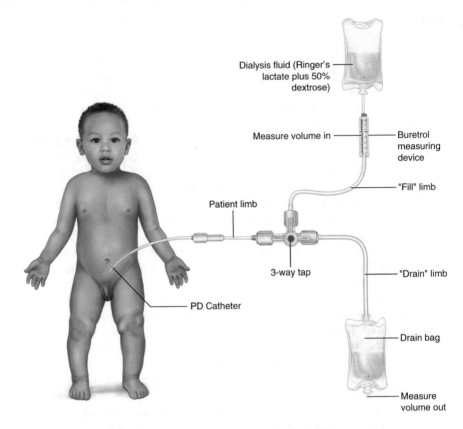

Dialysis fluid (Ringer's
lactate plus 50%
dextrose)

Measure volume in   Buretrol
                                                                     measuring
                                                                     device

                                                                     "Fill" limb

Patient limb

                                                                     "Drain" limb
                        3-way tap

PD Catheter   Drain bag

                                                                     Measure
                                                                     volume out

Fig. 35.1 Diagrammatic sketch of manual PD set-up with makeshift three-way tap

On the 'drain' cycle, this same three-way tap should then permit the dialysis fluid to drain into a drain bag, with the drained fluid measured (Diagram of Manual PD Set-up – see Fig. 35.1).

5. Commercially prepared dialysis fluids manufactured in a sterile manner and containing dextrose as the osmotic agent as well as electrolytes are the ideal fluids to be used for acute PD. If these dialysis fluids are not available, alternative fluids that could be used as 'home-made solutions' include Ringers lactate with added 50% dextrose (the addition of 20 ml of 50% dextrose results in a 1% glucose concentration – e.g. a 1.5% dextrose dialysis solution would require 30 ml 50% dextrose added to 1 l Ringers lactate). Caution should be taken when preparing these solutions with additives so as not to contaminate the preparation.

6. The basic principles of acute PD remain the same, regardless of whether the patient is located in a high- or low-resource location:

- Sterile technique for PD catheter insertion.
- Intravenous antibiotics should be provided at the time of PD catheter insertion to decrease the risk of post-operative infection.

- Secure the PD catheter to prevent it from being dislodged.
- Sterile set-up for manual dialysis (even for infants in developed countries who are often too small for PD cycler machines).
- Start with low dialysate dextrose concentration (e.g. 1.36–1.5% depending on the manufacturers) with close monitoring of fluid removal (e.g. ultrafiltration) and potential need for modification of dextrose concentration based upon the patient's overall fluid balance.
- Consider addition of heparin 500–1,000 u per 1,000 ml of PD fluid when initiating dialysis to reduce the likelihood of blood clots and fibrin obstructing the PD catheter.
- Attempt to limit the addition of additives to the PD fluid bags as this can increase the risk of infection; antibiotics such as cefotaxime/vancomycin or amikacin/vancomycin can be added when evidence of acute PD infection arises, with the specific agents chosen initially being broad spectrum and based on the antibiotic susceptibilities in the centre/region.
- In cases where PD needs to be initiated immediately, such as in the setting of AKI, start with small volumes of PD fluid, 10–20 ml/kg fill volume, to minimize the risk of dialysate leakage through the PD catheter insertion site, and increase as tolerated.
- Use the same fill, dwell and drain principles whether conducting manual or automated PD.

Clinical Pearls

1. Acute PD is a safe and effective treatment for acute kidney injury in children.
2. Whereas the "gold standard" is to have a PD catheter inserted by a surgeon in a dialysis facility, improvised techniques with 'make-shift' catheters and 'home-made' fluids can be used effectively in resource-limited locations.
3. The basic principles of peritoneal dialysis should be followed when conducting acute PD as treatment for AKI.

A new website on Open Pediatrics has a peritoneal dialysis simulator which has a training module consisting of a knowledge guide, tactics and case studies which are available and free of charge via the website. (https://www.openpediatrics.org).

References

1. Dellinger RP. The surviving sepsis campaign: where have we been and where are we going? Cleve Clin J Med. 2015;82(4):237–44.
2. Maitland K, Kiguli S, Opoka RO, Engoru C, Olupot-Olupot P, Akech SO, Nyeko R, Mtove G, Reyburn H, Lang T, Brent B, Evans JA, Tibenderana JK, Crawley J, Russell EC, Levin M,

Babiker AG, Gibb DM, FEAST Trial Group. Mortality after fluid bolus in African children with severe infection. N Engl J Med. 2011;364(26):2483–95.

3. Duke T. Elizabeth Mason WHO guidelines on fluid resuscitation in children with shock. Lancet. 2014;383(9915):411–2.

4. Axelrod DM, Anglemyer AT, Sherman-Levine SF, Zhu A, Grimm PC, Roth SJ, Sutherland SM. Initial experience using aminophylline to improve renal dysfunction in the pediatric cardiovascular ICU. Pediatr Crit Care Med. 2014;15(1):21–7.

5. Chadha V, Warady BA, Blowey DL, Simckes AM. Alon US.; Tenckhoff catheters prove superior to cook catheters in pediatric acute peritoneal dialysis. Am J Kidney Dis. 2000;35(6):1111–6.

6. Cullis B, Abdelraheem M, Abrahams G, Balbi A, Cruz DN, Frishberg Y, Koch V, McCulloch M, Numanoglu A, Nourse P, Pecoits-Filho R, Ponce D, Warady B, Yeates K, Finkelstein FO. Peritoneal dialysis for acute kidney injury. Perit Dial Int. 2014;34(5):494–517.

7. Auron A, Warady BA, Simon S, Blowey DL, Srivastava T, Musharaf G, Alon US. Use of the multipurpose drainage catheter for the provision of acute peritoneal dialysis in infants and children. Am J Kidney Dis. 2007;49(5):650–5.

Additional Resources

Callegari J, Antwi S, Wystrychowski G, Zukowska-Szczechowska E, Levin NW, Carter M. Peritoneal dialysis as a mode of treatment for acute kidney injury in sub-Saharan Africa. Blood Purif. 2013;36(3–4):226–30.

Esezobor CI, Ladapo TA, Lesi FE. Peritoneal dialysis for children with acute kidney injury in Lagos, Nigeria: experience with adaptations. Perit Dial Int. 2014;34(5):534–8.

Smoyer WE, Finkelstein FO, McCulloch M, Carter M, Brusselmans A, Feehally J. Saving Young Lives: provision of acute dialysis in low-resource settings. Lancet. 2015;386(10008):2056.

Smoyer WE, Finkelstein FO, McCulloch MI, Carter M, Brusselmans A, Feehally J. "Saving Young Lives" with acute kidney injury: the challenge of acute dialysis in low-resource settings. Kidney Int. 2016;89(2):254–6.

Chapter 36
Continuous Renal Replacement Therapy (CRRT) and Acute Kidney Injury (AKI)

Jordan M. Symons

Case Presentation

A 14-year-old girl with a history of recurrent high-risk acute lymphocytic leukemia undergoes hematopoietic stem cell transplant. Ten days after her conditioning regimen and transplant infusion, she develops watery diarrhea and fever; the patient is made NPO and broad-spectrum antibiotics are started. Later that evening she has a significant clinical change with abdominal pain and distension, followed by profound hypotension; she is transferred to the intensive care unit where she requires fluid resuscitation. Abdominal radiograph shows free air in the abdomen; CT scan shows edema and inflammation around the cecum. She is taken urgently to the operating room for cecostomy and drainage, after which she has further complications of hypotension requiring initiation of vasoactive infusions to support blood pressure; she is now on mechanical ventilation. Over the next 24 h, the patient receives numerous boluses of isotonic crystalloid and escalation of her vasoactive infusions to address hypotension; fluid input over this period is approximately 10 l. Her weight, initially 38 kg, is now 44 kg; serum creatinine, previously 0.7 mg/dL, has now climbed to 2.1 mg/dL. Urine output is now negligible. The critical care team contacts you for recommendations regarding this patient's acute kidney injury and options for renal replacement therapy.

After full evaluation of the patient, you recommend initiation of CRRT. The critical care team obtains vascular access with a 10 French double-lumen uncuffed hemodialysis catheter placed in the femoral position. Your initial prescription for CRRT is as follows:

- Polysulfone hemofilter with surface area of 1.1 m^2

J.M. Symons (✉)
Department of Pediatrics, University of Washington School of Medicine, Seattle, WA, USA

Division of Nephrology, Seattle Children's Hospital, Seattle, WA, USA
e-mail: jordan.symons@seattlechildrens.org

© Springer International Publishing AG 2017
B.A. Warady et al. (eds.), *Pediatric Dialysis Case Studies*,
DOI 10.1007/978-3-319-55147-0_36

- Standard tubing set; total extracorporeal volume (hemofilter and tubing) 165 ml
- Saline prime of extracorporeal circuit
- Blood flow rate of 150 ml/min
- Modality: continuous venovenous hemodiafiltration (CVVHDF)

  - Dialysate flow rate of 1,000 ml/h
  - Replacement fluid flow rate of 1,000 ml/h

- Citrate anticoagulation
- Ultrafiltration plan: even fluid balance to start

The patient is connected to the CRRT circuit and shows a mild drop in blood pressure at initiation which stabilizes with a small increase in the vasoactive infusions. During the initial 12 h of CRRT, the patient tolerates ultrafiltration of all infused volumes, maintaining a "net zero" fluid balance; the vasoactive infusions have been weaned. Blood testing reveals improved biochemical balance. In discussion with the critical care team, you develop a plan to increase the ultrafiltration rate to remove 20–30 ml/h with a goal to achieve a net fluid loss of 500 ml over the next 24 h.

Clinical Questions

1. Why would one choose CRRT in the setting of AKI?
2. What are the indications to initiate CRRT for AKI?
3. What are the clinical goals for CRRT when treating a patient with AKI?
4. How does one assure successful therapy with CRRT? What are the potential complications?
5. What criteria can one use to determine if it is time to transition off of CRRT?

Diagnostic Discussion

1. CRRT has become a well-established method of renal replacement therapy for pediatric patients. Literature describes pediatric-specific protocols and outcome data indicating usefulness of CRRT in treating critically ill children with AKI [1–4]. Choosing CRRT may offer several advantages for the critically ill patient with AKI:

   - *Slower, longer therapy.* Patients with AKI in the setting of critical illness often have concerns for cardiovascular instability. Intermittent hemodialysis provides renal replacement therapy over a relatively short period of time (e.g., 3–4 h/session); in a patient with hypotension receiving vasoactive infusions to support blood pressure, it may be challenging to achieve ultrafiltration goals within that session length. Short, rapid ultrafiltration may deplete the vascular compartment volume more quickly than it can be replaced by interstitial fluid, worsening hypotension; this effect may be exacerbated in critically ill patients with vascular leak syndromes. In contrast, CRRT sessions can extend over days, allowing slow, steady fluid removal which may be better tolerated by the critically ill patient.

- *Continuous therapy.* Since CRRT is provided continuously, fluid and metabolic balance can be maintained. This may simplify patient management (nutrition, medication infusion, blood product delivery, etc.) by allowing the critical care team to deliver therapies without concern for timing around an intermittent hemodialysis session. Wide swings in volume status are avoided, limiting unacceptable variation in blood pressure (see above) or pulmonary compromise.

Disadvantages of CRRT include relative complexity and the need for specialized equipment and highly trained staff, technical challenges associated with adapting CRRT devices designed for adults to use with pediatric patients, and limitations to patient mobility when undergoing continuous extracorporeal perfusion. Vascular access, a requirement for CRRT, may be difficult to achieve in some pediatric patients.

CRRT is well suited to address AKI in an ICU patient. Once vascular access is established, most CRRT devices permit initiation of therapy promptly. Through appropriate adjustment of the prescription, CRRT can address the metabolic and volume-related complications of AKI in a manner that may be better tolerated by the patient in the ICU (see above). AKI is often self-limited; CRRT can be discontinued with ease when the patient no longer requires the therapy (see below). In contrast, some patients with AKI in the setting of multi-organ dysfunction syndrome may have sustained AKI over many weeks; CRRT can provide appropriate metabolic and volume control over extended periods if necessary. CRRT can also be combined with other extracorporeal therapies that may be necessary for the care of the critically ill patient (e.g., ECMO, apheresis).

2. Renal replacement therapy would be indicated in a patient with AKI who demonstrates complications such as volume overload or metabolic imbalance that cannot be easily corrected or managed without compromising other aspects of care (e.g., limiting fluid input that also limits ability to provide nutrition) [5]. One may also consider initiating renal replacement in AKI to prevent fluid or metabolic imbalance from developing. Assessment of the patient should include careful history with attention to mechanisms of renal injury (nephrotoxin exposure, hypoperfusion, multi-organ dysfunction, etc.), depth of AKI (urine output, rapidity of metabolic changes secondary to renal dysfunction), daily therapeutic requirements (intravenous fluids, blood products, medications, etc.), and overall clinical status (hypotension, possible sepsis, mechanical ventilation, ECMO). Physical exam should concentrate on volume status, blood pressure, and level of cardiopulmonary compromise. Multidisciplinary coordination and discussion with all team members in the ICU (critical care physicians, nephrologists, consulting physicians, nurses, nutritionists, pharmacists) are necessary. This careful review will permit the clinician to make an assessment of the need for

renal replacement, the urgency of that need, and whether CRRT represents the best choice [4].

3. In the setting of AKI, the major clinical goals for the CRRT procedure are to regain and maintain fluid and metabolic balance, to permit other required treatments and therapies to occur, and to limit complications while awaiting recovery of renal function.

4. Having chosen to begin CRRT, one must develop a plan for the various components of the CRRT prescription:

- *CRRT device*. Several different devices designed specifically for CRRT are available around the world. A variation of CRRT, sometimes called slow low-efficiency dialysis (SLED), can be delivered with a standard hemodialysis machine modified for extended session length. The majority of devices have been developed for adult patients with varying levels of adaptation to permit use in pediatrics; recently, in selected locations, devices designed specifically for infants have undergone testing and are now becoming available [6]. When developing a CRRT program, one must carefully review the advantages and limitations of the available devices and consider the clinical needs of the program going forward, since CRRT machines require a significant investment of funds and programmatic support.

- *Hemofilter and tubing*. "Open" CRRT systems may permit a program to purchase hemofilters and tubing sets from other manufacturers; "closed" systems will use proprietary hemofilter and tubing sets designed specifically for a given device. When choosing for an individual patient, the clinician must consider the extracorporeal volume and whether this will be well tolerated by the patient; large volumes may require adjustments to the priming orders (see below). Variation in hemofilter surface area may have an impact on maximum ultrafiltration rates. Hemofilters can be made with various membrane materials; some materials are proposed to offer better outcomes in the setting of sepsis, but this remains controversial. No membrane material has proven superior for the overall treatment of AKI. Membrane composition has been implicated as a risk for a hypotensive reaction at initiation of CRRT (see below); this should be considered when choosing hemofilters for individual patients and for the program as a whole.

- *Priming of circuit*. Initial priming of the CRRT circuit is most often done with normal saline. This prime is commonly left in the circuit and delivered to the patient at therapy initiation when the patient's blood is perfused out into the circuit. Under varying clinical circumstances, the saline prime may be replaced with other fluids. The most common alternative in pediatrics is a blood prime, where a mix of packed red blood cells and either saline or 5% albumin, blended to a near-physiological hematocrit, replaces the pure saline prime at initiation. A blood prime may be considered when the patient has profound anemia at the time of initiation or if perfusion of the extracorporeal circuit may be expected to cause significant hypotension and cardiovascular collapse (e.g., when the extracorporeal volume is greater than 10% of the patient's blood volume).

- *Blood pump rate.* Several different equations and standards, based on patient size or weight, have been proposed to determine the blood pump rate for pediatric CRRT. Pragmatically, blood pump rate is often limited by the adequacy of the vascular access and the parameters available for the given CRRT device. As lower blood pump rate may increase the likelihood of circuit clotting and may limit clearance and ultrafiltration efficiency; choosing the fastest blood flow rate that can be easily and consistently delivered by the vascular access may be most reasonable.

- *Modality.* Controversy persists regarding the relative merits of convection, diffusion, or combination therapies for CRRT. No data show one modality to be superior when treating patients with AKI.

- *Infused fluids.* For CRRT devices that require pre-mixed solutions, commercially available products have largely replaced locally prepared solutions, reducing the burden in hospital pharmacies while providing quality control. Numerous products with varying formulations to address different clinical situations are available. Pediatric literature makes recommendations for the rate of infused fluids, balancing goals for effective clearance of molecular wastes with limitation on removal of beneficial substances; a commonly used formula to calculate delivered fluids for CRRT is 2,000–3,000 ml/h/1.73 m². There are no data to suggest the best rate in the setting of AKI. Fluid delivery may be divided between dialysate and replacement based on modality preference (see above). For programs using adapted hemodialysis machines to provide SLED or similar therapies, dialysate is prepared online from concentrates and dialysis water by the proportioning system; the choice for rate may be limited by the device.

- *Anticoagulation.* Delivery of CRRT requires sufficient anticoagulation of the circuit to permit ongoing extracorporeal perfusion without clotting. Critically ill patients with AKI may demonstrate coagulopathy that could conceivably permit CRRT without anticoagulation. Literature and experience suggest that this approach may not be successful; circuit life is often limited when no anticoagulation is used. The most commonly used agents for anticoagulation in CRRT are systemic heparin and regional citrate. Heparin has the advantage of relative simplicity and extensive experience, but carries risks of hemorrhage since the patient is also anticoagulated with systemic delivery of heparin. In regional citrate anticoagulation, citrate is infused into the arterial limb of the CRRT circuit, chelating calcium and thus preventing coagulation; the patient must receive a continuous infusion of calcium to maintain normocalcemia. Other options for CRRT anticoagulation also exist but are less commonly used. Further details regarding anticoagulation for CRRT are discussed in Chapter 38.

- *Fluid balance plan.* Many critically ill patients with AKI will have volume overload as part of their clinical picture. Literature and experience suggest that volume overload in this setting is associated with compromised cardiopulmonary status, leads to challenges in providing appropriate mechanical ventilator support, causes morbidity related to edema and total body water excess, and is correlated with mortality [5]. Addressing volume overload is therefore of paramount importance. Critically ill patients with AKI may, however have hypotension and vascular leak syndromes making ultrafiltration difficult. Large obligate daily fluid needs (parenteral nutrition, medications, blood products, etc.) add to the challenges. Initial ultrafiltration plans for critically ill patients initiating CRRT may, in turn, need to limit ultrafiltration rate to equal that of fluid delivery, keeping the patient at an "even" or "net zero" fluid balance. Such an approach will not improve the current level of volume overload but may limit exacerbation. At such time that vascular leak resolves and blood pressure stabilizes, the ultrafiltration rate may be increased with the goal of removing excess fluid and achieving euvolemia. Appropriate coordination with ICU teams is necessary to determine daily goals, adjusting based on the clinical condition of the patient.

- *Mitigation of complications.* Hypotension at initiation of CRRT is a common occurrence. Patients with hypotension may need vasoactive drugs to support blood pressure at initiation. Hypocalcemia should be addressed prior to initiation; this is especially true for those patients who will undergo blood priming or anticoagulation with citrate, as these interventions may further drop the patient's ionized calcium. Membrane reactions can cause hypotension and/or respiratory compromise; this has been reported most often with a specific membrane (AN-69) in the setting of a blood prime and profound acidosis, thought to be related to the release of bradykinin. Several mitigation procedures have been described to address this bradykinin release syndrome including pretreatment of the blood prime (pharmacologically, by addition of sodium bicarbonate, 5% albumin and occasionally calcium chloride according to a center-specific protocol, or by dialyzing the blood prime with the CRRT device itself), saline prime at initiation with simultaneous blood transfusion, or general avoidance of the implicated membrane. Hypotension may occur with errors in ultrafiltration rates; modern CRRT devices have safety systems designed to prevent accidental ultrafiltration errors, but vigilance at the bedside remains important. Biochemical, nutritional, or pharmacological imbalances may occur as a side effect of CRRT; careful review of laboratory trends and coordination with pharmacy and nutrition staff are required.

5. Return of urinary output, as an indication of resolving AKI, is the most commonly observed clinical marker suggesting that CRRT may be successfully discontinued. Daily urine output must be of a sufficiently high volume to provide clearance and fluid balance. Some patients may have clinical improvement before AKI resolves, demonstrating ongoing oliguria after resolution of cardiorespiratory complications or sepsis syndrome. Such patients may be candidates for transition to intermittent hemodialysis, which may be advantageous to simplify the daily regimen, permit mobilization, and allow transfer from the ICU to the general ward. When considering transition to intermittent hemodialysis, one must consider whether the oliguric patient can tolerate accumulation of a day's

worth of fluid and then further tolerate rapid ultrafiltration of that same volume in a relatively short (e.g., 4-h) hemodialysis session. Reduction of daily fluid delivery may be a necessary requirement for successful transition to intermittent hemodialysis.

Clinical Pearls

1. CRRT is a viable option to address AKI in pediatrics. There is established literature with published guidelines, extensive clinical experience, and evidence for successful outcomes.
2. CRRT is complex and requires special equipment and expertise. Advanced planning is necessary to develop a CRRT program, and careful coordination is needed between multiple disciplines for every case. Technical complexity of CRRT raises the risks for complications.
3. Advantages of CRRT over intermittent hemodialysis include its continuous nature, which permits steady maintenance of fluid and biochemical balance. Patients may receive their necessary daily fluids, medications, and nutrition with fewer biochemical or fluid shifts. The slow, steady nature of CRRT may be better tolerated by critically ill patients.
4. Obtaining vascular access and appropriate anticoagulation can be challenging aspects of CRRT, especially in smaller pediatric patients.
5. CRRT technology continues to advance, with dedicated devices that have greater capabilities to deliver more accurate and safer therapy. Most devices to date were designed for use with adult patients and have been adapted for pediatric use; newer devices designed specifically for small pediatric patients are now becoming available.
6. Close monitoring of fluid and biochemical balance is necessary when providing CRRT; one should suspect a technical error with sudden, unexpected changes and promptly evaluate.

References

1. Symons JM, Chua AN, Somers MJ, et al. Demographic characteristics of pediatric continuous renal replacement therapy: a report of the prospective pediatric continuous renal replacement therapy registry. Clin J Am Soc Nephrol CJASN. 2007;2(4):732–8.
2. Hayes LW, Oster RA, Tofil NM, Tolwani AJ. Outcomes of critically ill children requiring continuous renal replacement therapy. J Crit Care. 2009;24(3):394–400.
3. Askenazi DJ, Goldstein SL, Koralkar R, et al. Continuous renal replacement therapy for children <10 kg: a report from the prospective pediatric continuous renal replacement therapy registry. J Pediatr. 2013;162(3):587–92e3.
4. Modem V, Thompson M, Gollhofer D, et al. Timing of continuous renal replacement therapy and mortality in critically ill children. Crit Care Med. 2014;42(4):943–53.

5. Sutherland SM, Zappitelli M, Alexander SR, et al. Fluid overload and mortality in children receiving continuous renal replacement therapy: the prospective pediatric continuous renal replacement therapy registry. Am J Kidney Dis. 2010;55(2):316–25.
6. Ronco C, Garzotto F, Brendolan A, et al. Continuous renal replacement therapy in neonates and small infants: development and first-in-human use of a miniaturised machine (CARPEDIEM). Lancet. 2014;383(9931):1807–13.

Chapter 37
Continuous Renal Replacement Therapy (CRRT) for a Neonate

David J. Askenazi

Case Presentation

The patient was a male infant born after an uncomplicated labor and delivery to a 21-year-old G1P1, otherwise healthy mother at 31 weeks gestational age: birthweight was 1.4 kg. The infant did well for the first 49 days of life, on room air and feeding and growing normally. On day of life 50, he became acutely ill, developing severe abdominal distension with signs of sepsis, and was found to have a volvulus with intestinal perforation. He had emergent abdominal surgery with bowel resection and placement of a temporary colostomy. He continued to show signs of sepsis (although blood cultures remained negative) requiring continued broad-spectrum antibiotic coverage with ceftriaxone, gentamicin, and flagyl. He had cardiac dysfunction requiring cardiac support, respiratory dysfunction requiring ventilator support, and nutritional dysfunction requiring parenteral nutritional support. Over the coming days, his cardiorespiratory support escalated, and he received numerous blood products. During this time, he made 0.9–2.0 cc/kg/h of urine; yet due to his septic condition and third spacing of fluids, he progressively gained weight. His blood urea nitrogen (BUN) and serum creatinine increased over the ensuing days as shown in Table 37.1.

On day 55, Pediatric Nephrology was consulted to assist in the care of this patient. On examination the infant had BP 60/30 mmHg, HR 140/min on dopamine 5 mcg/kg/min and he was on conventional ventilation with a PEEP of 16 and FiO_2 at 85%. The infant had significant scalp, face, neck, chest, leg, feet, and hand edema. His abdomen was distended with diminished bowel sounds and a fluid wave. Review of electrolytes showed slowly progressive mild hyponatremia (serum Na:130 mmol/L), normokalemia, normal ionized calcium, elevated serum phosphorous at 7.1 mg/dL, uric acid normal, and serum albumin 1.9 g/dL. Several considerations

D.J. Askenazi, MD (✉)
Department of Pediatrics, University of Alabama at Birmingham, Children's Hospital of Alabama, Birmingham, AL, USA
e-mail: daskenazi@peds.uab.edu

© Springer International Publishing AG 2017   279
B.A. Warady et al. (eds.), *Pediatric Dialysis Case Studies*,
DOI 10.1007/978-3-319-55147-0_37

Table 37.1 Blood urea nitrogen (BUN) and serum creatinine

Day of life	1	49	50	51	52	53	54	55	56
Weight (kg)	1.4	3.0	3.5	4.1	4.5	4.7	4.9	5.1	5.1
BUN (mg/dL)	20	20	40	60	75	85	90	95	80
Cr (mg/dL)	1.0 mg/dl	0.3	0.4	0.5	0.6	0.6	0.6	0.6	0.5
Intake	140 cc	280	675	800	600	400	380	440	240
Urine output	50 cc	120	75	100	100	100	80	140	140

were raised: Is it time for dialysis? If so, what form of dialysis? If not, what are the indications to proceed to dialysis? What could help maximize medical management? Is he fluid overloaded, and if so, by how much?

Clinical Questions

1. Does this infant have acute kidney injury (AKI)?
2. Is renal support therapy indicated at this time? If not, what would you do instead?
3. Is renal support therapy now indicated? If so, what type would you choose?
4. Would you us a blood or saline prime? What are the risks associated with each? How can you make the blood prime more physiolgic?
5. What vascular access would you choose? In what location? Using what CRRT prescription?

Diagnostic Discussion

1. Previously referred to as acute renal failure, acute kidney injury (AKI) is characterized by a sudden impairment in kidney function, which results in retention of nitrogenous waste products (e.g., urea) and altered regulation of extracellular fluid volume, electrolytes, and acid-base homeostasis. The term "acute kidney injury" has replaced "acute renal failure" by most critical care and nephrology societies primarily to highlight the importance of recognition of this process at the time of "injury" as opposed to waiting until "failure" has occurred. Despite its limitations, serum creatinine (SCr) is the most commonly used measure to evaluate glomerular filtration in the clinical setting of AKI.

   Prior to 2009, the most common SCr cutpoint used to define neonatal AKI was set at an arbitrary cutoff of 1.5 mg/dL or greater, independent of day of life and regardless of the rate of urine output. In 2009, neonatal studies began to report AKI using a categorical staged definition similar to that used in pediatrics and adults, whereby an increase in SCr of 0.3 mg/dl or a 50% increase from baseline was used to define AKI. These studies suggest that AKI is common in critically ill neonates and that AKI is associated with mortality. At an NIH work-

Table 37.2 Neonatal acute kidney injury KDIGO classification

Stage	SCr	Urine output
0	No change in SCr *or* rise <0.3 mg/dL	≥0.5 ml/kg/h
1	SCr rise ≥ 0.3 mg/dl within 48 h *or* SCr rise ≥ 1.5–1.9 × reference SCr[a] within 7 days	<0.5 ml/kg/h for 6–12 h
2	SCr rise ≥ 2–2.9 × reference SCr[a]	<0.5 ml/kg/h for ≥12 h
3	SCr rise ≥ 3 × reference SCr[a] *or* SCr ≥ 2.5 mg/dl[b] *or* receipt of dialysis	<0.3 ml/kg/h for ≥24 h *or* anuria for ≥12 h

Reproduced with permission from Selewski DT, Charlton JR, Jetton JG, Guillet R, Mhanna MJ, Askenazi DJ, et al. Neonatal Acute Kidney Injury. *Pediatrics*. 2015;136(2):e463–73. Copyright © 2015 by the AAP
Differences between the proposed neonatal AKI definition and KDIGO include:
[a]Reference SCr will be defined as the lowest previous SCr value
[b]SCr value of 2.5 mg/dl represents GFR less than 10 ml/min/1.73 m^2

shop on neonatal AKI, experts agreed that a neonatal AKI definition that paralleled those currently used in adult and pediatric cohorts was a valid way to categorize neonatal AKI (Table 37.2). Several modifications were made to accommodate neonatal renal physiology related issues:

- Because SCr normally declines over the first week of life, each SCr is compared to the lowest previous value.
- As SCr of 2.5 mg/dl represents a glomerular filtration rate <10 ml/min/1.73 m^2 in neonates, this cutoff is used to define Stage 3 AKI (as opposed to 4.0 mg/dl in adults).

The group also agreed that studies to validate and improve how we define neonatal AKI (perhaps adding cystatin C) and urine biomarker-based AKI definitions are greatly needed.

The infant in this case met the AKI definition by creatinine criteria, but just barely. His primary problem was fluid overload. The degree of fluid overload is not a part of the AKI definition; yet, fluid overload is the most critical issue in optimizing medical management of the neonate and is the most common reason for initiation of renal support therapy in pediatric patients.

2. On day 55, the infant was 70% fluid overloaded (current weight – dry weight/ dry weight = 5.1–3.0 kg/3.0 kg = 0.7). Because he was making some urine and the low serum albumin suggested there was low oncotic pressure, we elected to maximize medical management by recommending the following:

   1. Insert bladder catheter to assure proper drainage.
   2. Increase blood pressure support to goals of at least SBP 80 mmHg and DBP 60 mmHg.
   3. Decrease fluids to insensible rate of 5 cc/h.
   4. Give 25% albumin 1 g/kg IV over 4 h.
   5. Give 2 mg/kg Lasix IV after albumin infusion once.
   6. Avoid additional nephrotoxic medications, if possible.

7. Consider changing from gentamicin to an antibiotic that is not nephrotoxic. If gentamicin is used, levels should be followed and the gentamicin level should be <2.0 before giving any additional doses.

8. Surgical consult for possible peritoneal dialysis catheter placement vs. vascular access for hemodialysis or CRRT.

In addition to these recommendations, we began to speak to the family, surgery team, and neonatologist about how we would assess a response to therapy and what targets we would use to determine when it was time for additional renal support beyond medical management.

The following day, although he made a bit more urine (see Table 37.1, day 55), his respiratory function deteriorated, and his ventilator settings were progressively increased to FiO2 of 100% and PEEP of 16. His BUN improved slightly; his creatinine remained the same.

3. After deliberation, the NICU, surgery, and nephrology teams and the family agreed that because he did not have a significant increase in UOP despite aggressive diuretic therapy and due to his worsening respiratory failure, the potential risks of waiting for him to diurese on his own outweighed the potential risks that come with renal support therapy. We chose to dialyze him using CRRT as he had abdominal drains, a colostomy, and recent surgical exploration of his abdomen, all of which made peritoneal dialysis not only high risk, but technically challenging. Intermittent hemodialysis (IHD) was also rejected because he was too hemodynamically unstable to tolerate the aggressive fluid removal that is unavoidable with IHD when ultrafiltration is restricted to several hours of IHD each day. This is in contrast to the 24 h of slow, continuous fluid removal provided by CRRT. We estimated that his total blood volume was 70 ml/kg × 3.0 kg = 210 cc. The smallest CRRT circuit we had available was a circuit of 100 ml; thus, the CRRT extracorporeal volume (ECV) for this patient on this circuit would be 100 ml/210 ml = 48% of estimated blood volume.

4. The risk to perform a saline prime for this infant is substantial as almost 50% of his blood volume would need to be removed to prime the CRRT machine (for a 70 kg adult, it would be like removing approximately 2.5 Liters of blood to prime the machine). We elected to prime the circuit with pRBCs according to our hospital protocol, which states that children with an extracorporeal circuit volume >10% of estimated blood volume should have the circuit primed with pRBCs. It is important to consider the risk of the blood priming procedure (pRBCs from the blood bank can have a HCT >70%, pH < 7.0 and an ionized calcium <0.3, as citrate is used to bind calcium in blood products to prevent clotting). There are several ways to make the blood prime more physiologic during the blood prime procedure. Our protocol calls for blood to be given 1:1 with sodium bicarbonate to dilute and make the blood pH more physiologic. In addition, we give calcium chloride 1 mL/kg of 100 mEq/mL $CaCl_2$ – at the time of the blood prime to the baby to counteract the possible effects of hypocalcemic blood.

Other centers have also found good results with other blood prime procedures, but all essentially address the potential issues of low pH, high HCT, and low ionized Ca. The blood prime can be made more physiologic by "normalizing" it with the addition of 5% albumin, $CaCl_2$, sodium bicarbonate, and heparin (to avoid clotting the pRBCs when $CaCl_2$ is added) prior to infusing it to the circuit (similar to what is done with extracorporeal membrane oxygenation). Some centers will prime the circuit and dialyze the blood in the CRRT system for a given period of time to make it more physiologic prior to the start of CRRT.

It is important to note that there are no coagulation factors or platelets in pRBCs. Thus, a blood prime will dilute out the other components in the blood. One should expect a drop in platelet count and coagulation factors after blood prime by any method. Careful attention is needed for those patients who require serial blood primes in a short time period and in those who are already at risk for bleeding.

Fortunately, new machines and filters which have much smaller extracorporeal volumes have been adapted/developed for newborns. These machines promise to decrease the challenges and complication of initiating CRRT in small children, which will change the risk/benefit balance such that earlier support for neonates who could benefit from renal support therapy can be instituted.

5. (a) Access: The surgeons placed a 7F, 10 cm double lumen catheter in the right internal jugular vein.
   (b) Modality: We chose to run CRRT as CVVHDF (continuous veno-venous hemodiafiltration) as per our hospital protocol.
   (c) Clearance, fluids, and rates: We ran dialysis plus replacement fluids at 2,000 mL/1.73 m^2/h, which approximates 30 mL/kg/h body weight for an adult. We use identical fluids for dialysis and replacement fluids (Prismasol 2 K/3.5 Ca with 1 meq KCl/L and 1 meq KPhos/liter and 0.5 meq/L MgCl).
   (d) Anticoagulation: We use heparin anticoagulation at our center. We give 20 units/kg bolus of heparin and start a heparin infusion at 20 units/kg/h and titrate the heparin for a goal of PTT = 50–70 s, measured in the circuit at the post-filter port of the CRRT machine. (For a discussion of heparin vs. citrate anticoagulation of CRRT circuits, see Chap. 38.)
   (e) Net ultrafiltration rates: We set the net ultrafiltration hourly rate as follows: every hour we calculate the amount of fluid in, subtract the amount of fluid out in urine and take this balance off in addition to taking off 10 cc/h extra (with a goal to remove around 240 cc/day =8% of dry weight per day).

Epilogue

During the initiation of therapy, our patient's blood pressure decreased from 90/50 mmHg to around 70/30 mmHg, and HR increased from 140/min to 160/min. He responded to an increase in dopamine from 15 to 20 units/kg/h. He was dialyzed at the above settings for 7 days, although we adjusted the fluid removal rate daily or twice daily with the goal to remove fluid fast enough to wean the ventilator support, but slow enough to avoid hypotension and oliguria. We were able to steadily remove fluid such that 6 days after starting CRRT, his weight had decreased from 5.1 to 3.8 kg. We were able to steadily wean the settings on his ventilator, and he was successfully extubated. His urine output remained intact during the week of CRRT. He recovered from his surgical procedures over the coming weeks. Following hospital discharge, he was seen one month after hospitalization in the AKI follow-up clinic and intermittently for the first 2 years of life, where he continued to have acceptable renal function indices (serum creatinine = 0.4 mg/dl; normal electrolytes, normal blood pressure and normal urine protein).

Clinical Pearls

1. Early recognition of AKI in neonates requires careful attention to rising creatinine, changes in urine output, and fluid homeostasis.
2. Ideally, early consultation with nephrology can help maximize medical management (with the goal to maximize kidney perfusion, maintain adequate fluid/electrolyte homeostasis, assure adequate bladder drainage, avoid nephrotoxic medications) and may limit the morbidity and mortality ascribed to AKI.
3. The decision to embark on renal support therapy should not be based on the same principles that are used to start dialysis for ESRD. Just like blood pressure support, ventilator support and nutritional support are instituted when the demands of the child exceed the organ's ability to support the child, renal support should be instituted when the kidney is not doing its job appropriately and the child is being affected in a negative way. Fluid overload is the most common indication for RRT in children.

Bibliography

1. Askenazi D, Ingram D, White S, Cramer M, Borasino S, Coghill C, et al. Smaller circuits for smaller patients: improving renal support therapy with Aquadex. Pediatr Nephrol (Berlin, Germany). 2016;31(5):853–60.
2. Askenazi DJ, Koralkar R, Hundley HE, Montesanti A, Patil N, Ambalavanan N. Fluid overload and mortality are associated with acute kidney injury in sick near-term/term neonate. Pediatr Nephrol (Berlin, Germany). 2013;28(4):661–6.
3. Askenazi DJ, Goldstein SL, Koralkar R, Fortenberry J, Baum M, Hackbarth R, et al. Continuous renal replacement therapy for children </=10 kg: a report from the prospective pediatric continuous renal replacement therapy registry. J Pediatr. 2013;162(3):587–92.e3.
4. Bridges BC, Askenazi DJ, Smith J, Goldstein SL. Pediatric renal replacement therapy in the intensive care unit. Blood Purif. 2012;34(2):138–48.
5. Chaturvedi S, Ng KH, Mammen C. The path to chronic kidney disease following acute kidney injury: a neonatal perspective. Pediatr Nephrol (Berlin, Germany). 2017;32(2):227–41.
6. Coulthard MG, Crosier J, Griffiths C, Smith J, Drinnan M, Whitaker M, et al. Haemodialysing babies weighing <8 kg with the Newcastle infant dialysis and ultrafiltration system (Nidus):

comparison with peritoneal and conventional haemodialysis. Pediatr Nephrol (Berlin, Germany). 2014;29(10):1873–81.

7. Jetton JG, Askenazi DJ. Update on acute kidney injury in the neonate. Curr Opin Pediatr. 2012;24(2):191–6.

8. Lee ST, Cho H. Fluid overload and outcomes in neonates receiving continuous renal replacement therapy. Pediatr Nephrol (Berlin, Germany). 2016;31(11):2145–52.

9. Lorenzin A, Garzotto F, Alghisi A, Neri M, Galeano D, Aresu S, et al. CVVHD treatment with CARPEDIEM: small solute clearance at different blood and dialysate flows with three different surface area filter configurations. Pediatr Nephrol (Berlin, Germany). 2016;31(10):1659–65.

10. Nishimi S, Ishikawa K, Sasaki M, Furukawa H, Takada A, Chida S. Ability of a novel system for neonatal extracorporeal renal replacement therapy with an ultra-small volume circuit to remove solutes in vitro. Pediatr Nephrol (Berlin, Germany). 2016;31(3):493–500.

11. Piggott KD, Soni M, Decampli WM, Ramirez JA, Holbein D, Fakioglu H, et al. Acute kidney injury and fluid overload in neonates following surgery for congenital heart disease. World J Pediatr Congenit Heart Surg. 2015;6(3):401–6.

12. Selewski DT, Charlton JR, Jetton JG, Guillet R, Mhanna MJ, Askenazi DJ, et al. Neonatal acute kidney injury. Pediatrics. 2015;136(2):e463–73.

Chapter 38
Anticoagulation and Continuous Renal Replacement Therapy (CRRT)

Timothy E. Bunchman

Case Presentations

Case 1

A 7-year-old (23 kg) child develops multi-organ system failure due to sepsis. At the time of nephrology consultation, he is intubated on high ventilator settings (80% FIO2, PEEP of 12 mmHg), on norepinephrine and dopamine for vasopressor support (BP of 84/37 mmHg) and has evidence of disseminated intravascular coagulation on labs (PT 23, INR of 2.7, PTT of 59). He is oligoanuric with 12% fluid overload. Due to his tenuous blood pressure and need for solute and fluid clearance, CRRT is initiated.

Clinical Questions

1. What vascular access should be placed and where?
2. What are options for anticoagulation

   (a) Heparin
   (b) Citrate

3. If heparin is used, what protocol should be followed and how should it be monitored?
4. If citrate is used, what protocol should be followed and how should it be monitored?
5. What are the risks of heparin in this setting?
6. What are the risks of citrate in this setting?

T.E. Bunchman (✉)
Department of Pediatric Nephrology, Virginia Commonwealth University,
Richmond, Virginia, USA
e-mail: timothy.bunchman@vcuhealth.org

© Springer International Publishing AG 2017
B.A. Warady et al. (eds.), *Pediatric Dialysis Case Studies*,
DOI 10.1007/978-3-319-55147-0_38

Diagnostic Discussion

1. The proper choice of a vascular access must take into consideration the size of the access as well as optimal location for placement to maximize blood flow. Work by Hackbarth and colleagues has addressed this by looking at the database of the prospective pediatric CRRT (ppCRRT) registry [1]. In his work evaluating a cohort of greater than 300 children, he demonstrated that the optimal vascular access size in a child of this age and weight would be in the range of an 8–10 French double lumen catheter. Presently, there is no triple lumen catheter that would be available in this smaller French size. Companies such as Covidien, MedComp, and Arrow have accesses in this size in North America. Outside of North America, Vygon has accesses of this size. Optimal placement would be in the right internal jugular vein unless contraindicated based upon coagulopathy or ventilation management. Blood flow rates of 100 to 150 ml/minute can be easily obtained with this type of access and location. Whereas recirculation is a discussion in chronic hemodialysis, in CRRT due to its continuous nature, recirculation is not a concern. Access information can be found at www.pcrrt.com.

2. Style of practice as well as comfort will determine the type of anticoagulation. Historically, heparin had been utilized commonly in the 1990s and early 2000s. In 1989, Ward and Mehta published the first work on the use of citrate in adults who were treated with CRRT [2]. This protocol delivers a hypertonic sodium solution with the citrate, requiring a low sodium dialysate or replacement fluid to avoid sodium excess. In 2002, we published the first experience in pediatric CRRT with the use of a lower sodium containing citrate solution (ACD-A (Baxter)) [3]. The simplicity of this protocol has caught on making it a standard of practice at many institutions. Brophy and colleagues, using the ppCRRT database, published data in children showing similar CRRT circuit patency using heparin or citrate [4]. A recent study by Zaoall et al. in pediatric CRRT comparing citrate to heparin demonstrated superior circuit integrity and life in the citrate arm [5].

3. Heparin protocols are commonly based upon an initial bolus of heparin followed by a continuous infusion to titrate to either a PTT of twice normal or a bedside ACT (activated clotting time) of approximately 200 seconds [6]. Work by our group two decades ago demonstrated the efficacy of this approach. Protocols for heparin can be found at www.pcrrt.com.

4. Citrate works by binding calcium from the blood which, in turn, inhibits clotting. The best example of this is that blood bank blood comes in a liquid due to the fact that citrate is added to the bag of blood, lowering the ionized calcium (Ica) to an average of 0.2 mmol/l (normal is 1.1–1.3 mmol/l). Protocols exist that are based on two components. First, the citrate solution (commonly ACD-A) is infused post patient but pre-CRRT filter at a rate linked to the blood flow rate. Then an Ica is measured post-CRRT filter with a target to be approximately 1/3 physiologic or a level between 0.25 and 0.5 mmol/l. The ACD-A infusion is adjusted up if the circuit Ica is greater than 0.5 mmol/l or lowered if it is less than 0.25 mmol/l. The second component is a calcium (chloride or gluconate) infusion back to the patient, preferably independent of the CRRT circuit in a central

line to target the patient to a normal Ica of 1.2–1.3 mmol/l. If the patient has an Ica less than 1.1 mmol/l, the calcium infusion is adjusted upward; if it is greater than 1.3 mmol/l, it is adjusted downward. The sieving coefficient (clearance) of citrate is identical (equal to 1) using either convection (CVVH) or diffusion (CVVHD) making this simple for either approach [7]. A typical protocol would be a dialysate or replacement rate of 2,000–2,500 ml/h/1.73 m², a BFR of 100 ml/min, an ACD-A infusion to begin at 1.5× the BFR on an IV pump at 150 ml/h (not per minute), and the calcium infusion initiated at 0.4× the ACD-A rate or in this case around 60 ml/h (not per minute). CaCl 8 g or Ca gluconate 23.5 g can be mixed in 1 liter of normal saline for this protocol. Adjustment of the Ica of the circuit and the patient would be done hourly for a few hours until steady state is achieved and then measured, and if needed, adjusted on a q4–6 h time interval. Protocols for ACD-A citrate can be found at www.pcrrt.com.

5. The risks associated with the use of heparin are that of bleeding and rarely heparin-induced thrombocytopenia (HIT). As opposed to citrate, with heparin both the circuit and the patient will undergo anticoagulation. In turn, attention to the infusion rate coupled with the target PTT or ACT will allow for minimal risk to the child. HIT is a rare event in children, but is associated with an acute drop in the platelet count that may predispose to excessive bleeding or in some unusual cases cause a rebound hypercoagulable state with an increased risk of clotting.

6. Citrate side effects are common, but not life threatening. The most common side effect is that of a metabolic alkalosis that can occur due to metabolism of the citrate to bicarbonate by the liver. The metabolic alkalosis may be exaggerated with the use of high bicarbonate containing dialysate or replacement solutions and other sources of alkali (e.g., TPN acetate) or other sources of citrate (blood products). In the face of a metabolic alkalosis, one can lower the bicarbonate in the dialysate or replacement solution. Another option is to add normal saline (pH of 5.4) as a separate infusion to the patient and filter off the infused volume with CRRT. Normal saline can also be given as the replacement fluid (in a CVVHD mode) or as dialysate fluid (in a CVVH mode) to add back acid to offset the alkalosis. The other side effect is a term that is coined "citrate lock" which occurs when the total calcium from the chemistry lab is elevated in the face of a normal simultaneously drawn Ica of the patient. An example of this is a patient Ica of 1.25 mmol/l and a total calcium from the chemistry lab of 14 mg/dl (with a normal albumin). This "gap" is calcium bound to citrate giving the false appearance of hypercalcemia. This is the result of excessive citrate accumulating in the patient. One treats this by dropping the citrate infusion rate or by increasing the dialysate or replacement rate to increase citrate clearance.

Case 2

A young teen had chronic liver failure due to a congenital etiology. At the time of a viral illness, he developed vomiting and dehydration. As he was volume reconstituted, he showed evidence of deterioration of liver function (acute on chronic liver failure) with evidence of acute kidney injury (AKI) and progressive oliguria. Further investigation demonstrated an elevated ammonia (>200 mic mol/L) as well as a deterioration of his coagulation status with a PT of 47, PTT of 93, and an INR of 4.7. Due to a progressive encephalopathy as a result of his fulminant hepatic failure (FHF), he was intubated for airway protection, and mannitol was administered. Lactulose was begun to lower the ammonia, and workup for causes of deterioration of liver function and discussions of liver transplantation were begun. Due to the need for ammonia clearance, treatment of fluid overload, as well as overall solute clearance, high-volume CRRT was begun.

Clinical Questions

1. What vascular access should be in place and where?
2. What are options for anticoagulation?

   (a) Heparin vs citrate vs prostacyclin

3. If heparin is used, what protocol should be followed and how should it be monitored?
4. If citrate is used, what protocol should be followed and how should it be monitored?
5. If prostacyclin is used, what protocol should be followed and how should it be monitored?
6. What are the potential complications associated with the use of heparin in this setting?
7. What are the potential complications associated with the use of citrate in this setting?
8. What are the potential complications associated with the use of prostacyclin in this setting?

Diagnostic Discussion

Many of the questions in case 2 are redundant with case 1 so that they will not be repeated:

1. Redundant with case 1.
2. The temptation in FHF is to avoid anticoagulation due to the underlying coagulopathy. Whereas this may be effective initially, the use of fresh frozen plasma (FFP) to correct the coagulopathy may result in rebound clotting. Heparin and citrate can both be used in FHF but are fraught with unique risks (see sections below). Prostacyclin is an alternative for anticoagulation, especially in patients with liver disease [8]. Its mechanism is at the level of inducing platelet dysfunction. Little data is available regarding its use in the CRRT literature; a recent paper by Deep's group has demonstrated its use in liver failure. Protocols for prostacyclin are available at www.pcrrt.com

3. Heparin is relatively contraindicated in patients with FHF due to the already present coagulopathy. Despite that statement, low-dose heparin at a dose of 5 units/kg/h has been used effectively in this population with minimal impact upon the PTT or INR while maintaining circuit patency (personal experience). This needs to be used with great caution to avoid exacerbating the underlying risk of bleeding.
4. Citrate can be used in FHF, utilizing the same protocol that is used in non-FHF, with one exception. The dose of citrate is approximately 30–50% of the regular infusion rate due to citrate accumulation in liver failure. Citrate excess (citrate lock) is more commonly seen in this setting, not only due to the lack of metabolism, but also due to increased citrate exposure from blood products (packed red blood cells and FFP). If citrate lock occurs, a reduction in the citrate dose may be needed to avoid citrate excess.
5. Prostacyclin protocols for FHF can be found at www.pcrrt.com. A constant infusion ranging from 2 to 8 ng/kg/min can be infused post patient and prefilter for circuit anticoagulation. The way to monitor efficacy is by circuit life, for there is no strict monitoring similar to that of heparin or citrate. At times, the prostacyclin may need to be combined with low-dose heparin (5 units/kg/h) to improve circuit life. Future work by Akash Deep's group at King's College in London, UK, is in progress using this approach to anticoagulation (personal communication).
6. The use of heparin in the setting of FHF can be complicated by bleeding and over anticoagulation and mandates very careful monitoring to avoid the potential for lethal bleeding.
7. The use of citrate in the setting of FHF can be complicated by the development of a metabolic acidosis (citrate has a pH of 5.4) due to the lack of hepatic metabolism as well as citrate lock. Both of these affects are manageable and reversible with removal of the citrate. Additionally, as opposed to heparin and prostacyclin, citrate is dialyzed off easily; accordingly, if signs of complications arise, increasing the dialysis prescription will result in improved clearance.
8. The use of prostacyclin in the setting of FHF may result in excess bleeding (due to platelet dysfunction) as well as vasodilation. The vasodilatation may result in hypotension, flushing with headache, tachycardia, bradycardia, or ventilation mismatch with hypoxia. If this occurs, stop the drug and the effect will resolve quickly due to its short half-life. If needed for future anticoagulation, restarting the drug at a lower dose is recommended.

Clinical Pearls

1. Vascular access size and location will have a significant effect upon CRRT circuit life and therapy. The right IJ is the best location for placement.
2. Citrate anticoagulation can be performed with no systemic risk of bleeding. The development of metabolic alkalosis can be treated with normal saline that has a pH of 5.4.
3. Citrate lock or excess can be treated by increasing the clearance of citrate (sieving coefficient of 1) or by decreasing the citrate infusion rate.

4. Prostacyclin may be used in settings in which there is a severe risk of bleeding (with heparin) or citrate excess. Protocols suggest acceptable CRRT circuit life with no risk of bleeding or hypotension.

References

1. Hackbarth R, Bunchman TE, Chua AN, et al. The effect of vascular access location and size on circuit survival in pediatric continuous renal replacement therapy: a report from the PPCRRT registry. In J Artif Organs. 2007;30:1116–21.
2. Mehta RL, McDonald BR, Aguilar MM, Ward DM. Regional citrate anticoagulation for continuous arteriovenous hemodialysis in critically ill patients. Kidney Int. 1990;38(5):976–81.
3. Bunchman TE, Maxvold NJ, Barnett J, et al. Pediatric hemofiltration: Normocarb® dialysate solution with citrate anticoagulation. Pediatr Nephrol. 2002;17:150–4.
4. Brophy PD, Somers MJ, Baum MA, et al. Multi-centre evaluation of anticoagulation in patients receiving continuous renal replacement therapy (CRRT). Nephrol Dial Transplant. 2005;20:1416–21.
5. Zaoral T, Haldik M, Zapletalova J, et al. Circuit lifetime with citrate vs heparin in pediatric continuous venovenous hemodialysis. Pediatr Crit Care Med. 2016;17(9):e399–405.
6. Bunchman TE, Donckerwolcke RA. Continuous arterial-venous diahemofiltration and continuous veno-venous diahemofiltration in infants and children. Pediatr Nephrol. 1994;8:96–102.
7. Chadha V, Garg U, Warady BA, et al. Citrate clearance in children receiving continuous venovenous renal replacement therapy. Pediatr Nephrol. 2002;17(10):819–24.
8. Goonaskeera CD, Wang J, Bunchman TE, Deep A. Factors affecting circuit life during continuous renal replacement therapy in children with liver failure. Ther Apher Dial. 2015;19(1):16–22.

Chapter 39
Extracorporeal Liver Dialysis in Children

Betti Schaefer and Rainer Büscher

Case Presentation

The hitherto healthy 10-year-old Melanie presented to her general practitioner with watery diarrhea for 2 days. Within 1 week her condition worsened and she developed icterus and pale stools. On admission she was somnolent and had blurry speech, skin and scleral jaundice for >72 h, facial petechiae, hematomas, and limb edema. Her condition required immediate intensive care unit treatment.

Liver enzymes were elevated with a total and direct serum bilirubin of 15.2 and 8 mg/dl, respectively. Serum ammonia was high (94 µmol/l) and serum albumin level was low (23 g/l). Platelet count was 155 G/l and INR was elevated up to 3.0. Melanie's blood showed mild hemolysis with a low level of serum hemoglobin (7.2 g/dl) and elevated lactate dehydrogenase. Serum ceruloplasmin level was low (7 mg/dl). Virological screenings for hepatitis types A, B, and C, herpes simplex virus, human herpesvirus 6, Epstein-Barr virus, and cytomegalovirus did not reveal any pathology. Left ventricular function remained normal with marginal pericardial fluid. Abdominal sonography showed a large amount of ascites and an enlarged pancreas without signs of liver cirrhosis.

Due to the rapidly increasing INR and a thrombocyte count of only 90 G/l, fresh frozen plasma (FFP) was repeatedly administered. Due to a low serum ceruloplasmin level, a test dose of D-penicillamine (250 mg) was administered, resulting in an increased excretion of urine copper (up to 4 mg/day). The D-penicillamine dose had to be reduced to 150 mg/day, due to onset of hematuria and proteinuria. Her

B. Schaefer (✉)
Division of Pediatric Nephrology, Center for Pediatrics and Adolescent Medicine,
University of Heidelberg, Heidelberg, Germany
e-mail: Betti.Schaefer@med.uni-heidelberg.de

R. Büscher
Department of Pediatric Nephrology, University Children's Hospital, Essen, Germany

© Springer International Publishing AG 2017
B.A. Warady et al. (eds.), *Pediatric Dialysis Case Studies*,
DOI 10.1007/978-3-319-55147-0_39

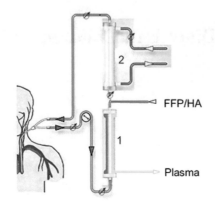

1 = Plasma filter
2 = High-flux HD filter
⊘= Pressure control
FFP: Fresh Frozen Plasma
HA: Human Albumin

Fig. 39.1 Tandem plasma exchange and hemodialysis

general condition worsened, and she developed hepatic encephalopathy grade 3 requiring high urgency listing for liver transplantation (LTx).

Plasma exchange (PE) combined with hemodialysis (HD) was performed as a bridging therapy to LTx. Before the first tandem plasma exchange and hemodialysis (tPE/HD) session could be started, low blood pressure (78/39 mm Hg) occurred despite volume and vasopressor therapy. Total serum bilirubin reached 30 mg/dl (direct serum bilirubin was 15 mg/dl), INR was 4.1, and serum ammonia increased to 140 μmol/l. Following the first tPE/HD treatment, total and direct bilirubin levels decreased (14 mg/dl, 7 mg/dl); INR and serum ammonia levels dropped almost to the normal range (1.3 and 63 μmol/l). Regional citrate was used for anticoagulation. No treatment-related adverse events occurred during the rapid (2 h PE and 3.3 h HD) tPE/HD session. Additional standard medical therapy (SMT) consisted of low-protein parenteral nutrition, intestinal sterilization, diuretics, and transfusion of coagulation factors, erythrocyte, and platelet concentrates. The subsequent tPE/HD sessions performed every 12–24 h were similarly effective with 50% decreases of total and direct bilirubin, serum ammonia, and urea levels, which maintained the patient in a good clinical condition until successful liver transplantation (see Fig. 39.1).

Clinical Questions

1. What is the diagnosis? What is the etiology of acute liver failure? What is the rationale for high urgency listing for liver transplantation?
2. What are possible therapeutic options?
3. When should extracorporeal liver support (ELS) be initiated? What are absolute and relative indications for this treatment?

4. What are the advantages and disadvantages of individual extracorporeal liver support systems? What are the clinical outcomes and patient survival rates? What is the level of evidence supporting the efficacy of ELS?
5. Is combined plasma exchange and hemodialysis a rational choice for extracorporeal liver support?
6. What are the advantages and possible drawbacks of simultaneous/tandem plasma exchange and hemodialysis?

Diagnostic Discussion

1. Shortly after admission, Melanie's clinical status and medical history raised suspicion of acute liver failure (ALF), which is a rare and often life-threatening clinical condition. The etiology of ALF varies with age. In 40% of infants, ALF is due to inherited errors of metabolism, such as neonatal hemochromatosis. Forty percent of affected older children have viral infections, and only ten percent are diagnosed with drug intoxication, such as acetaminophen. Under the age of 35 years, Wilson's disease (incidence rate 1:30,000) should always be considered even if there is no prior history of liver, neurologic, or psychiatric abnormalities. Wilson's disease causes ALF in ~5% of cases and usually manifests with neurological symptoms during adolescence. The etiology of ALF remains unexplained in almost 50% of all cases [1].

    While laboratory findings confirmed abnormally high liver enzymes, screenings for viral infections and toxic agents were negative. At the time of admission, the plasma ceruloplasmin level was already low (normal range > 20 mg/dl). The fulminant course of liver failure and the suspicion of Wilson's disease prompted a trial of D-penicillamine therapy. A test dose of D-penicillamine yielded significantly increased urine copper excretion, confirming the hypothesis that ALF was due to Wilson's disease, a copper storage disorder. Fulminant liver failure due to Wilson's disease is irreversible; long-term adequate liver function is unlikely and LTx is the only feasible therapeutic option. While deceased donor organ availability for LTx is severely limited, children are preferred recipients. High urgency listing usually allows LTx within 1 week.
2. One third of the children with ALF recover with standard medical therapy. This includes low-protein intake, close monitoring of serum glucose and electrolytes, intestinal sterilization to minimize the risk of gram-negative infection and endotoxemia, stabilization of blood pressure, reduced volume intake, diuretic therapy, and transfusion of FFP, clotting factors, platelets, and erythrocytes. Chelation therapy and a low-copper diet might improve the general status of the patient with Wilson's disease, but cannot restore the deficient specific functions of the liver.

    Extracorporeal liver support systems can be used to bridge the critical time interval to either recovery of liver function or successful LTx. Available ELS treatment modalities include: plasma exchange combined with hemodialysis, applied either sequentially or simultaneously ("tandem" PE/HD therapy), molecular adsorbent recirculating system (MARS), single-pass albumin dialysis (SPAD), and the Prometheus(R) Therapy System are available treatment methods. Due to the high toxin accumulation rate in ALF, frequent intermittent sessions or continuous treatment is required. In addition to ALF, possible indications for ELS include acute-on-chronic liver failure, primary liver graft rejection or dysfunction, hepatobiliary surgery, and hepatogenic pruritus.

3. Indications for ELS in ALF in children have mainly been adopted from adults [2, 3]. Hepatic encephalopathy ≥ grade 3 is an urgent indication for liver support therapy since it can lead to irreversible central nervous system damage. Coagulation failure is only poorly manageable by repeated infusions of coagulation factor concentrates and fresh frozen plasma. Since this is expensive and rapidly results in excessive volume and nitrogen overload with consequent cerebral edema, coagulation failure represents an absolute indication for ELS. Serum ammonia >200 µmol/l and indirect serum bilirubin in excess of 25 mg/dl are generally considered ELS indications. ELS should also be considered in cases of hepatic cardiopathy, hemodynamic instability, hepatorenal and hepatopulmonary syndromes, increased intracranial pressure, and hepatic encephalopathy grade 2. Due to the rapid dynamics of clinical deterioration in ALF, early rather than late institution of ELS is usually practiced in experienced units.

4. The advantages and disadvantages of ELS treatment modalities are summarized in Table 39.1 [4, 5]. The widespread availability and expertise with plasma exchange and hemodialysis are an unquestionable advantage of their combined use in ALF. Although none of the ELS treatment modalities have been systematically evaluated in pediatric cohorts, the accumulated evidence in adults and positive experience in pediatric case series justify their case-specific use in children as well. In adults most randomized clinical trials demonstrated improved outcomes in patients treated with ELS compared to SMT. ELS resulted in improved systemic and cerebral perfusion [6–8], reduced portal hypertension [9], improved renal function [10], reduced intracranial pressure [7], and attenuated hepatic encephalopathy [11, 12]. Moreover, randomized trials with small numbers of patients suggested improved short-term survival of adults with hepatorenal syndrome [13] and acute-on-chronic liver failure [14]. However, four large trials did not confirm any survival benefit of MARS compared to SMT [8, 15–17].

Coagulation capacity is critically compromised in patients with ALF, due to reduced hepatic synthesis, splenic decomposition of thrombocytes, and factor depletion due to bleeding and/or coagulation failure. Deterioration of coagulation failure with MARS has repeatedly been described [18–22], which is likely explained by mechanical platelet sequestration during blood passage through the filter and membrane-induced immune-mediated coagulation factor consumption [19–22]. Similar effects should occur with Prometheus and SPAD. Furthermore, unlike regional citrate anticoagulation, heparin anticoagulation further increases the bleeding risk in children with acute kidney/liver injury. However, citrate anticoagulation tends to be avoided in some centers for patients with ALF due to concerns for citrate accumulation/toxicity in this setting [23, 24].

Table 39.1 Advantages and disadvantages of extracorporeal liver support therapies

	PE/HD	Prometheus	SPAD	MARS
Advantages	High detoxification capacity Efficient compensation of liver synthesis failure, reduced bleeding risk Neutral volume and nitrogen balance Less expensive Widely available	No exogenous protein delivery, no infectious and allergic risk Continuous administration feasible	No exogenous protein delivery, no infectious or allergic risk Continuous administration feasible Relatively easy to perform and less expensive in small children	No exogenous protein delivery, no infectious or allergic risk Continuous administration feasible Good clinical tolerability
Disadvantages	Intermittent therapy Infectious and allergic risks related to exogenous protein load	Additional bleeding risk Plasma substitution is associated with volume and nitrogen load High costs and workload (system exchange every 8–12 h) High extracorporeal volume	Additional bleeding risk Plasma substitution is associated with volume and nitrogen load High amounts of albumin required for extended treatment and in children with larger body surface area	Additional bleeding risk Plasma substitution is associated with volume and nitrogen load High costs and workload (system exchange every 8–12 h)

PE/HD plasma exchange in combination with hemodialysis, *SPAD* single-pass albumin dialysis, *MARS* molecular adsorbent recirculating system

Unlike MARS, SPAD, and Prometheus, combined hemodialysis and plasma exchange not only achieve efficient detoxification but also restore plasma coagulation factors in patients with ALF. This effect is achieved without any net volume and nitrogen load, avoiding the toxicity of frequent plasma transfusions which are still required with the other ELS modalities. Moreover, PE and HD are widely available, relatively inexpensive, and much less challenging to perform technically than the specific ELS technologies. In our center we treated ten children suffering from ALF with MARS and eight of them also with combined PE and HD. Whereas MARS treatment reduced serum bilirubin and ammonia only slightly and did not prevent coagulation failure, combined PE/HD reduced serum bilirubin, ammonia, and INR levels by more than one third, supporting the superior efficacy of this approach [18].

5. In a recent survey, 92% of pediatric nephrology centers surveyed reported the use of tandem PE/HD treatment [25]. The feasibility and clinical tolerability of the procedure have been demonstrated in two case series [26, 27].

6. An evident advantage of performing PE and HD in tandem via a single extracorporeal system is the reduction of total extracorporeal treatment time (and cost), with less staff time spent for system setup and treatment monitoring. We confirmed a time-saving effect of tandem PE/HD when comparing 92 combined and 113 sequential PE/HD treatments in children with comparable clinical conditions [26]. Furthermore, performing tandem PE/HD within a single circuit might be associated with better patient fluid volume and body temperature control by individual adjustment of ultrafiltration rate and dialysate fluid temperature.

Another potential benefit of tandem PE and HD should be the reduced cumulative heparin load. However, in our study, the total heparin dose did not differ substantially, since a 2–3-fold higher initial heparin bolus was given for the tandem sessions [26].

Uncontrolled observational studies in adults have shown a 10% rate of minor adverse events with tandem HD/PE [28–30]. We observed higher incidence rates of dialysis-related adverse events (i.e., clotting, hemolysis, and blood leakage) with tandem vs. sequential PE/HD (14% vs. 7%), which might be related to the relatively higher extracorporeal volume in children compared to adults [26]. Thus, the benefits of rapid purification by combining PE and HD within a single session must be balanced against an increased risk of technical adverse events, which mandates a stringent protocol of tight monitoring of system pressures and coagulation status.

Clinical Pearls

1. Pediatric ALF is a rare and usually rapidly progressive disease. With clinical practice guidlines limited to suggestions on how to assess disease severity and progression, diagnostic and therapeutic approaches remain largely individualized.
2. The clinical manifestation of Wilson's disease ranges widely from asymptomatic up to fulminant liver failure, with or without neurological symptoms, and is usually associated with Coombs-negative hemolytic anemia.
3. While extracorporeal liver support systems efficiently remove water-soluble and protein-bound toxins associated with liver failure, the survival benefit of ELS over standard medical treatment is controversial.
4. In view of its relatively good clinical tolerability, ELS seems to be justified in the pediatric population. Plasmapheresis combined with hemodialysis is widely available, relatively inexpensive, and easy to perform and is the only ELS system combining detoxification with volume- and nitrogen-neutral replacement of albumin and coagulation factors.
5. PE and HD might be performed sequentially or in a tandem setting for critically ill patients to provide rapid and effective intervention. The potentially higher procedure-related adverse event risk of the latter mandates meticulous control of coagulation status and system pressures.

References

1. Cochran JB, Losek JD. Acute liver failure in children. Pediatr Emerg Care. 2007;23:129–35.
2. Nadalin S, Heuer M, Wallot M, Auth M, Schaffer R, Sotiropoulos GC, et al. Paediatric acute liver failure and transplantation: the University of Essen experience. Transpl Int. 2007;20:519–27.
3. Markiewicz-Kijewska M, Szymczak M, Ismail H, Prokurat S, Teisseyre J, Socha P, et al. Liver transplantation for fulminant Wilson's disease in children. Ann Transplant. 2008;13:28–31.
4. Schaefer B, Schmitt CP. The role of Molecular Adsorbents Recirculating System (MARS) dialysis for extracorporeal liver support in children. Pediatr Nephrol. 2013;28:1763–9.
5. Auth MK, Kim HS, Beste M, Bonzel KE, Baumann U, Ballauff A, et al. Removal of metabolites, cytokines and hepatic growth factors by extracorporeal liver support in children. J Pediatr Gastroenterol Nutr. 2005;40:54–9.
6. Sorkine P, Ben Abraham R, Szold O, Biderman P, Kidron A, Merchav H, et al. Role of the molecular adsorbent recycling system (MARS) in the treatment of patients with acute exacerbation of chronic liver failure. Crit Care Med. 2001;29:1332–6.
7. Schmidt LE, Svendsen LB, Sørensen VR, Hansen BA, Larsen FS. Cerebral blood flow velocity increases during a single treatment with the molecular adsorbents recirculating system in patients with acute on chronic liver failure. Liver Transpl. 2001;7:709–12.
8. Schmidt LE, Wang LP, Hansen BA, Larsen FS. Systemic hemodynamic effects of treatment with the molecular adsorbents recirculating system in patients with hyperacute liver failure: a prospective controlled trial. Liver Transpl. 2003;9:290–7.
9. Sen S, Mookerjee RP, Cheshire LM, Davies NA, Williams R, Jalan R. Albumin dialysis reduces portal pressure acutely in patients with severe alcoholic hepatitis. J Hepatol. 2005;43:142–8.
10. Mitzner SR, Klammt S, Peszynski P, Hickstein H, Korten G, Stange J, et al. Improvement of multiple organ functions in hepatorenal syndrome during albumin dialysis with the molecular adsorbent recirculating system. Ther Apher. 2001;5:417–22.
11. Sen S, Davies NA, Mookerjee RP, Cheshire LM, Hodges SJ, Williams R, et al. Pathophysiological effects of albumin dialysis in acute-on-chronic liver failure: a randomized controlled study. Liver Transpl. 2004;10:1109–19.
12. Hassanein TI, Tofteng F, Brown Jr RS, McGuire B, Lynch P, Mehta R, et al. Randomized controlled study of extracorporeal albumin dialysis for hepatic encephalopathy in advanced cirrhosis. Hepatology. 2007;46:1853–62.
13. Mitzner SR, Stange J, Klammt S, Risler T, Erley CM, Bader BD, et al. Improvement of hepatorenal syndrome with extracorporeal albumin dialysis MARS: results of a prospective, randomized, controlled clinical trial. Liver Transpl. 2000;6:277–86.
14. Heemann U, Treichel U, Loock J, Philipp T, Gerken G, Malago M, et al. Albumin dialysis in cirrhosis with superimposed acute liver injury: a prospective, controlled study. Hepatology. 2002;36:949–58.
15. El Banayosy A, Kizner L, Schueler V, Bergmeier S, Cobaugh D, Koerfer R. First use of the Molecular Adsorbent Recirculating System technique on patients with hypoxic liver failure after cardiogenic shock. ASAIO J. 2004;50:332–7.
16. Banares R, Nevens F, Larsen FS, Jalan R, Albillos A, Dollinger M. Extracorporeal liver support with MARS in patients with acute-on-chronic liver failure. The RELIEF trial. J Hepatol. 2010;52:459.
17. Saliba F, Camus C, Durand F, Mathurin P, Delafosse B, Barange K, et al. Predictive factors of transplant free survival in patients with fulminant and subfulminant hepatic failure: results from a randomized controlled multicenter trial. J Hepatol. 2009;50:89–90.
18. Schaefer B, Schaefer F, Engelmann G, Meyburg J, Heckert KH, Zorn M, et al. Comparison of Molecular Adsorbents Recirculating System (MARS) dialysis with combined plasma exchange and haemodialysis in children with acute liver failure. Nephrol Dial Transplant. 2011;26:3633–9.

19. Meijers BK, Verhamme P, Nevens F, Hoylaerts MF, Bammens B, Wilmer A, et al. Major coagulation disturbances during fractionated plasma separation and adsorption. Am J Transplant. 2007;7:2195–9.

20. Faybik P, Bacher A, Kozek-Langenecker SA, Steltzer H, Krenn CG, Unger S, et al. Molecular adsorbent recirculating system and hemostasis in patients at high risk of bleeding: an observational study. Crit Care. 2006;10:24.

21. Bachli EB, Schuepbach RA, Maggiorini M, Stocker R, Müllhaupt B, Renner EL. Artificial liver support with the molecular adsorbent recirculating system: activation of coagulation and bleeding complications. Liver Int. 2007;27(4):475–84.

22. Doria C, Mandalà L, Smith JD, Caruana G, Scott VL, Gruttadauria S, et al. Thromboelastography used to assess coagulation during treatment with molecular adsorbent recirculating system. Clin Transpl. 2004;18:365–71.

23. Kreuzer M, Bonzel KE, Büscher R, Offner G, Ehrich JH, Pape L. Regional citrate anticoagulation is safe in intermittent high-flux haemodialysis treatment of children and adolescents with an increased risk of bleeding. Nephrol Dial Transplant. 2010;25:3337–42.

24. Brophy PD, Somers MJ, Baum MA, Symons JM, McAfee N, Fortenberry JD, et al. Multi-centre evaluation of anticoagulation in patients receiving continuous renal replacement therapy (CRRT). Nephrol Dial Transplant. 2005;20:1416–21.

25. Filler G, Clark WF, Huang SH. Tandem hemodialysis and plasma exchange. Pediatr Nephrol. 2014;29:2077–82.

26. Schaefer B, Ujszaszi A, Schaefer S, Heckert KH, Schaefer F, Schmitt CP. Safety and efficacy of tandem hemodialysis and plasma exchange in children. Clin J Am Soc Nephrol. 2014;9:1563–70.

27. Paglialonga F, Ardissino G, Biasuzzi A, Testa S, Edefonti A. Tandem plasma-exchange and haemodialysis in a paediatric dialysis unit. Pediatr Nephrol. 2012;27:493–5.

28. Dechmann-Sültemeyer T, Linkeschova R, Lenzen K, Kuril Z, Grabensee B, Voiculescu A. Tandem plasmapheresis and haemodialysis as a safe procedure in 82 patients with immune-mediated disease. Nephrol Dial Transplant. 2009;24:252–7.

29. Farah M, Levin A, Kiaii M, Vickars L, Werb R. Combination hemodialysis and centrifugal therapeutic plasma exchange: 18 years of Canadian experience. Hemodial Int. 2013;17:256–65.

30. Pérez-Sáez MJ, Toledo K, Ojeda R, Crespo R, Soriano S, Alvarez de Lara MA, et al. Tandem plasmapheresis and hemodialysis: efficacy and safety. Ren Fail. 2011;33:765–9.

Chapter 40
Therapeutic Apheresis

Stuart L. Goldstein

Case Presentations

Case 1

A 5-year-old male presents to a tertiary medical center emergency department (ED) following a 20 min generalized tonic-clonic seizure. In the ED, he was found to be afebrile and have a heart rate of 86/min, a respiratory rate of 32/min, and a blood pressure of 160/100 mmHg. The boy had a 7-day history of painless gross hematuria that was described as "cola-colored." His primary pediatrician was concerned about a urinary tract infection, obtained a clean-catch urine culture, and initiated trimethoprim-sulfamethoxazole empirically. Past medical history was negative for trauma or recent infections. His family history was also negative for relevant kidney disease including chronic kidney disease, end-stage kidney disease, and nephrolithiasis.

In the ED, the patient was postictal and was assessed as pale and to have periorbital edema and 3+ lower extremity edema to the pretibial level. The remainder of the physical exam was unremarkable, with relevant negative findings for skin rashes, purpura, petechiae, or joint swelling. Laboratory findings included the following: white blood cell count 15,500 per mcL, hemoglobin 9.8 g/dL, hematocrit 31%, platelet count 175,000 per mcL, serum sodium 134 meq/L, potassium 5.4 meq/L, chloride 105 meq/L, total carbon dioxide 19 meq/L, blood urea nitrogen 75 mg/dL, serum creatinine 1.9 mg/dL, glucose 254 mg/dL, calcium 8.9 mg/dL, phosphorus 5.7 mg/dL, and serum albumin 2.8 g/dL.

S.L. Goldstein, MD (✉)
Center for Acute Care Nephrology, Pheresis Service,
Cincinnati Children's Hospital Medical Center, Cincinnati, OH, USA

University of Cincinnati College of Medicine, Cincinnati, OH, USA
e-mail: Stuart.Goldstein@cchmc.org

© Springer International Publishing AG 2017
B.A. Warady et al. (eds.), *Pediatric Dialysis Case Studies*,
DOI 10.1007/978-3-319-55147-0_40

He was transferred to the intensive care unit where he was started on a continuous infusion of nicardipine and twice daily intermittent furosemide with a resultant improvement in blood pressure to 125/85 and urine output of 1.5 L over the first day of admission. On ICU day 2, his serum creatinine had increased to 2.9 mg/dL. He then received an empiric pulse dose of methylprednisolone and a renal biopsy with the initial light microscopy reading of 50% of the glomeruli containing cellular crescents. The immunofluorescence and electron microscopy results weren't available until the next day. That evening, he developed hemoptysis, worsening respiratory status requiring intubation, and invasive mechanical ventilation. His hemoglobin decreased to 5.4 g/dL, necessitating packed red blood cell transfusion. You are called to evaluate for the indications for therapeutic plasma exchange (TPE) and provide recommendations regarding the TPE prescription and course.

Clinical Questions

1. What factors should be considered in the rationale for initiating a course of TPE?
2. How is the "dose" of TPE prescribed?
3. How is the duration of a TPE treatment course determined for this patient?
4. What are the risks of TPE?

Diagnostic Discussion

1. TPE should be considered when there is a known or presumed pathogenic substance in the circulating plasma volume that can be removed at a rate that is faster than it can be removed in the body. In most cases, this is an IgG antibody, as is likely the case in this patient whose main differential diagnoses are anti-glomerular basement membrane antibody disease (aka, Goodpasture syndrome) and systemic autoimmune vasculitis (e.g., Wegener's granulomatosis). The goal of TPE is the mechanical removal of the offending pathogenic substance, which usually needs to be combined with some pharmacological immunosuppression management to decrease its production.
2. The dose of TPE is quantified in terms of the "total plasma volume" exchanged. Formulae for estimation of TBV (in liters) and plasma volume (PV, in liters) are based on the patient's height (H, in meters), weight (W, in kilograms), and venous Hct (in %)

   Male: $BV = 0.3669 \times H^3 + 0.03219 \times W$ [1]
   Female: $BV = 0.3561 \times H^3 + 0.03308 \times W$
   $PV = BV \times (1 - Hct/100)$

   The association between volumes exchanged and pathogenic substance removal generally follows first-order kinetics, where the efficiency of removal is greatest early in the procedure and decreases progressively during the exchange (Table 40.1). While the optimal plasma volume exchange depends on the clinical

Table 40.1 Efficiency of antibody reduction by plasma exchange volume

Plasma volume exchange (L)	Percent plasma removed
0	0
0.5	39.3
1.0	63.2
1.5	77.7
2.0	86.5
2.5	91.8
3.0	95.0

scenario, a standard practice of a 1.0–1.5 volume exchange establishes a lower threshold of removal while minimizing longer treatment times with diminished efficacy.

The other prescription factor to consider is the composition of the plasma replacement fluid. In most cases, 5% albumin is chosen as the replacement fluid. However, in certain conditions where important blood proteins may be beneficial, such as coagulation factors or ADAMTS-13 (in TTP), fresh frozen plasma may be preferable as replacement fluid.

3. This boy has rapidly progressive glomerulonephritis secondary to, as noted above, anti-glomerular basement membrane antibody disease (aka Goodpasture syndrome) or a systemic autoimmune vasculitis (e.g., Wegener's granulomatosis). In some conditions, such as Goodpasture syndrome, there is a marker to follow (i.e., anti-glomerular basement membrane antibody level). But it is not always the case that a measurable antibody titer correlates with disease activity. In most diseases, a measurable pathogenic factor is not available, so the clinician must look for secondary clinical features such as resolution of signs (improvement in inflammatory or hematological markers, improvement in kidney function) or symptoms (resolution of hemoptysis). In 2010, the American Society for Apheresis published guidelines on "The Use of Therapeutic Apheresis in Clinical Practice" for nearly 60 conditions [2]. This guideline provides information on the typical plasma exchange dose and expected treatment course based on the literature available at the time. The recommendations should be taken as an initial treatment plan and modified as needed based on the individual patient course. The current recommendations are considered daily procedures in fulminant cases or those with diffuse alveolar hemorrhage, then every 2–3 days for a total of six to nine procedures. The total plasma volume exchange should be 1–1.5, and in patients with diffuse alveolar hemorrhage, replacement with plasma is recommended to avoid dilutional coagulopathy.

4. The risks of TPE are similar to the risk associated with any extracorporeal therapy including blood loss, hypotension, hypertension, and vascular access infection. In addition, since many pheresis circuits are anticoagulated with citrate, hypocalcemia resulting from citrate toxicity can result in cardiac arrhythmias. Successive daily TPE procedures using albumin for replacement fluid can lead to a dilutional coagulopathy. Therefore, many centers check a pre-procedure fibrinogen level and will use fresh frozen plasma as part of the replacement fluid

volume for concentrations less than 100–150 mg/dL. Finally, since patients receive a large volume of blood products as replacement fluid over the short period of procedure time, they can be at risk for transfusion-related acute lung injury (TRALI), which is characterized by the rapid onset of non-cardiogenic pulmonary edema. Patients who exhibit respiratory distress during a TPE procedure with blood products as replacement fluid should have the procedure terminated and receive supplemental oxygen and corticosteroids.

Clinical Pearls

1. The decision to initiate a course of TPE for patients with acute glomerulonephritis or other systemic disease should be based on the plausibility of a pathogenic substance that can be removed from the plasma.
2. The TPE prescription and duration of course can be based on the time frame expected for improvement based on case series in the literature and the ASFA guidelines.
3. The clinical team should determine which marker(s) they will follow at the outset to assess for treatment response or lack thereof.

Case 2

A 12-year-old African-American girl with end-stage kidney disease (ESKD) secondary to focal segmental glomerulosclerosis (FSGS) is being maintained on hemodialysis and is active on the deceased donor kidney transplant list. The kidney transplant team receives a call that a suitable donor has been identified and starts to mobilize the team to provide the transplant.

Clinical Questions

1. What is the risk of FSGS recurrence after kidney transplantation?
2. What factors should determine initiation and the duration of the TPE course in patients who develop FSGS recurrence after kidney transplantation?
3. Should prophylactic TPE be provided to patients with FSGS in the peri-transplant period?

Diagnostic Discussion

1. The FSGS recurrence rate after kidney transplantation ranges from 30 to 50%, with increased recurrence risk associated with younger age at presentation with primary FSGS and a more rapid progression to ESKD. The presence of a patho-

genic circulating factor was reported in 1996, where serum from patients with FSGS recurrence, but not from patients without recurrence, lead to increased permeability of albumin in isolated rat glomeruli [3]. The albumin permeability of the rat glomeruli was reduced when exposed to serum from patients who had undergone TPE with subsequently diminished proteinuria. Thus, the biological plausibility of a circulating factor leading to FSGS recurrence after kidney transplantation, and the rationale for TPE in such patients, was established.

2. The efficacy of TPE in leading to decreased proteinuria in FSGS recurrence is well established, with a 70–80% reported response rate [4]. However, there is no consensus as to the optimal TPE regimen. A meta-analysis of 12 case series in 2001 revealed that 11 different protocols were used among them [5]. Nonetheless, this meta-analysis showed that 32/44 patients responded, with a shorter time from recurrence to TPE initiation in responders vs. nonresponders (10 days vs. 19 days). In addition, the pooled data suggested a higher rate of secondary relapse in patients who received fewer than ten total TPE procedures.

3. Recurrence of FSGS after renal transplantation has important clinical implications for children. Data from the North American Pediatric Renal Trials and Collaborative (NAPRTCS) demonstrate FSGS recurrence that leads to a reduction in the expected 5-year allograft survival rate from living related donors compared to deceased donors [6]. Given the high rate of recurrence and the negative effect on allograft survival, small studies have looked at the effect of prophylactic TPE in the peri-transplant period [7]. These studies suggest a decrease in recurrence rate from 60% to 33% in high-risk patients, which were defined as patients who had a previous renal transplant with FSGS recurrence or high-grade proteinuria going into transplant.

Clinical Pearls

1. Patients should be monitored closely for recurrence of FSGS in the early post-transplant period.
2. TPE should be started promptly, preferably within 10 days of the onset of proteinuria. A minimum treatment course should be 10 days, and TPE should be continued until the urine protein/creatinine ratio is <0.5.
3. The role of empiric prophylactic TPE is uncertain, but there may be a benefit in patients deemed at high risk. High-risk pediatric patients include those who had rapid progression of their native FSGS, who have a previous FSGS recurrence, or who have active proteinuria at the time of transplantation.

References

1. Nadler SB, Hidalgo JH, Bloch T. Prediction of blood volume in normal human adults. Surgery. 1962;51(2):224–32.

2. Szczepiorkowski ZM, Winters JL, Bandarenko N, Kim HC, Linenberger ML, Marques MB, et al. Guidelines on the use of therapeutic apheresis in clinical practice – evidence-based approach from the apheresis applications Committee of the American Society for apheresis. J Clin Apher. 2010;25(3):83–177.
3. Savin VJ, Sharma R, Sharma M, McCarthy ET, Swan SK, Ellis E, et al. Circulating factor associated with increased glomerular permeability to albumin in recurrent focal segmental glomerulosclerosis. N Engl J Med. 1996;334(14):878–83.
4. Keith DS. Therapeutic apheresis rescue mission: recurrent focal segmental glomerulosclerosis in renal allografts. Semin Dial. 2012;25(2):190–2.
5. Davenport RD. Apheresis treatment of recurrent focal segmental glomerulosclerosis after kidney transplantation: re-analysis of published case-reports and case-series. J Clin Apher. 2001;16(4):175–8.
6. Baum MA, Stablein DM, Panzarino VM, Tejani A, Harmon WE, Alexander SR. Loss of living donor renal allograft survival advantage in children with focal segmental glomerulosclerosis. Kidney Int. 2001;59(1):328–33.
7. Ohta T, Kawaguchi H, Hattori M, Komatsu Y, Akioka Y, Nagata M, et al. Effect of pre-and post-operative plasmapheresis on posttransplant recurrence of focal segmental glomerulosclerosis in children. Transplantation. 2001;71(5):628–33.

Chapter 41
Neonatal Hyperammonemia

Hui-Kim Yap

Case Presentation

A newborn female presented at 36 h of life with a poor suck. She was born to first-degree consanguineous parents at 38 weeks gestation following a normal pregnancy and normal vaginal delivery, with a birth weight of 3,260 g. Apgar scores were 9 at 1 and 5 min. On examination, she was noted to be quiet. Her temperature was 34.6 °C. She was noted to be tachypneic and grunting, with a respiratory rate of 60 breaths per minute. Pulses were palpable with a capillary refill time of 3 s. Cardiac and respiratory examination was unremarkable. The anterior fontanelle was normal. The liver was palpable 2 cm below the right subcostal margin, but there was no splenomegaly. Oxygen saturation was 100% on hood box. As the maternal high vaginal swab had heavy growth of Group B Streptococcus, she was initially investigated for sepsis and started on empiric intravenous crystalline penicillin and gentamicin after blood cultures were taken. A complete blood count showed a total white count of 20.3×10^9/L with neutrophilia. Hemoglobin was 24.5 g/dL with a hematocrit of 65.8% and a platelet count of 433×10^9/L. C-reactive protein was <20 mg/L. A lumbar puncture was performed and showed normal cerebrospinal fluid cell counts and biochemistry. Chest X-ray was normal.

At 45 h of life, her condition deteriorated. She was noted to be frothing from the mouth, with a depressed sensorium and reacting only to pain. Her muscle tone was increased, with an incomplete Moro response. Her pupils were 2 mm bilaterally and equally reactive to light. An arterial blood gas on FiO_2 of 30% showed the presence of respiratory alkalosis, with pH of 7.563, pCO_2 of 22 mmHg, pO2 of 62 mmHg,

H.-K. Yap (✉)
Department of Pediatrics, Yong Loo Lin School of Medicine, National University of Singapore, Singapore, Singapore
e-mail: hui_kim_yap@nuhs.edu.sg

© Springer International Publishing AG 2017
B.A. Warady et al. (eds.), *Pediatric Dialysis Case Studies*,
DOI 10.1007/978-3-319-55147-0_41

and a standard bicarbonate level of 20 mmol/L. Blood glucose was 4.3 mmol/L (77.4 mg/dL). She subsequently (48 h of life) developed an episode of apnea with oxygen desaturation down to 70%, associated with facial twitching. She was immediately intubated and ventilated, and intravenous phenobarbitone (25 mg/kg) was administered to control the seizures. The serum ammonia level was high at 881 umol/L (1,234 ug/dL), with a venous blood lactate of 2.6 mmol/L (23.4 mg/dL). A diagnosis of hyperammonemia secondary to a presumed urea cycle defect was made, and she was transferred to the pediatric intensive care unit for further management at 52 h of life. She was hydrated with intravenous 10% dextrose solution and intravenous sodium benzoate, and arginine chloride (sodium phenylacetate was not available) therapy was initiated. In addition, pediatric nephrology was consulted for acute hemodialysis.

A double-lumen 6.5 French catheter was inserted into the patient's right femoral vein. Hemodialysis was commenced 2 h after transfer using a 0.4 m² polysulfone dialyzer (Hemoflow F3, Fresenius, Homburg, Germany) and neonatal lines with blood priming of the circuit which had a total priming volume of 72 mL (~27% of patient's blood volume). The initial blood flow rate was 30 mL/min, and the dialysate flow rate was 500 mL/min, with a dialysate bath containing bicarbonate 35 mmol/L, potassium 2 mmol/L, and calcium 1.75 mmol/L. Heparin anticoagulation was used, maintaining the activated clotting time between 150 and 200 s. Intravenous 20% mannitol, 1 g/kg, was infused over the first hour of dialysis. Her blood ammonia at the time of dialysis initiation had increased to 2,091 umol/L (2,928 ug/dL), and her general condition was noted to have worsened, as she was not responding to pain. Her fontanelle was full and her pupils were fixed at 3 mm. During the dialysis procedure, her blood pressure remained stable ranging from 80/60 to 95/70 mmHg. After 4 h of dialysis, her blood ammonia had decreased to 1,853 umol/L (2,596 ug/dL). At this point, the dialyzer clotted and hemodialysis was discontinued. As the patient's neurological status remained poor as reflected by flaccid tone and fixed/dilated pupils, her parents opted not to continue with dialysis, and the patient died 12 h later. Postmortem liver biopsy enzyme analysis confirmed complete carbamoyl phosphate synthetase I deficiency.

Clinical Questions

1. What are the causes of neonatal hyperammonemia?
2. What is the recommended approach to the diagnostic assessment of a neonate with hyperammonemia?
3. What is the recommended initial clinical management of the neonate with hyperammonemia?
4. What is the dialytic modality of choice for the neonate with hyperammonemia?
5. What are the outcomes of dialytic therapy in neonatal hyperammonemia?

Diagnostic Discussion

1. Neonatal hyperammonemia is a clinical condition characterized by marked elevation of the serum ammonia level resulting in neurologic abnormalities including drowsiness, poor feeding, vomiting, hypotonia, posturing, seizures, and coma [1, 2]. It can result in cerebral edema with severe damage to the developing brain leading to cognitive impairment, epilepsy, cerebral palsy, and even death, if left untreated. The international prevalence of neonatal hyperammonemia ranges from 1:8,000 to 1:44,000 live births [3].

   The causes of neonatal hyperammonemia include urea cycle defects, organic acidemias, fatty acid oxidation defects, disorders of pyruvate metabolism, hyperammonemia-hyperornithinemia-hypocitrullinemia, lysinuric protein intolerance, carbonic anhydrase VA deficiency, hyperinsulinism-hyperammonemia, transient hyperammonemia of the newborn, severe dehydration, and liver failure. Urea cycle disorders are due to a deficiency of enzymes that convert nitrogen to urea for excretion, and these include carbamoyl phosphate synthetase I deficiency, ornithine transcarbamylase deficiency, argininosuccinate synthetase deficiency (type I citrullinemia) and argininosuccinate lyase deficiency (argininosuccinic aciduria), N-acetyl glutamate synthetase deficiency, and arginase deficiency (argininemia).

2. Newborn infants with hyperammonemia typically appear well initially but present between 24 and 48 h after birth with drowsiness, poor suck, hypothermia, and tachypnea, following the introduction of dietary protein intake in the form of milk feeds. A major differential diagnosis is sepsis, and this should be promptly evaluated and excluded. In this setting, metabolic emergencies must always be considered in the absence of risk factors or evidence of sepsis, and the patient evaluation should include measurement of arterial pH and pCO2, serum bicarbonate, glucose, ammonia, electrolytes, lactate, amino acids, and urine organic acids and orotic acid [3]. The concomitant presence of a high anion gap metabolic acidosis with hyperlactatemia, ketosis, and hypoglycemia suggests organic acidemias, defects of pyruvate metabolism, or liver disease; the presence of respiratory alkalosis and a normal lactate suggests urea cycle disorders such as hyperammonemia-hyperornithinemia-hypocitrullinemia, lysinuric protein intolerance, or transient hyperammonemia of the newborn; the presence of mixed metabolic acidosis and respiratory alkalosis and hypoglycemia suggests fatty acid oxidation defects (with hypoketosis) and carbonic anhydrase VA deficiency (with ketosis). Concomitant elevation of liver enzymes suggests the presence of liver failure. Further diagnostic evaluation such as tissue enzyme activity assays or DNA sequencing, in conjunction with array comparative genomic hybridization, is required to establish the specific enzyme deficiency.

3. The severity and duration of hyperammonemia in the neonate significantly correlate with the subsequent degree of neurological damage and cognitive impairment. Early intervention may improve survival [4]. Initial management should include the provision of glucose at 10 mg/kg/min in order to minimize protein

catabolism [3]. Close patient monitoring is important to avoid fluid overload which may worsen any preexistent cerebral edema. Intubation and assisted ventilation should be performed if the patient's respiratory status deteriorates so as to minimize the work of breathing, thus reducing caloric demands and nitrogen catabolism. Protein intake should be stopped for at least 24–48 h and until there is initial patient stabilization; thereafter, it can be restarted at 1.5–1.75 g/kg per day with intravenous amino acids to prevent protein catabolism and with close monitoring of the serum ammonia level at least every 3 h.

Prompt removal of ammonia is imperative in order to limit the severity of the neurological dysfunction. Ammonia is removed by pharmacologic interventions and dialysis. In urea cycle disorders, a combination of sodium phenylacetate and sodium benzoate at a dose of 250 mg/kg, each diluted in 25–35 mL 10% dextrose and infused over 90 min, is used as nitrogen scavengers [5]. The conjugation products, phenylacetylglutamine and hippurate, are water soluble and are excreted in the urine; hence, there must be adequate renal function for these compounds to be removed to avoid toxicity [6].

Except in the case of congenital arginase deficiency, the presence of arginine deficiency associated with a urea cycle disorder results in a catabolic state; therefore, intravenous arginine hydrochloride (200 mg/kg) is added to the infusion empirically, and the maintenance dose is subsequently adjusted once a definitive diagnosis of the enzyme deficiency is identified.

Dialysis should be started in the neonate with hyperammonemia when the serum ammonia level is greater than 500 umol/L (700 ug/dL) and at lower levels between 350 and 400 umol/L (490–560 ug/dL) if the response to medical management after 4 h is inadequate [3, 7].

4. Extracorporeal dialysis is the modality of choice for removal of ammonia, as diffusion of ammonium occurs readily across synthetic dialysis membranes [2]. Diffusion of ammonia is slower across the peritoneal membrane resulting in lower ammonium clearances with peritoneal dialysis. Intermittent hemodialysis (IHD) using blood flow rates of 10–12 mL/kg per minute and a dialysate flow rate of 500 mL/min is an efficient modality for removal of small molecules compared to conventional continuous venovenous hemodiafiltration (CVVHDF) at a clearance of 2 L/h per 1.73m^2 [2]. By removing amino acids such as citrulline, glycine, and glutamine, IHD also enhances the efficiency of nitrogen removal. However, CVVHDF, which utilizes both diffusive and convective transport, is preferred in the hemodynamically unstable neonate in whom low systemic blood pressure and the use of drugs such as arginine that causes vasodilatation through nitric oxide release preclude the higher blood flow rates required for IHD [8]. In addition, although IHD can rapidly reduce very high serum ammonium levels with the potential for resultant improved neurological outcomes, the procedure is unfortunately associated with a high risk of ammonia rebound [2]. This occurs because of ongoing catabolism, especially if there is accompanying infection, and also as a result of a delay in the effect of the pharmacologic nitrogen scavengers which may take up to 48 h to reverse the catabolic process. In turn, continuing with CVVHDF after the initial IHD may be useful to keep the ammonia

levels stable during this period of potential rebound. Moreover, CVVHDF provides the advantage of being able to maintain a normal electrolyte profile in terms of potassium and phosphate in the metabolically unstable infant. To improve the efficacy of CVVHDF in clearing ammonia, a high-dose prescription consisting of a blood flow rate of 10 ml/kg/min and a dialysate flow rate ranging from 3 to 5 L/h may be used [2].

Extracorporeal membrane oxygenation (ECMO) together with HD has high blood flow rates of 170–200 mL/min, and has been used in some centers to rapidly reduce markedly elevated ammonia levels [9]. However, this modality is associated with higher morbidity as it requires surgical vascular access and may not be necessary with the advent of the combined modalities of IHD and high-dose CVVHDF.

Although peritoneal dialysis is not the modality of choice for the dialytic treatment of neonatal hyperammonemia, it is easier to perform in sick neonates compared to the extracorporeal techniques and may be initiated earlier while awaiting transport to a specialized center for extracorporeal dialysis. Even in centers where extracorporeal dialysis is available, significant therapy downtime secondary to technical issues related to the ability of the HD catheter to attain adequate blood flow rates and circuit clotting can negate the advantages of higher ammonia clearance by these modalities [10, 11]. Moreover, peritoneal dialysis can provide additional benefits in terms of an intraperitoneal glucose load to minimize catabolism, as well as removal of albumin and amino acids to achieve a negative nitrogen balance, thus reducing the ammonia load [11]. If peritoneal dialysis is the only modality available, the dialysis prescription should, in turn, be optimized to include 1.5% glucose dialysis solution with a fill volume of 40–50 mL/kg and hourly cycles for greater than 48 h in order to remove the ammonia load. Of course, it should be noted that peritoneal dialysis in neonates can be fraught with technical problems as well, such as poor catheter function, dialysate leakage, and infection, all of which could have a negative impact on ammonia management.

Based on the principles noted above, in the presence of severe hyperammonemia with a serum ammonia concentration of greater than 1,500 umol/L (2,101 ug/dL), *many centers prescribe* IHD initially to rapidly reduce the ammonia load to less than 200 umol/L (280 ug/dL), followed by CVVHDF to prevent ammonia rebound. In contrast, *other centers prefer* high-dose CVVHDF, using a blood flow rate of at least 10 ml/kg/min and a dialysate flow rate of 2–3 times the blood flow rate, especially for those patients with a serum ammonia concentration of 500–1,500 umol/L (700–2,101 ug/dL) (Fig. 41.1). Once dialysis has been initiated, the serum ammonia levels should be monitored on an hourly basis until the levels are sustained below 200 umol/L (280 ug/dL), at which time dialysis can be stopped with control of protein catabolism dependent on the provision of adequate nutrition and the activity of nitrogen scavengers. Unfortunately, both IHD and CVVHDF also remove the pharmacological agents sodium phenylacetate and sodium benzoate, both of which are small molecules and readily dialyzable; hence, dose adjustments may have to be made to maintain the serum ammonia level below 200 umol/L (280 ug/dL) [12].

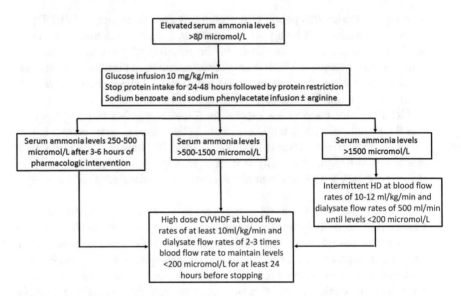

Fig. 41.1 Algorithm showing indications for dialysis in neonates with urea cycle disorder and hyperammonemia. *HD* hemodialysis, *CVVHDF* continuous venovenous hemodiafiltration

5. Earlier reports on survival rates for neonatal hyperammonemia due to urea cycle disorders were dismal, with survival at about 20% [13]. Thankfully, this has improved, and survival rates have been about 80% over the past 20 years due to better nutritional and pharmacologic management and better dialytic options [1, 2, 4, 13]. However, despite these advances, the prognosis in terms of neurodevelopmental outcome for neonates with urea cycle disorders is still guarded, especially when the serum ammonia is greater than 350 umol/L(490 ug/dL) [13]. Neurodevelopmental complications include cerebral palsy, intellectual disability, learning problems, seizure disorders, speech disorders, and attention-deficit hyperactivity disorders. Other studies have shown that the neurological outcome may not be related to peak ammonia levels but to the duration of severe hyperammonemia, with better cognitive outcomes in those whose exposure was less than 24 h [2, 4].

Clinical Pearls

1. Newborns with hyperammonemia typically present as a metabolic emergency between the ages of 24 and 48 h.
2. Early management including glucose infusion, protein restriction, and pharmacologic intervention with nitrogen scavengers is important to limit neurological

damage. Dialysis is required to urgently remove ammonia if pharmacologic intervention is insufficient to remove the ammonia load.

3. The severity of the neurological outcome appears to be related to the duration of severe hyperammonemia and not to the peak ammonia levels.

References

1. Gropman AL, Summar M, Leonard JV. Neurological implications of urea cycle disorders. J Inherit Metab Dis. 2007;30:865–9.
2. Auron A, Brophy PD. Hyperammonemia in review: pathophysiology, diagnosis, and treatment. Pediatr Nephrol. 2012;27:207–22.
3. Häberle J, Boddaert N, Burlina A, Chakrapani A, Dixon M, Huemer M, Karall D, Martinelli D, Crespo PS, Santer R, Servais A, Valayannopoulos V, Lindner M, Rubio V, Dionisi-Vici C. Suggested guidelines for the diagnosis and management of urea cycle disorders. Orphanet J Rare Dis. 2012;7:32. doi:10.1186/1750-1172-7-32.
4. Emms GM. Nitrogen sparing therapy revisited 2009. Mol Genet Metab. 2010;100:565–71.
5. Summar M. Current strategies for the management of neonatal urea cycle disorders. J Pediatr. 2001;138:S30–9.
6. Brusilow SW, Valle DL, Batshaw M. New pathways of nitrogen excretion in inborn errors of urea synthesis. Lancet. 1979;2(8140):452–4.
7. Schaefer F, Straube E, Oh J, Mehls O, Mayatepek E. Dialysis in neonates with inborn errors of metabolism. Nephrol Dial Transplant. 1999;14:910–8.
8. Fakler CR, Kaftan HA, Nelin LD. Two cases suggesting a role for the L-arginine nitric oxide pathway in neonatal blood pressure regulation. Acta Paediatr. 1995;84:460–2.
9. Summar M, Pietsch J, Deshpande J, Schulman G. Effective hemodialysis and hemofiltration driven by an extracorporeal membrane oxygenation pump in infants with hyperammonemia. J Pediatr. 1996;128:379–82.
10. Picca S, Dionisi-Vici C, Bartuli A, De Palo T, Papadia F, Montini G, Materassi M, Donati MA, Verrina E, Schiaffino MC, Pecoraro C, Iaccarino E, Vidal E, Burlina A, Emma F. Short-term survival of hyperammonemic neonates treated with dialysis. Pediatr Nephrol. 2015;30:839–47.
11. Bunchman TE. The complexity of dialytic therapy in hyperammonemic neonates. Pediatr Nephrol. 2015;30:701–2.
12. Bunchman TE, Barletta GM, Winters JW, Gardner JJ, Crumb TL, McBryde KD. Phenylacetate and benzoate clearance in a hyperammonemic infant on sequential hemodialysis and hemofiltration. Pediatr Nephrol. 2007;22:1062–5.
13. Kido J, Nakamura K, Mitsubuchi H, Ohura T, Takayanagi M, Matsuo M, Yoshino M, Shigematsu Y, Yorifuji T, Kasahara M, Horikawa R, Endo F. Long-term outcome and intervention of urea cycle disorders in Japan. J Inherit Metab Dis. 2012;35:777–85.

Chapter 42
Primary Hyperoxaluria

Stefano Picca, Elisa Colombini, and Pierre Cochat

Case Presentations

Case 1

An Italian 6-month, 7 kg female child presented at a local hospital with acute, severe dehydration and renal failure requiring urgent hemodialysis (HD). She was put on a four sessions/week HD schedule. At 8 months of age, she was transferred to our hospital for further investigation. Abdomen X-rays and US showed bilateral nephrolithiasis and nephrocalcinosis. The patient was anuric. Urinary (oxaluria/creatininuria 196 μmol/mmol [normal: 12–55 μmol/mmol]) and blood tests (plasma oxalate 233 mol/mmol (normal: 10–70 μmol/mmol)) demonstrated hyperoxaluria and high plasma oxalate levels (pOx). Bone X-ray showed reduced bone density and radiopaque bands in the distal metaphyseal radius, ulna, femurs, proximal tibia, and radius. There was no evidence of flecked retinopathy. Genetic testing revealed two heterozygous mutations (p.Val 139del; pGly170Arg) confirming the diagnosis of primary hyperoxaluria type 1 (PH1). Intensive bicarbonate HD with six 4-h sessions/week was adopted. The dry weight was 7.4 kg, and a 0.3 m² polysulfone filter was used with Qb 80 mL/min and Qd 500 mL/min.

Peritoneal dialysis was not considered due to the rapidly expected liver and kidney transplantation from a related living donor.

S. Picca (✉) • E. Colombini
Dialysis Unit, Department of Pediatrics, "Bambino Gesù" Children's Research Hospital, Rome, Italy
e-mail: stefano.picca@opbg.net

P. Cochat
Reference Center for Rare Renal Diseases Nephrogones, Hospices Civils de Lyon & Université Claude-Bernard Lyon 1, Lyon, France

© Springer International Publishing AG 2017   315
B.A. Warady et al. (eds.), *Pediatric Dialysis Case Studies*,
DOI 10.1007/978-3-319-55147-0_42

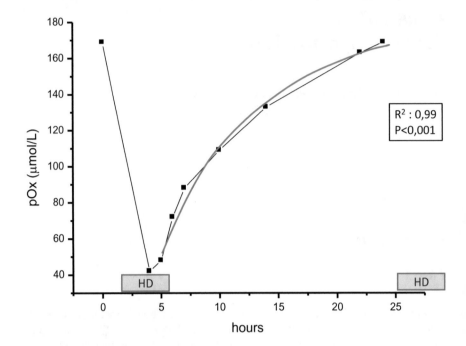

Fig. 42.1 Patient #1: Curvilinear best-fit line of pOx rebound. Although there is an 84% pre-post-HD oxalate reduction ratio, pOx regains values >50 µmol/L in 1 hr post-HD. The quick bending of the curvilinear course of pOx suggests rapid Ox tissue deposition

pOx was measured during HD (Fig. 42.1), and the oxalate (Ox) generation rate (G_{Ox}), Ox distribution volume (V_{Ox}), and Ox mass removal (MR) were calculated (see methods below). Plasma oxalate was 169 µmol/L pre-HD and 42 µmol/L post-HD, respectively. G_{Ox} was 13.62 µmol/L per hour (29.9 mmol/week/1.73 m²). V_{Ox} was 2.79 L (39.9% of BW), and weekly MR was 2.9 mmol (13.8 mmol/week per 1.73 m²). HD Ox clearance was 19.4 mL/min (130.3 L/week per 1.73 m²), and Ox tissue deposition resulted in 3.45 mmol/week (16.13 mmol/week per 1.73 m²).

Case 2

A 6-year-old 17.5 kg female child from Morocco presented at a local hospital with abdominal pain and vomiting. Abdominal ultrasound showed small kidneys with poor corticomedullary differentiation, multiple stones, severe renal failure (plasma creatinine 21.4 mg/dL), and high pOx. The patient was transferred to our hospital for further investigation. Genetic testing showed two heterozygous mutations (pIle244hr; pVal326Tyr) and confirmed a diagnosis of PH1. The patient was anuric. Bicarbonate HD with 3-h sessions four times per week was initiated. A 0.7 m² polysulfone filter was adopted with Qb 150 mL/min and Qd 500 mL/h. Simultaneously, automated

Oxalate levels during combined transplantation

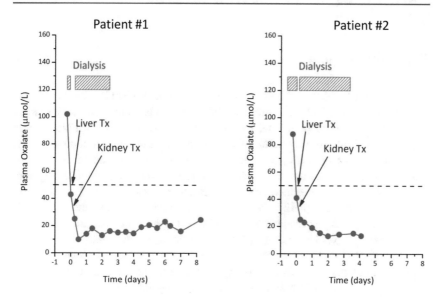

Fig. 42.2 Dialysis in combined liver-kidney transplantation: HD during the anhepatic phase of liver transplantation followed by CRRT in the first days after transplantation

peritoneal dialysis (APD) was added with daily nocturnal APD of 9 h with 600 mL exchange volume, total daily dialysate volume 5,000 mL, and 12 cycles per session. pOx was evaluated during both HD and PD (Fig. 42.2), and G_{Ox}, V_{Ox}, and MR were calculated (see below). Pre-HD pOx was 175 μmol/L and post-HD 28 μmol/L.

In a 44-h inter-HD period, two 9-h PD sessions were performed. Pre-PD pOx was 107 μmol/L and 153 μmol/L and post-PD values were 116 μmol/L and 166 μmol/L, respectively. G_{Ox} was 14.1 μmol/L per hour; (19.9 mmol/week/1.73 m²). V_{Ox} was 4.0 L (22.6% of BW). Total weekly MR with combined HD and PD was 3.89 mmol (8.1 mmol/week per 1.73 m²); MR was 3.09 mmol with HD alone. PD Ox removal accounted for 21% of total removal. Ox clearance was 31.74 mL/min (63.5 L/week per 1.73 m²) by HD and 1.5 mL/min (12 L/week per 1.73 m²) by PD. With this HD and PD schedule, Ox tissue deposition was 24.8 mmol/week (51.7 mmol/week per 1.73 m²).

Clinical Questions

1. What is the genetic basis of primary hyperoxaluria?
2. What is the pathophysiology of kidney damage in PH?
3. Why is dialysis an inadequate long-term treatment for PH?
4. When is dialysis indicated and what is the goal of therapy?

5. How can dialysis therapy be modeled in pediatric patients?
6. What is the role of kidney and liver transplantation?

Diagnostic Discussion

1. PH1 is a rare autosomal recessive disease of Ox metabolism leading to increased renal excretion of Ox, recurrent urolithiasis, nephrocalcinosis, and systemic deposition of Ox in peripheral tissues (named "oxalosis") [1]. There are three types of PH due to a mutation of one of at least three genes coding for liver enzymes, resulting in enzymatic activity deficiency. PH1 is caused by mutations in the alanine/glyoxylate aminotransferase (AGT) gene, leading to the dysfunction of vitamin B6-dependent liver-specific peroxisomal enzyme. Primary hyperoxaluria type 2 (PH2) is caused by mutations in the glyoxylate reductase-hydroxypyruvate reductase (GRHPR) gene catalyzing the reduction of glyoxylate to glycolate and of hydroxypyruvate to D-glycerate.

   In both PH1 and PH2, enzyme deficiency leads to increased conversion of the small intermediary metabolite glyoxylate to the metabolic end-product oxalate. Primary hyperoxaluria type 3 (PH3) is caused by mutations in a liver-specific mitochondrial enzyme gene, 4-hydroxy-2-oxoglutarate aldolase (HOGA) that is important for metabolism of hydroxyproline [2].

2. PH1 is the most frequent cause of oxalosis. The prevalence of PH1 is 1–3 per million and the incidence is 1:100,000 live births in Europe. The prevalence increases to 10–13% in countries where consanguineous marriages are common, like Kuwait and Tunisia [2]. Ox is a dicarboxylic acid with a molecular weight of 90 g/mol, produced by the liver and completely excreted by the kidney in healthy subjects. Urinary excretion is less than 45 mg/day or 0.5 mmol/1.73 m^2 [3]. In PH1, as renal function decreases, Ox begins to accumulate in kidney tubules and in the interstitium leading to nephrocalcinosis. Subsequently, as glomerular filtration rate (GFR) decreases, Ox accumulates mainly in the bone [1], heart [4], and retina [1], finally leading to systemic oxalosis.

3. Ox is a small molecule ($C_2O_4^{-2}$), easily diffusible through dialysis membranes. However, Ox generation (G_{Ox}) by the liver has been estimated to be 4–7 mmol/1.73 m^2 per day, while dialysis removal approximates 1–2 mmol/1.73 m^2 per day in adult patients (and 3–4 mmol/1.73 m^2 per day in children) [2]. The consequence is a continuous Ox accumulation in body stores that explains the commonly accepted inadequacy of dialysis as a chronic therapy for oxalosis.

4. However, dialysis is needed in a few peculiar scenarios: (1) awaiting transplantation; (2) when small patient size does not allow transplantation; (3) in preparation for kidney transplantation, whether before or after liver transplantation, in order to deplete oxalate from the body; (4) following isolated kidney or combined liver-kidney transplantation with any delay in achieving optimal renal function; and (5) in any condition in which the only alternative is absolute withdrawal of all therapy (e.g., in

developing countries) [5]. The relative level of plasma calcium oxalate (CaOx) saturation (β_{CaOx}) is considered the most important factor for the development of CaOx tissue deposition (TD). It expresses the state of saturation as the factor of the calculated free calcium and Ox concentration, divided by the actual solubility product at the actual ionic strength of the plasma sample [6]. There is a strict correlation between the pOx and β_{CaOx}. Hoppe et al. demonstrated that a pOx level over 30 μmol/L is associated with a $\beta_{CaOx} > 1$. The latter is indicated as the cutoff point above which CaOx supersaturation occurs [7]. Therefore, the theoretical goal of dialysis treatment is considered to keep the pOx below 30–50 μmol/L [2].

Early studies on Ox dialysis were performed on adult patients. Marangella et al. first described Ox kinetics in adult patients affected by PH1. In these patients, pOx decreased to 80% of the initial value: during HD, pOx decreased to less than 50 μmol/L. However, after HD, pOx increased linearly above 50 μmol/L within 3–6 h, reaching a plateau after 6–9 h [8]. This trend was quite different from the linear increase of small molecules (i.e., urea) described in the interdialysis period. These authors hypothesized that this could be due to the achievement of the Ox saturation threshold [2, 6] with further precipitation and rapid deposition of crystals of calcium oxalate (CaOx) in peripheral tissues [9].

In the study of Yamauchi et al., G_{Ox} was calculated in one adult patient using the approach of Marangella et al. [8] according to a single-pool model. pOx was evaluated for the first 2 h after HD completion, and linear regression calculated was assumed as G_{Ox}. Using both standard HD and hemodiafiltration (HDF) with high permeable triacetate membranes, these authors demonstrated that 2–5 mmol of Ox per day can be removed, while 4–6 mmol per day are generated. No significant differences in Ox removal were found between HD vs. HDF. Conversely, weekly Ox removal significantly increased by increasing the number of dialysis sessions per week from three to six [10].

Jamieson et al. studied 127 liver transplants in 117 patients affected by PH1. Posttransplantation survival was better in patients in which the time spent on dialysis was less than 5 years compared with those who experienced dialysis for more than 5 years; in addition, the length of the dialysis treatment period negatively impacted the clinical status of patients during the course on dialysis and at transplantation [11]. Conversely, in the study of Bergstralh et al., no correlation was found between the time on dialysis and transplant outcome in 203 patients from the International Primary Hyperoxaluria Registry [12].

The most significant attempt to individualize dialysis therapy in PH1 was by Tang et al., on adult patients treated by HD. Eight out of 14 adult patients were treated by HD six times/week, two patients five times/week, and three patients three times/week. One patient was on home HD and underwent daily 4-h HD. G_{Ox} was assumed as the historical daily Ox production estimated by the 24-h urine Ox determination of a given patient when the GFR was >50 mL/min per 1.73 m^2. Mean reduction in pOx was 78.4 ± 7.7% after one HD session, with a mean pre- and post-HD pOx of 70.6 ± 38.4 μmol/L and 13.3 ± 5.9 μmol/L, respectively. These authors also found a poor correlation between Ox Kt/V and

MR. This probably indicates equilibration of pOx with extravascular compartments (thus suggesting a multi-pool model) or different G_{Ox} among patients. However, by comparing Ox MR and historical G_{Ox}, the authors were able to model dialysis strategy in order to overcome endogenous oxalate production and obtain a significant reduction of pre-HD pOx in 1–29 months. This was achieved by increasing the number of HD sessions per week. Most importantly, 10 out of 13 patients could reduce pre-HD pOx below 50 µmol/L, thus theoretically avoiding Ox tissue deposition [13].

5. In children, such a model is not always applicable. There are at least two issues that differentiate oxalosis dialysis treatment in children from that in adult patients. First, G_{Ox} is generally higher in children than in adult patients, due to a more severe PH1 phenotype. This high G_{Ox} may impair the benefit of even the most efficient dialysis schedule [14]. Secondly, a number of children present at diagnosis with oligoanuria, making historical daily Ox production unavailable. Therefore, the only possible dialysis strategy in children remains that of maximization of Ox removal, given the unpredictability of G_{Ox} [9].

In children, HD and PD have both been used for the removal of Ox. HD is more effective than PD [15–17]. In 1994, Bunchman and Swartz demonstrated in a 7-year-old patient that using combined continuous cycling peritoneal dialysis (CCPD) plus high-efficiency HD at 6 sessions /week resulted in total Ox removal of 1,480 mg/week, with CCPD accounting for nearly 10% of the total removal. However, in this study, CCPD was performed far from its highest efficiency (1.5 L q6 hours) [18]. In the same study, intra-HD urea and Ox kinetics were compared. While both urea and Ox levels monitored during the 3–3.5 h of HD demonstrated a similar 60% reduction, the Ox arterial-venous difference across the dialyzer and the clearance so determined were 30–50% smaller than those for urea. The authors concluded that the distribution volume of Ox is smaller than that for urea, ranging from 35% to 55% of the total body water. These findings were explained by the poor solubility of Ox deposits in tissues and the limited ability to mobilize Ox during treatment.

In the study of Illies et al., six children treated with renal replacement therapy (RRT) were studied to evaluate pOx, Ox clearance, and Ox removal with different dialyzers and blood flow rates with HD, and adapting dwell time and the number of daily exchanges according to peritoneal equilibration tests with PD. A high-flux hemodialyzer (0.7 m^2) and a maximal blood flow rate (150 mL/min) were most efficient in Ox MR, as was more cycles/exchange (10 cycles at night and one or two exchanges during the day) per day and increased dwell time (60 min/cycle). In patients with residual urinary output, urinary removal of Ox was between 5.6 and 12.4 mmol/week per 1.73 m^2. In HD-treated patients, Ox dialysance was between 158 and 444 L/week per 1.73 m^2, while in those treated with PD, Ox clearances of 66 and 103 L/week per 1.73 m^2 were found. One patient received combined HD and PD, reaching a total Ox MR between 10.1 and 24.1 mmol/week per 1.73 m^2. The authors concluded that in children with oxalosis, as much dialysis as the patient and the family can tolerate should be prescribed and stressed the importance of an early start of treatment in order to preserve residual renal function that, in their patients, accounted for a significant portion of Ox elimination [9].

In the two cases described in the introduction, no residual urine output was present. In these cases, Ox removal is provided only by dialysis, and optimization of dialysis efficacy on Ox accumulation becomes of paramount importance. In our cases, Ox kinetics was calculated by a single-pool model adapted from Marangella and Yamauchi [8, 10]. In case 1, for HD, pOx was evaluated at the start (C_0) and end of the session (C_t); then at 1, 2, 3, 6, 10, and 18 h after HD completion; and at the start of the next session (C_{02}). In case 2, similar measurements of pOx were performed for HD and for PD, at 1, 4, and 6 h and at the start of PD. For PD, pOx was evaluated at the start and at the end of dialysis. In both cases, Ox was measured in dialysate. In HD, dialysate Ox was measured in dialysate collected at time 0, 5, 30, 60, 90, 120, 150, 180, 210, and 240 min.

In HD, MR was calculated as MR = C_dOx $* Q_d$, where C_dOx is Ox concentration in dialysate and Q_d dialysate flow (500 mL/min), during the session.

In PD, MR was calculated as MR = C_dOx $* V_{PD}$, where V_{PD} was the total volume of the drain bag.

G_{Ox} was calculated as

$$G_{Ox}(\mu mol / l per h) = (a + b * T_{id} - C_t) / T_{id},$$

where a and b are intercept and slope of the equation of linear regression built with the first three points of pOx after HD completion, T_{id} is interdialysis time (hours), and C_t is the pOx at the end of T_{id}.

Ox distribution volume (V_{Ox}) (liters) was calculated as

$$V_{Ox} = MR / (C_0 - C_t) + (G_{Ox} * T_d),$$

where T_d is dialysis time (hours).

Ox tissue deposition (TD) was calculated as

$$TD(\mu mol / 24 h) = (G_{Ox} * V_{Ox} * 24) - MR.$$

Our results show that a six-time per week HD schedule is necessary to limit Ox deposition to the least possible extent. In addition, reducing HD frequency is harmful even in the presence of daily PD, which accounted for one third of total Ox removal in case 2. It is noteworthy that in the two described cases, G_{Ox} indexed to BSA was much higher in case 1 while TD was much lower compared with case 2, due to the higher Ox clearance and consequent MR.

Most of the studies on dialysis in oxalosis in children have been mainly focused on dialysis efficiency. Conclusions are generally univocal and lead to the adoption of an intensified dialysis schedule including both HD and PD [2, 9, 18]. In the two described cases, the analysis of the inter-HD pOx course illustrates well the key issues of oxalosis dialysis treatment in small children. Firstly, Ox rebound occurs earlier than in adult patients [10], probably due to the generally more severe phenotype of the metabolic defect. Secondly, as in adults, the curvilinear best-fit line of pOx rebound may tend to plateau earlier than in adults, suggesting rapid tissue deposition. Lastly, this rebound induces an almost constant pOx level above 50 µmol/L, even in the presence of a 75% pOx reduction with HD (per se, this suggests a CaOx supersaturation ($\beta_{CaOx} > 1$) with consequent constant risk of tissue deposition (see Fig. 42.1).

6. The liver is the only organ responsible for glyoxylate detoxification. Preemptive liver transplantation (LT) would appear a logical approach, but there are ethical issues and a risk of death associated with the procedure. Isolated kidney transplantation (KT) is accompanied by a high risk of recurrence [3]. Combined liver-kidney transplantation (CLKT) is the optimal treatment for ESRD caused by severe forms of PH1, but not in those who benefit from vitamin B6 therapy and/or favorable mutations [19]. Another option is a sequential procedure that is LT, followed by a period of dialysis to reduce oxalate load from the body, with subsequent KT [2]. In this case, remobilization of oxalate from the tissues to plasma and urine is a slow event leading to a high pOx level for up 3–4 years after transplantation [19]. Recurrent nephrocalcinosis is a risk in these patients and may lead to reduced kidney graft function. During sequential CLKT, HD or continuous renal replacement therapy (CRRT) may be required in the OR following the LT phase or following CLKT when delayed renal graft function occurs. In the future, the treatment of such PH patients will probably rely on i-RNA therapy targeting enzyme blockade.

Epilogue

In our two patients who underwent combined LKT, dialysis was performed during the anhepatic phase of the operation and then stopped and restarted after anastomosis completion. In the following days, dialysis was continued as CVVHDF (see Fig. 42.2) and stopped when pOx was stable at <50 µmol/L.

Clinical Pearls

1. No form of dialysis is able to prevent oxalate accumulation in patients with primary hyperoxaluria type 1, so that reliance on its use should therefore be avoided or at least limited.
2. When mandatory, dialysis frequency and continuity (more than efficiency) is the key issue in the treatment of patients with oxalosis.
3. The most intensive dialysis regimen (HD + PD) is the best available option.
4. Limitation of Ox stores is probably the best achievable result with the presently available dialysis modalities.

5. The analysis of pOx concentration in the interdialytic period provides essential information on generation, distribution volume, and tissue deposition of Ox.
6. HD followed by CRRT is important in combined LKT in order to keep pOx below the saturation threshold and avoid early Ox deposition and resultant injury to the transplanted kidney.

References

1. Coulter-Mackie MB, White CT, Lange D, Chew BH. Primary hyperoxaluria type 1. GeneReviews® [internet]. Seattle: University of Washington, Seattle; 1993–2016. 2002 Jun 19 [updated 2014 Jul 17].
2. Cochat P, Hulton SA, Acquaviva C, Picca S, et al. Primary hyperoxaluria type 1: indications for screening and guidance for diagnosis and treatment. Nephrol Dial Transplant. 2012;27:1729–36.
3. Cochat P, Rumsby G. Primary hyperoxaluria. N Engl J Med. 2013;369:649–58.
4. Mookadam F, Smith T, Jiamsripong P, et al. Cardiac abnormalities in primary hyperoxaluria. Circ J. 2010;74:2403–9.
5. Cochat P, Liutkus A, Fargue S, Basmaison O, Ranchin B, Rolland M-O. Primary hyperoxaluria type 1: still challenging! Pediatr Nephrol. 2006;21:1075–81.
6. Hoppe B, Kemper MJ, Bokenkamp A, Langman CB. Plasma calcium-oxalate saturation in children with renal insufficiency and in children with primary hyperoxaluria. Kidney Int. 1998;54:921–5.
7. Hoppe B, Kemper MJ, Bökenkamp A, Portale AA, Cohn RA, Langman CB. Plasma calcium oxalate supersaturation in children with primary hyperoxaluria and end-stage renal failure. Kidney Int. 1999;56:268–74.
8. Marangella M, Petrarulo M, Cosseddu D, Vitale C, Linari F. Oxalate balance studies in patients on hemodialysis for type I primary hyperoxaluria. Am J Kidney Dis. 1992;19:546–53.
9. Illies F, Bonzel K-E, Wingen A-M, Latta K, Hoyer PF. Clearance and removal of oxalate in children on intensified dialysis for primary hyperoxaluria type 1. Kidney Int. 2006;70:1642–8.
10. Yamauchi T, Quillard M, Takahashi S, Nguyen-Khoa M. Oxalate removal by daily dialysis in a patient with primary hyperoxaluria type 1. Nephrol Dial Transplant. 2001;16:2407–11.
11. Jamieson NVA. 20-year experience of combined liver/kidney transplantation for primary hyperoxaluria (PH1): the European PH1 transplant registry experience 1984–2004. Am J Nephrol. 2005;25:282–9.
12. Bergstrahl EJ, Monico CG, Lieskeb JC, Hergesa RM, LangmanCB HB, Milliner DS. Transplantation outcomes in primary hyperoxaluria. Am J Transpl. 2010;10:2493–501.
13. Tang X, Voskoboev NV, Wannarka SL, Olson JB, Milliner SD, Lieske JC. Oxalate quantification in hemodialysate to assess dialysis adequacy for primary hyperoxaluria. Am J Nephrol. 2014;39:376–82.
14. Cochat P. Primary hyperoxaluria. Kidney Int. 1999;55:2533–47.
15. Harambat J, van Stralen KJ, Espinosa L. Characteristics and outcome of children with primary oxalosis requiring renal replacement therapy. Clin J Am Soc Nephrol. 2012;7:458–65.
16. Watts RW, Veall N, Purkiss P. Oxalate dynamics and removal rates during haemodialysis and peritoneal dialysis in patients with primary hyperoxaluria and severe renal failure. ClinSci (Lond). 1984 May;66:591–7.
17. Dell'Aquila R, Feriani M, Mascalzioni E, Ronco C, La Greca G. Oxalate removal by differing dialysis techniques. ASAJO. 1992;38:797–800.
18. Bunchman TE, Swartz RD. Oxalate removal in type I hyperoxaluria or acquired oxalosis using HD and equilibration PD. Perit Dial Int. 1994;14:81–4.
19. Jalanko H, Pakarinen M. Combined liver and kidney transplantation in children. Pediatr Nephrol. 2014;29:805–14.

Chapter 43
Intoxications

Vimal Chadha

Case Presentation

A 17-year-old previously healthy boy was brought to the emergency room with symptoms of nausea, vomiting, and lethargy. His parents had found him in his room with an empty unlabeled medicine bottle. His girlfriend with whom he had been going steady for several months had reportedly left him recently. On examination, he was febrile (101 °F) and diaphoretic, with a rapid pulse (120/min). He had rapid and deep breathing (38/min), and his pupils were round and equal in size and reactive to light. He was confused and became agitated during the examination. He was suspected of having an acute intoxication. Initial serum chemistries revealed sodium 142 mEq/L, potassium 3.4 mEq/L, chloride 100 mEq/L, bicarbonate 14 mEq/L, urea nitrogen 30 mg/dL, creatinine 1.2 mg/dL, calcium 9.8 mg/dL, glucose 72 mg/dL, and albumin 3.8 g/dL. An arterial blood gas revealed pH 7.46 and $PaCO_2$ 22 mmHg. Based on the "toxidrome," he was suspected of experiencing salicylate intoxication. A plasma salicylate level was obtained and revealed a value of 85 mg/dL. After receiving a fluid bolus (20 mL/kg of lactated Ringer's solution), he was transferred to the intensive care unit for further management. A Foley catheter was placed for accurate recording of urine output, and the intravenous fluids were changed to D5%, 0.45% saline with 40 mEq/L of sodium bicarbonate and were given at twice the maintenance rate. Two hours later, he became more combative. Serum chemistries revealed worsening acidosis, and the serum salicylate level had increased to 96 mg/dL. A nephrology consult was requested to help with the management of his acute intoxication. Hemodialysis was subsequently initiated because of the severity of the intoxication as reflected by worsening clinical symptoms despite adequate supportive measures, worsening acidosis, and a rising serum

V. Chadha, MD (✉)
Division of Pediatric Nephrology, University of Missouri, Kansas City School of Medicine, Children's Mercy Hospital, Kansas City, MO, USA
e-mail: vchadha@cmh.edu

© Springer International Publishing AG 2017
B.A. Warady et al. (eds.), *Pediatric Dialysis Case Studies*,
DOI 10.1007/978-3-319-55147-0_43

salicylate level. After a 4 h hemodialysis session, there was marked improvement in the patient's sensorium, the serum bicarbonate level improved to 21 mEq/L, and the salicylate level was 47 mg/dL. The alkaline diuresis was continued, and 6 h later the serum salicylate level had decreased to 24 mg/dL. IV fluids were then changed to D5%, 0.9% saline with 20 mEq/L of potassium chloride at the maintenance rate, and the patient was transferred out of the ICU.

Clinical Questions

1. How common are intoxications in children?
2. What is the general approach for the management of a patient with evidence of an acute intoxication?
3. What are the indications for initiating dialysis therapy for the management of intoxications?
4. Which physical properties of the ingested toxin and associated pharmacokinetic principles determine the effectiveness of dialysis therapy?
5. Which dialysis modality/extracorporeal therapy is best suited for the management of acute intoxications?

Diagnostic Discussion

1. Intoxications are a significant cause of morbidity and mortality; the 2014 Annual Report of the American Association of Poison Control Centers (AAPCC) published information on 2,165,142 cases of human exposures, and nearly half (47.7%) were in children <6 years of age [1]. The top five substance classes involved in all human exposures were analgesics (11.3%), cosmetics/personal care products (7.7%), household cleaning substances (7.7%), sedatives/hypnotics/antipsychotics (5.9%), and antidepressants (4.4%). Most (79.4%) intoxications were unintentional; suicidal intent was suspected in 11.2% of cases. As is the case with our patient, intentional exposures were more commonly seen in patients aged 13–19 years.

   The management of intoxications is a significant burden on healthcare resources. According to the 2014 Annual Report, 6,12,184 (28.3%) cases were managed in a healthcare facility; 1,01,141 of those patients (16.5%) were admitted to a critical care unit. While the overall number of fatalities from intoxications is relatively low (total of 1,173 reported in 2014), a greater frequency of serious outcomes are seen in those with intentional exposures.

2. All patients presenting with clinical evidence of an acute intoxication should be evaluated for the severity of exposure, and attempts should be made to identify the likely toxin(s) from the patient history and circumstances surrounding the intoxication, presentation (toxidrome), urine drug screen, and blood levels in

Table 43.1 Common emergency antidotes

Toxin	Antidote
Acetaminophen	*N-acetylcysteine*
Atropine	*Physostigmine*
Benzodiazepines	*Flumazenil*
B-blockers	*Glucagon*
Calcium channel blockers	*Calcium chloride*
Carbon monoxide	*Oxygen*
Cyanide	*Amyl nitrite* *Sodium nitrite* *Sodium thiosulfate*
Digoxin	*Digoxin antibody fragments*
Ethylene glycol	*Ethanol* *Fomepizole*
Methanol	*Ethanol* *Fomepizole*
Nitrites	*Methylene blue*
Opiates	*Naloxone*
Organophosphates	*Atropine*
Carbamates	*Pralidoxime*
Tricyclic antidepressants	*Sodium bicarbonate*

specific situations. The following general principles of management are utilized based on the severity of the intoxication and the suspected toxin:

I. Patient stabilization (maintenance of the airway, ventilation, and hemodynamic status)
II. Decontamination (removal of poison from the site of absorption such as the GI tract or skin)
III. Administration of antidotes, if applicable
IV. Supportive care (treatment of hypotension, arrhythmias, respiratory failure, acid-base and electrolyte imbalance, and seizures)
V. Elimination of poison by manipulation of urine volume and pH
VI. Removal of poison by extracorporeal therapies

It is important to note that the majority of patients can be managed by approaches I through V with excellent results. It should also be noted that some of the routine standard therapies, such as the use of ipecac syrup and gastric lavage, have come under scrutiny and are not advocated as standard of care [2].

Antidotes: The availability of several specific antidotes has assumed an increasingly important role in the management of certain intoxications. However, antidotes are useful in only a fraction of intoxications and need to be administered as early as possible, often within the first few hours of exposure. The list of commonly used antidotes and indications is provided in Table 43.1.

Table 43.2 Criteria for extracorporeal therapy as treatment for acute intoxication

Potentially lethal plasma concentration of intoxicant known to be cleared effectively from blood by extracorporeal therapy
Significant quantity of circulating toxin that is metabolized to a more noxious substance (e.g., methanol, ethylene glycol)
Ingestion and probable absorption of a potentially lethal dose
Severe clinical intoxication with abnormal vital signs
Impairment of normal route of excretion
Progressive clinical deterioration despite careful medical management
Prolonged coma with its potential hazards (e.g., aspiration pneumonia, septicemia).
Need for prolonged assisted ventilation
Persistent hypotension or need for vasoactive therapy
Poisoning by agents with delayed toxicity (e.g., paraquat).

Reprinted with permission from Ref. [5]

Urine volume and pH manipulation: Several toxins that are filtered through the glomerulus can be reabsorbed in the proximal convoluted tubule (PCT). The reabsorption from the PCT can be decreased by increasing the urinary volume which lowers the urinary concentration of the filtered toxin, thereby decreasing the urine-tubular cell concentration gradient. In addition, toxins such as salicylates and phenobarbital that are weak acids are maximally non-ionized in an acidic environment which facilitates their absorption across the cell membranes and hence reabsorption in the PCT. With urine alkalization (pH > 7.5), salicylates and phenobarbital are predominantly in the ionized form and are thus trapped in the tubule and excreted in the urine.

While infusing large volumes of intravenous fluids containing sodium bicarbonate, one should carefully monitor the patient for electrolyte disorders such as hypokalemia, hypocalcemia, and hypernatremia and for the development of cerebral and/or pulmonary edema.

3. Extracorporeal therapy for removal of a toxin is required in <2.5% of patients presenting with an intoxication. In general, this approach should be instituted when the rate of toxin removal by an extracorporeal method is deemed to be significantly greater than the spontaneous rate of elimination by hepatic and/or renal excretion. It may also be recommended when the intrinsic clearance is impaired by the disease process and the extracorporeal method is the only means by which effective clearance can be provided. The list of toxic substances that have been subjected to extracorporeal therapies is quite long, and information is available on more than 200 substances [3, 4]. However, the ability to remove a toxic substance by extracorporeal therapy is not equivalent to an indication for these procedures. One must take into account the patient's underlying health (including any comorbidities), the toxicity of the absorbed substance, the presence of or likelihood of advancing to severe illness, and the availability of acceptable alternatives (good supportive care, antidotes). The broadly agreed upon criteria for initiating extracorporeal therapy are shown in the Table 43.2.

In the patient described in the vignette, the decision to perform dialysis was made based on clinical parameters such as worsening mental status, mild acute kidney injury, and a refractory acid-base balance, in addition to the plasma salicylate concentration. While sole reliance on the plasma salicylate concentration to determine the need for extracorporeal therapy is not advised, serious consideration for hemodialysis should be given for acutely poisoned patients with salicylate concentrations of at least 100 mg/dL or patients with chronic salicylate concentrations of at least 60 mg/dL.

4. The most common physical properties and pharmacokinetic principles that determine the effectiveness of dialysis therapy for treatment of intoxications are molecular weight, volume of distribution (V_d), protein binding, water permeability, lipid solubility, and intercompartmental transfer.

Toxins with a molecular weight of <500 Da are easily removed by hemodialysis (currently available high-efficacy dialyzers can provide useful clearance for substances with a molecular weight of up to 2,000 Da).

The volume of distribution (V_d) is an imaginary space that represents the volume of fluid in which a known amount of drug would have to be diluted to yield the measured serum concentration. A V_d that is significantly larger than actual body water reflects a high degree of tissue concentration, while a small V_d suggests concentration within the intravascular space. V_d is one of main factors that determines the accessibility of a drug/toxin to removal by dialysis therapy; a large V_d implies that the amount of drug present in the plasma represents only a small fraction of the total body load. Thus, even if a hemodialysis session extracts most of the drug present in blood flowing through the circuit, the amount of drug removed represents only a small percentage of the total body drug burden. The volume of distribution of some of the common substances involved in poisoning is listed in Table 43.3.

Many substances bind with varying affinity to plasma proteins, such as albumin, or to intracellular proteins in the tissues. Thus, in addition to dissolving in fat, substances can accumulate in tissues according to their degree of protein binding. Protein binding limits the amount of free drug available for removal across dialysis membranes. Highly protein-bound substances are therefore not amenable to therapy with extracorporeal modalities. However, at toxic levels the protein-binding sites are usually saturated, resulting in a higher percentage of unbound drug that can be effectively removed by dialysis therapy.

Similarly, lipid-soluble drugs can accumulate extensively in the adipose tissue that acts as a reservoir with poor accessibility due to decreased vascular perfusion.

Salicylates, in particular, have a low molecular weight (138 Da) and a low V_d (0.2 L/kg) that makes this class of drugs amenable to effective removal by dialysis. Although the protein binding is high (80–90%), the free fraction that is available for removal by dialysis is increased with toxic doses.

Finally, the efficacy of any extracorporeal therapy is assessed by the accurate determination of the amount of drug removed from the body. Several

Table 43.3 Properties of substances frequently involved in poisonings

Substance	Molecular weight (Da)	Volume of distribution (L/kg)	Protein binding (%)
Acetaminophen	151	0.95	25
Aminoglycoside	*	0.2–0.3	< 5
Amphotericin B	924	4.0	90
Benzodiazepine	*	0.3–6.6	85–98
Carbamazepine	228	0.8–1.6	75
Digoxin	765	5–8	20–30
Ethanol	46	0.7	0
Ethylene glycol	62	0.6	0
Indomethacin	327	0.12	99
Isopropyl alcohol	60	0.7	0
Lithium	7	0.5–0.9	0
Methanol	32	0.7	0
Methotrexate	456	0.76	45–50
Narcotic	*	3–16	*
Phenobarbital	232	0.7–1.0	40–60
Phenytoin	252	0.6–0.7	90
Salicylate	138	0.1–0.2	80–90
Theophylline	*	0.4–0.7	55
Tricyclic antidepressants	*	6–50	90–97
Valproate	144	0.19–0.23	90

Reprinted with permission from Ref. [5]
*Variable depending on the specific drug in that class

parameters such as clearance, efficiency ratio, extraction ratio, mass removal, and decrease in half-life are commonly utilized to scientifically assess drug removal from the body in an attempt to determine the success or failure of the intervention.

5. Hemodialysis is widely available, and there is an extensive experience associated with its use for detoxification purposes. Hemodialysis is an effective modality for removal of toxins such as methanol, ethylene glycol, salicylates, acetaminophen, barbiturates, carbamazepine, and valproic acid, all of which have a low molecular weight and a small V_d.

In patients with hemodynamic instability, continuous renal replacement therapy (CRRT) can be used. While the rate of clearance is slower with CRRT, this modality has the advantage of being able to remove substances that distribute in multiple compartments with slow equilibration. CRRT thus mitigates the rebound phenomenon seen after a session of hemodialysis. Lithium is a substance known for its intracellular distribution. Although it is not highly protein bound, its relatively large V_d coupled with its slow transcellular diffusion makes CRRT the preferred modality for its elimination.

In hemoperfusion, blood is percolated through a cartridge packed with activated charcoal or another resin coated with a semipermeable membrane. Toxins are adsorbed onto the charcoal or polystyrene resin despite protein binding, making this modality a better choice for highly protein-bound poisons. These cartridges can also absorb lipid-soluble substances and substances with a molecular weight up to 40,000 Da. Despite the theoretical appeal of hemoperfusion for the treatment of intoxications, its use remains quite limited. The cartridges are not freely available in all hospitals, and modern dialyzers with highly porous membranes and large surface areas characteristically achieve clearance rates approaching those achieved with hemoperfusion.

In peritoneal dialysis, the clearance kinetics are dependent on the intrinsic characteristics of the peritoneal membrane and the mesenteric circulation and are not amenable to significant external adjustments. Overall, peritoneal dialysis is only 10–25% as effective as hemodialysis in terms of clearance, and its efficacy is further compromised if the patient is hypotensive. Thus, the role of peritoneal dialysis in detoxification is limited to situations where extracorporeal modalities are not available, contraindicated, or not possible due to the lack of vascular access.

In infants and toddlers, exchange transfusion can be used to successfully remove toxins that are protein bound and present in the vascular compartment.

When confronted with a case of intoxication, the physician must consider many parameters in choosing the appropriate therapeutic modality. A simplified decision-making approach is provided in the algorithm (Fig. 43.1).

Clinical Pearls

1. Most intoxications are mild and can be managed outside of the healthcare facility. Intentional intoxications usually involve a pharmaceutical agent(s) with an associated greater frequency of serious outcomes.
2. The majority of intoxicated patients can be managed with general supportive measures and effective symptomatic treatment.
3. Extracorporeal therapies are required for a select group of patients who experience moderate to severe intoxication with a substance that is easily dialyzable.
4. Toxins with a low molecular weight (<500 Da), low volume of distribution (V_d), and low protein binding are easily cleared by extracorporeal therapies. Additional pharmacokinetic properties such as water permeability, lipid solubility, and intercompartmental transfer also influence clearance.

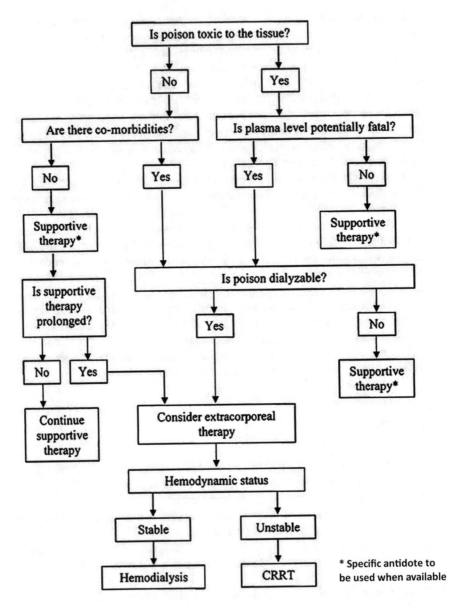

Fig. 43.1 Simplified approach to a patient with poisoning (Reprinted with permission from Ref. [5])

References

1. Mowry JB, Spyker DA, Brooks DE, McMillan N, Schauben JL. Annual report of the American Association of Poison Control Centers' national Poison data System (NPDS): 32nd annual Report. 2014. http://www.aapcc.org.
2. Hojer J, Troutman WG, Hoppu K, Erdman A, Benson BE, Megarbane B, Thanacoody R, Bedry R, Caravati EM. Position paper update: ipecac syrup for gastrointestinal decontamination. Clin Toxicol. 2013;51:134–9.
3. Winchester JF. Dialysis and hemoperfusion in poisoning. Adv Ren Replace Ther. 2002;9(1):26–30.
4. Shannon MW, Borron SW, Burns M, editors. Haddad and Winchester's clinical management of poisoning and drug overdose. 4th ed. Philadelphia: W. B. Saunders; 2007.
5. Chadha V. Extracorporeal therapy for drug overdose and poisoning. In: Warady BA, Schaefer F, Alexander SR, editors. Pediatric dialysis. 2nd ed. New York: Springer; 2012.

Chapter 44
Acquired Cystic Kidney Disease

Eugene Y.H. Chan and Bradley A. Warady

Case Presentation

A 17-year-old Chinese girl first presented with steroid-resistant nephrotic syndrome at age 8 years, secondary to focal segmental glomerulosclerosis (FSGS). Despite the use of multiple immunosuppressive agents and treatment with ACE inhibitors, she remained unresponsive to therapy and rapidly progressed to end-stage renal disease (ESRD). Peritoneal dialysis (PD) was initiated at age 10 years, and she was subsequently transitioned to hemodialysis (HD) following several episodes of peritonitis. After 4 years of chronic dialysis, she received a deceased donor kidney transplant.

Unfortunately, her primary disease recurred during the immediate postoperative period with resultant massive proteinuria. Multiple therapeutic approaches, including plasmapheresis and rituximab, were attempted without success. Eventually, HD had to be resumed 1 month posttransplant, followed by graft nephrectomy. She remained dialysis dependent for 3 years and was inactive on the transplant waiting list due to the high risk of disease recurrence. Of note, she retained her native kidneys.

Nine years following her initial presentation with FSGS, an abdominal ultrasound (US) was performed as part of the evaluation of nonspecific abdominal pain. To the surprise of her nephrologist, the US study revealed multiple small cysts in bilaterally small, echogenic kidneys, consistent with the diagnosis of acquired cystic kidney disease (ACKD). Of concern, one of the cysts (2 cm) in the left kidney

E.Y.H. Chan, MRCPCH, FHKAM(Paed) (✉)
Princess Margaret Hospital, Hong Kong, China
e-mail: genegene.chan@gmail.com

B.A. Warady, MD
Division of Pediatric Nephrology, University of Missouri, Kansas City School of Medicine,
Children's Mercy Hospital, Kansas City, MO, USA

© Springer International Publishing AG 2017
B.A. Warady et al. (eds.), *Pediatric Dialysis Case Studies*,
DOI 10.1007/978-3-319-55147-0_44

appeared complex in nature with internal echogenicity. A non-contrast-enhanced MRI characterized the complex cyst as Bosniak category III. Due to the risk of malignancy within the kidneys, bilateral nephrectomies were performed and confirmed the diagnosis of ACKD. Histologic examination of the 2 cm mass from the left kidney demonstrated a papillary proliferation of large atypical cells with abundant eosinophilic cytoplasm. In the setting of ACKD, the diagnosis was acquired cystic kidney disease-associated renal cell carcinoma (RCC).

As she was determined to have early local disease (T1N0M0), she did not require adjuvant therapy, and she is currently being followed by oncology with regular assessments per computer tomography (CT) of the thorax and magnetic resonance imaging (MRI) of her abdomen/pelvis, the latter without contrast enhancement.

Clinical Questions

1. What is ACKD? How is it different from hereditary cystic kidney disease?
2. How is the diagnosis of ACKD made?
3. How common is ACKD in children with ESRD?
4. What is the single most serious consequence of ACKD?
5. How should dialysis patients and transplant recipients be screened for ACKD?

Diagnostic Discussion

1. First described by Dunnill et al. in 1977, ACKD is characterized by the presence of multiple small cysts in bilaterally small kidneys of patients with ESRD, without hereditary or congenital cystic disease [1]. In the same report, nearly half of the patients on chronic HD showed ACKD on autopsy [1]. In contrast to ACKD, inherited cystic kidney disease such as autosomal dominant polycystic kidney disease (ADPKD) typically presents with large cysts and enlarged kidneys. Whereas cysts in ADPKD occur in extrarenal locations, ACKD is an intrarenal condition, and cyst formation is limited to the kidneys [2].

   The pathogenesis of ACKD remains poorly understood. Uremia, tubular obstruction, and ischemia have long been speculated to be the key mediators of cyst development [3]. Since the composition of the cyst fluid is similar to that of glomerular filtrate, and the histology reveals tubular epithelial cells, cysts in ACKD likely arise from proximal renal tubules [2, 3]. More recently, several growth factors (e.g., hepatocyte growth factor) and proto-oncogenes (e.g., c-Jun) have been implicated in the pathogenesis of ACKD [4, 5]. Male gender and African-American race have inconsistently been identified as risk factors for ACKD [3, 6].

   Although ACKD was initially described in those on chronic HD, subsequent reports have revealed that it also occurs in patients with all stages of chronic kidney disease (CKD), from pre-dialysis patients to transplant recipients.

2. To date, there is no consensus on the diagnostic criteria for ACKD. Variable recommendations have been made regarding the required number of cysts, in adults from as little as three to more than five cysts in each kidney. Nonetheless, the requirement for multiple cysts is strictly adhered to in adults because the presence of a solitary renal cyst is common in the general adult population. In contrast, in pediatric patients with ACKD, US evaluation may reveal only 1–2 renal cysts during the early course of chronic dialysis, findings which do not satisfy the adult diagnostic criteria for ACKD [7]. Therefore, de novo cyst formation has been proposed as an additional criterion for the pediatric CKD/ESRD population [7].

3. The lack of consensus regarding a case definition has led to a variable reported incidence of ACKD in adult patients. Narasimhan et al. investigated 130 patients with CKD (30 pre-dialysis and 100 on maintenance dialysis) with US and/or CT. Seven percent of pre-dialysis patients and 22% of those on dialysis were diagnosed with ACKD [6]. In the same study, patients with ACKD experienced a significantly longer duration of dialysis therapy (49.8 months), compared to those patients with a solitary cyst or no cysts who were dialyzed for 28 months and 15 months, respectively [6]. Matson et al. reported that the prevalence of ACKD in adults was 8% at dialysis initiation, more than 40% after 3 years of dialysis, and 90% after 5-10 years [8].

   Data pertaining to the frequency of ACKD in children is scarce [7, 9–12]. Only four pediatric reports are identified, and most series have included a limited number of patients, short observation periods, as well as young adult patients [7, 10–12]. Overall, the incidence of ACKD in children has been reported to be from 21.6% to 45.8%. Findings of these studies are presented in Table 44.1.

   In the largest pediatric series, Sieniawska et al. examined 21 pre-dialysis children with CKD and 28 patients on chronic dialysis, with ages ranging from 1 month to 15.8 years [7]. Two (9.8%) of the pre-dialysis patients and 6 (21.6%) children on dialysis were diagnosed with ACKD. No particular primary renal disorder in children has been determined to be associated with ACKD in any of the published reports [11].

   While ACKD has been described in pediatric and adult renal transplant recipients with concern that the use of a calcinerurin inhibitor may predispose to the disorder [13], interestingly, regression of ACKD following kidney transplantation has also been reported [6, 12].

4. The single most serious consequence of ACKD is malignant transformation. Although RCC can occur in ESRD patients without cystic changes of the kidneys, the development of ACKD substantially increases the risk of neoplasia, with an odds ratio of 6 [14]. Denton et al. examined 260 adult patients in a center where ipsilateral native nephrectomy was routinely performed in all kidney transplant recipients [14]. During a 6-year observation period, 33% and 4.2% of patients developed ACKD and RCC, respectively. Of note, 91% of patients with RCC had underlying ACKD [14]. Being the most common subtype of RCC in the ESRD population, ACKD-associated RCC was recently recognized as a distinct entity in the 2012 Vancouver Classification of Renal Neoplasia, published

Table 44.1 ACKD in children and young adults with CKD

Author	Pediatric patients only	Number of patients	Mean Age (years)	Observation period (months)	Incidence of ACKD	Incidence of neoplasia
Leichter et al. [10]	No	15	15.9 ± 4.5	37.8 ± 13.1	5/15 (33%)	1 (6%)
Sieniawska et al. [7]	Yes	Pre-RRT: 21 RRT: 28	Pre-RRT: 5.45 ± 3.99 RRT: 9.92 ± 4.39	Pre-RRT: 23.4 ± 12.6 RRT: 15.2 ± 10.4	Pre-RRT: 2/21(9.8%) RRT: 6/28 (21.6%)	No
Querfeld et al. [12]	No	48	17 ± 5.1	68.4 ± 45.6	12/42 (29%)	1 (2%)
Mattoo et al. [11]	No	24	19.8 ± 5.3	77.8 ± 44.3	11/24 (45.8%)	2 (8%)

ACKD acquired cystic kidney disease, *CKD* chronic kidney disease, *RRT* renal replacement therapy including peritoneal dialysis, hemodialysis, and kidney transplantation

by the International Society of Urological Pathology [15]. These tumors occur as nodules over the cyst wall and have various histological appearances [16]. Acinar, solid-alveolar, tubular, papillary, microcystic and macrocystic, and solid sheetlike patterns have been reported in different proportions and combination [15]. Most importantly, when compared with the general population, RCC in adult patients with ESRD (with and without ACKD) is generally less symptomatic, smaller in size, diagnosed earlier, and is of a lower stage at diagnosis [17–19]. A potential explanation for this observation is the benefit of a routine surveillance program.

The true incidence of RCC in children with ACKD is unclear, varying from 0% to 8% [7, 10–12]. Mattoo et al. described two out of 24 (8%) patients on chronic dialysis with RCC, after a relatively long period of follow-up (mean 77.8 ± 44.2 months) [11]. In this cohort, both patients diagnosed with RCC had underlying ACKD [11]. It is also worth mentioning that since most cases of RCC in children have been identified only when renal cysts have had suspicious radiological findings or the patients became symptomatic, there is likely an underestimation of the aforementioned incidence of RCC. Prospective studies with a long duration of follow-up, possibly carried out by national or international registries such as the International Pediatric Dialysis Network (IPDN) and the North American Renal Trials and Collaborative Studies (NAPRTCS), will be required to better define the incidence of ACKD and RCC in children with CKD/ESRD.

5. Most pediatric and adult patients with ACKD are asymptomatic. Thus, routine surveillance is important for early ACKD and RCC detection, with the hope of improving the patient's long-term outcome. Unfortunately, there is currently no consensus recommendation regarding ACKD and RCC surveillance in children with CKD prior to renal replacement therapy, on dialysis or following kidney transplantation. However, the suggestion has been made by some that annual screening ultrasound evaluation of native kidneys be conducted in all children on dialysis, as well as of the native kidneys and allograft of transplant recipients.

More definitive recommendations have been made for adults. It has been recommended that adult patients on dialysis for more than 3–5 years undergo annual screening with CT and US [2, 3]. In the transplant population, the widely endorsed KDIGO guidelines suggest that it is unnecessary to screen for renal malignancy, while the European Association of Urology recommends annual US screening of both native and graft kidneys [20].

Ultrasound is an important screening tool for ACKD, due to its noninvasive nature, low cost, and lack of radiation exposure and nephrotoxicity. In ACKD, the associated cysts may be simple or complex. Features of simple cysts on US include (1) absence of internal echoes, (2) posterior enhancement, (3) round or oval in shape, and (4) sharp, thin posterior walls. Cysts that do not meet these criteria are considered complex cysts and require further characterization.

CT and MRI are secondary diagnostic tools to be used to differentiate between benign and potentially malignant lesions. The Bosniak renal cyst classification scheme is a useful tool in assessing the risk of RCC and to help guide subsequent management. Complex cysts characterized as Bosniak IIF (F for follow-up), III, and IV are associated with a progressively higher prevalence of malignancy. The risk of malignancy is <1%, 0–3%, 5–20%, 40–60%, and 76–100% for renal cysts of Bosniak I, II, IIF, III, and IV, respectively [21, 22]. In general, renal cysts of Bosniak IIF require close surveillance and those of Bosniak III and IV require nephrectomy. When contrast is contraindicated (GFR < 30 ml/1.73 m²/min), as is the case in most patients with ACKD, the American College of Radiology recommends US with Duplex Doppler or MRI rather than CT for further evaluation of suspicious renal cysts, as non-contrast-enhanced CT has limited ability to identify malignant lesions [23]. At the same time, MRI studies should be conducted without contrast because of concerns for systemic nephrogenic fibrosis. Accurate classification based on Bosniak categories will guide subsequent nonsurgical or surgical management.

Clinical Pearls

1. De novo cyst development should be considered as an important diagnostic criterion of ACKD in children. Thorough communication with radiologists, who may not be familiar with this pediatric disorder, is crucial to making an accurate diagnosis.
2. Children on dialysis may be at particular risk for ACKD with an incidence of the disorder that is likely comparable to that experienced by adult patients.
3. The incidence of ACKD is directly proportional to the duration of dialysis therapy. This suggests that extra attention to the possible development of ACKD is required in centers where the average waiting time for kidney transplantation is long.
4. Renal cell carcinoma (RCC) is the most serious complication of ACKD.
5. A routine surveillance program, which includes an annual US evaluation, should be considered for early ACKD and RCC detection.

References

1. Dunnill M, Millard P, Oliver D. Acquired cystic disease of the kidneys: a hazard of long-term intermittent maintenance haemodialysis. J Clin Pathol. 1977;30(9):868–77.
2. Grantham JJ. Acquired cystic kidney disease. Kidney Int. 1991;40(1):143–52.
3. Ishikawa I, editor. Acquired cystic disease: mechanisms and manifestations. Semin Nephrol. 1991;11(6):671–84. Elsevier.
4. Konda R, Sato H, Hatafuku F, Nozawa T, Ioritani N, Fujioka T. Expression of hepatocyte growth factor and its receptor C-met in acquired renal cystic disease associated with renal cell carcinoma. J Urol. 2004;171(6):2166–70.
5. Oya M, Mikami S, Mizuno R, Marumo K, Mukai M, Murai M. C-jun activation in acquired cystic kidney disease and renal cell carcinoma. J Urol. 2005;174(2):726–30.
6. Narasimhan N, Golper TA, Wolfson M, Rahatzad M, Bennett WM. Clinical characteristics and diagnostic considerations in acquired renal cystic disease. Kidney Int. 1986;30(5):748–52.
7. Sieniawska M, Roszkowska-Blaim M, Welc-Dobies J. Acquired cystic kidney disease in renal insufficiency. Child Nephrol Urol. 1990;11(1):20–4.

8. Matson MA, Cohen EP. Acquired cystic kidney disease: occurrence, prevalence, and renal cancers. Medicine. 1990;69(4):217–26.
9. Hogg RJ. Acquired renal cystic disease in children prior to the start of dialysis. Pediatr Nephrol. 1992;6(2):176–8.
10. Leichter HE, Dietrich R, Salusky IB, Foley J, Cohen AH, Kangarloo H, et al. Acquired cystic kidney disease in children undergoing long-term dialysis. Pediatr Nephrol. 1988;2(1):8–11.
11. Mattoo TK, Greifer I, Geva P, Spitzer A. Acquired renal cystic disease in children and young adults on maintenance dialysis. Pediatr Nephrol. 1997;11(4):447–50.
12. Querfeld U, Schneble F, Wradzidlo W, Waldherr R, Tröger J, Schärer K. Acquired cystic kidney disease before and after renal transplantation. J Pediatr. 1992;121(1):61–4.
13. Lien Y-HH, Hunt KR, Siskind MS, Zukoski C. Association of cyclosporin A with acquired cystic kidney disease of the native kidneys in renal transplant recipient. Kidney Int. 1993;44(3):613–6.
14. Denton MD, Magee CC, Ovuworie C, Mauiyyedi S, Pascual M, Colvin RB, et al. Prevalence of renal cell carcinoma in patients with ESRD pre-transplantation: a pathologic analysis. Kidney Int. 2002;61(6):2201–9.
15. Srigley JR, Delahunt B, Eble JN, Egevad L, Epstein JI, Grignon D, et al. The International Society of Urological Pathology (ISUP) Vancouver classification of renal neoplasia. Am J Surg Pathol. 2013;37(10):1469–89.
16. Delahunt B, Srigley JR, Montironi R, Egevad L. Advances in renal neoplasia: recommendations from the 2012 International Society of Urological Pathology Consensus Conference. Urology. 2014;83(5):969–74.
17. Cheung CY, Lam MF, Lee KC, Chan GSW, Chan KW, Chau KF, et al. Renal cell carcinoma of native kidney in Chinese renal transplant recipients: a report of 12 cases and a review of the literature. Int Urol Nephrol. 2011;43(3):675–80.
18. Mehra R, Smith SC, Divatia M, Amin MB. Emerging entities in renal neoplasia. Surg Pathol Clin. 2015;8(4):623–56.
19. Chen K, Huang HH, Aydin H, Tan YH, Lau WK, Cheng CW, et al. Renal cell carcinoma in patients with end-stage renal disease is associated with more favourable histological features and prognosis. Scand J Urol. 2015;49(3):200–4.
20. Karam G, Kälble T, Alcaraz A, Aki F, Budde K, Humke U. Guidelines on renal transplantation of the European Association of Urology (EAU). 2014. https://www.dropbox.com/s/xxuyvtt561cimt0/EAU%20Renal%20Transplatnation%20guideline.pdf?dl=0.
21. Frascà GM, Sandrini S, Cosmai L, Porta C, Asch W, Santoni M, et al. Renal cancer in kidney transplanted patients. J Nephrol. 2015;28(6):659–68.
22. Weibl P, Klatte T, Kollarik B, Waldert M, Schüller G, Geryk B, et al. Interpersonal variability and present diagnostic dilemmas in Bosniak classification system. Scand J Urol Nephrol. 2011;45(4):239–44.
23. Heilbrun ME, Remer EM, Casalino DD, Beland MD, Bishoff JT, Blaufox MD, et al. ACR Appropriateness Criteria indeterminate renal mass. J Am Coll Radiol. 2015;12(4):333–41.

Index

© Springer International Publishing AG 2017
B.A. Warady et al. (eds.), *Pediatric Dialysis Case Studies*,
DOI 10.1007/978-3-319-55147-0